Ultrasound-Guided Procedures

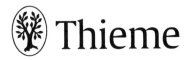

Ultrasound-Guided Procedures

Edited by

Vikram S. Dogra, MD
Professor of Radiology, Urology, and Biomedical
    Engineering
Associate Chair for Education and Research
Department of Imaging Sciences
University of Rochester Medical Center
Rochester, New York

Wael E.A. Saad, MBBCh
Associate Professor of Radiology
Division of Vascular Interventional Radiology
Department of Radiology
University of Virginia Medical System
Charlottesville, Virginia

Thieme
New York · Stuttgart

Thieme Medical Publishers, Inc.
333 Seventh Ave.
New York, NY 10001

Executive Editor: Timothy Hiscock
Managing Editor: J. Owen Zurhellen IV
Editorial Director: Michael Wachinger
Editorial Assistant: Adriana di Giorgio
International Production Director: Andreas Schabert
Production Editor: Heidi Grauel, Maryland Composition
Medical Illustrator: Anthony M. Pazos
Vice President, International Marketing and Sales: Cornelia Schulze
Chief Financial Officer: James W. Mitos
President: Brian D. Scanlan
Compositor: Thomson Digital
Printer: Sheridan Books, Inc.

Library of Congress Cataloging-in-Publication Data

Ultrasound-guided procedures / edited by Vikram S. Dogra, Wael E.A. Saad.
     p. ; cm.
  Includes bibliographical references and index.
  ISBN 978-1-60406-170-3
  1. Diagnostic ultrasonic imaging. I. Dogra, Vikram. II. Saad, Wael E. A.
  [DNLM: 1. Ultrasonography, Interventional—methods. WN 208 U47425 2009]
  RC78.7.U4U4464 2009
  616.07'543—dc22

                                             2009019406

Important note: Medical knowledge is ever-changing. As new research and clinical experience broaden our knowledge, changes in treatment and drug therapy may be required. The authors and editors of the material herein have consulted sources believed to be reliable in their efforts to provide information that is complete and in accord with the standards accepted at the time of publication. However, in view of the possibility of human error by the authors, editors, or publisher of the work herein or changes in medical knowledge, neither the authors, editors, nor publisher, nor any other party who has been involved in the preparation of this work, warrants that the information contained herein is in every respect accurate or complete, and they are not responsible for any errors or omissions or for the results obtained from use of such information. Readers are encouraged to confirm the information contained herein with other sources. For example, readers are advised to check the product information sheet included in the package of each drug they plan to administer to be certain that the information contained in this publication is accurate and that changes have not been made in the recommended dose or in the contraindications for administration. This recommendation is of particular importance in connection with new or infrequently used drugs.

Some of the product names, patents, and registered designs referred to in this book are in fact registered trademarks or proprietary names even though specific reference to this fact is not always made in the text. Therefore, the appearance of a name without designation as proprietary is not to be construed as a representation by the publisher that it is in the public domain.

Printed in the United States

978-1-60406-170-3

This book is dedicated to all those teachers who have persevered to achieve excellence.

—VSD

To my thoughtful father who enriched my life; my mother and grandparents
and their endless affection and love; and to my loving wife, for her support
and patience through the labors of my work.

—WEAS

Contents

Preface

Ultrasound provides a safe multiplanar real-time survey of human anatomy and pathology. In well-trained hands it is an invaluable and relatively inexpensive guidance modality. As a result, image-guidance utilizing ultrasound for invasive procedures is now commonplace. In numerous complex procedures, ultrasound provides the initial imaging for percutaneous access, which is the first step in such percutaneous procedures. This book encompasses numerous ultrasound-guided procedures as well as ultrasound-guided access for more complex procedures. Postaccess details of the more complex procedures are beyond the scope of this book; however, details of ultrasound-guided access are provided. Even if a particular procedure is not included in the contents, the reader should be able to extrapolate the appropriate ultrasound-guided access technique from procedures applied to similar anatomy.

In this book we provide a point-by-point, practical how-to checklist for ultrasound-guided interventions and percutaneous access. Exemplary images and illustrations have been utilized to aid in the teaching and understanding of the ultrasound-guided procedures presented. We hope that this book provides a valuable contribution to the literature on percutaneous procedures and pleasant read at all levels during and after diagnostic and/or interventional radiology training.

Acknowledgments

We would like to thank Margaret Kowaluk, Katherine Tower, and Anthony M. Pazos for their artistic work and dedication. They have helped make this book unique; without them, this book would not have been possible.

Vikram S. Dogra, MD
Professor of Radiology, Urology and Biomedical Engineering
Associate Chair for Education and Research
Department of Imaging Sciences
University of Rochester Medical Center
Rochester, New York

Wael E.A. Saad, MBBCh
Associate Professor of Radiology
Division of Vascular Interventional Radiology
Department of Radiology
University of Virginia Medical System
Charlottesville, Virginia

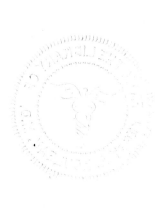

Contributors

Monzer M. Abu-Yousef, MD
Department of Radiology
University of Iowa Hospitals and Clinics
Iowa City, Iowa

Daniel B. Brown, MD
Professor of Radiology
Chief, Interventional Radiology and Interventional
    Oncology
Department of Radiology
Thomas Jefferson University
Philadelphia, Pennsylvania

Vikram S. Dogra, MD
Professor of Radiology, Urology, and Biomedical
    Engineering
Associate Chair for Education and Research
Department of Imaging Sciences
University of Rochester Medical Center
Rochester, New York

Beth S. Edeiken-Monroe, MD
MD Anderson Cancer Center
Houston, Texas

Bruno D. Fornage, MD
MD Anderson Cancer Center
Houston, Texas

Jennifer A. Harvey, MD
Division of Breast Imaging
Department of Radiology
University of Virginia
Charlottesville, Virginia

Christine O. Menias, MD
Associate Professor of Radiology
Mallinckrodt Institute of Radiology
Washington University
St. Louis, Missouri

Brett J. Monroe, MD
Surgical Resident
The Michael E. Debakey Department of General Surgery
Baylor College of Medicine
Houston, Texas

Dean A. Nakamoto, MD
Department of Radiology
University Hospitals of Cleveland Case Medical Center
Cleveland, Ohio

Chiou Li Ong, MBBS, FRCR
Department of Diagnostic Imaging
KK Women's and Children's Hospital
Singapore

Suhas G. Parulekar, MD
MD Anderson Cancer Center
Houston, Texas

Wael E.A. Saad, MBBCh
Associate Professor of Radiology
Division of Vascular Interventional Radiology
Department of Radiology
University of Virginia Medical System
Charlottesville, Virginia

Ralf Thiele, MD
Division of Allergy/Immunology and Rheumatology
University of Rochester
Rochester, New York

Ahmet Tuncay Turgut, MD
Department of Radiology
Ankara Training and Research Hospital
Ankara, Turkey

Sudhir Vinayak, MD
Consultant Radiologist
Section Head Ultrasound
The Aga Khan University Hospital
Nairobi, Kenya

I Ultrasound-Guided Biopsies

1 Liver Biopsy

Wael E.A. Saad

Classification and Indications

Liver biopsies are classified into random liver biopsies and target-specific liver lesion biopsies.

Random Liver Biopsy

A random liver biopsy is a liver tissue sample that is obtained to evaluate diffuse liver disease such as

- Liver cirrhosis
- Liver fibrosis
- Hemachromatosis
- Wilson's disease (Hepatolenticular degeneration)
- Steatosis (fatty liver, nonalcoholic steatohepatitis [NASH])
- Viral hepatitis baseline/surveillance
- Primary sclerosing cholangitis (PSC)
- Liver transplant rejection
- Liver transplant ischemia

There are two types of random liver biopsies (**Table 1.1**):

- Transjugular random liver biopsies (**Fig. 1.1**)
- Percutaneous random liver biopsies
  - Intercostal random right hepatic lobe biopsy
  - Subcostal random right hepatic lobe biopsy
  - Subxyphoid random left lobe biopsy

Target-selected Liver Biopsy/Liver Lesion Biopsy

A liver lesion biopsy is a liver tissue sample that is obtained to evaluate a specific focal liver lesion such as

- Hepatic metastasis
- Atypical hemangiomas
- Hepatocellular carcinoma (HCC; hepatoma)
- Adenoma
- Focal nodular hyperplasia
- Regenerative nodule

Table 1.1   Comparison Between Transjugular Liver Biopsy and Percutaneous Liver Biopsy

	Transjugular Liver Biopsy	Percutaneous Liver Biopsy

Skill Set Required	Requires a specialized skill set
	  Vascular access
	  Transcatheter skills
		Requires a less specialized skill set
		However, requires good command of ultrasound guidance

Diagnostic Yield	Generally less pathologic diagnostic yield due to no parenchymal imaging/image guidance Needle caliber smaller than 18-gauge (20–21 gauge)	Generally higher pathologic diagnostic yield due to Parenchymal imaging/image guidance Needle caliber can be 18-gauge or higher
Additional Diagnostic Yield	Additional information on hepatic disease evaluation can be obtained Pathologic appearance of hepatic venography in advanced cirrhosis Hepatic venous pressures can be obtained to diagnose portal hypertension	Can identify unknown superadded focal liver disease Can provide additional diagnostic information on known focal liver disease

Coagulopathy Thresholds*	Higher threshold for coagulopathy
	Suggested thresholds:
	  ∎ INR: ≤1.7–1.9
	  ∎ PLT: ≥50,000
	  ∎ aPTT: ≤60 s
		Lower threshold for coagulopathy
		Suggested thresholds:
		  ∎ INR: ≤1.4–1.5
		  ∎ PLT: ≥50,000–70,000
		  ∎ aPTT: ≤45–50 s

*Coagulopathy thresholds are suggestions. Variations of set thresholds among institutions and individual operators are typical. Safe thresholds are difficult to set (prove based on evidence-based science) due to numerous clinical variables.

Abbreviations: INR, international normalized ratio; PLT, platelets; aPTT, active prothrombin time.

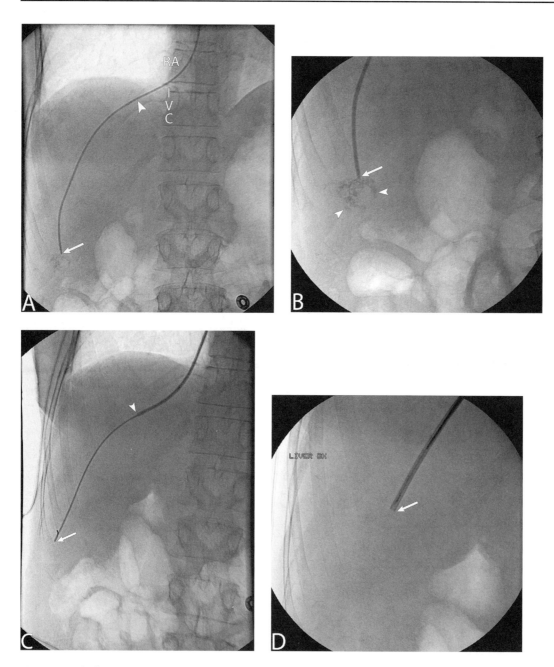

Fig. 1.1 Single fluoroscopic image in the first step of a transjugular liver biopsy. The first step is selective catheterization of one of the hepatic veins. The right hepatic vein is preferable because it provides the greater wire and catheter purchase. **(A)** On a frontal projection the right hepatic vein usually starts (its caval orifice: *arrowhead*) near the vertebro-phrenic angle, which is close to the junction. A 5-French catheter has been passed down the superior vena cava, through the right atrium (RA) and into the inferior vena cava (IVC). A right turn is made and the catheter is passed all the way down near the periphery (subhepatic capsule: *arrow*). **(B)** Single fluoroscopic image, which is a magnified view of the periphery of the liver at the end of the 5-French catheter seen in **Fig. 1.1A**. Contrast is injected very gently through the catheter tip (*arrow*), which stains the hepatic parenchyma (*arrowheads*). This proves that the catheter is wedged and a wedged hepatic pressure can be obtained. The result obtained when the wedged hepatic pressure is subtracted from the central venous pressure (CVP) is helpful in determining the porto-systemic gradient to help diagnose portal hypertension. **(C)** Single fluoroscopic image where a 0.035-inch wire is passed down the catheter (*arrow*). The 5-French catheter has been removed and a curved-tip metal introducer sheath is being passed down the wire. The tip of the curved-tip introducer sheath is at the arrowhead. **(D)** Single fluoroscopic image that is a magnified view of the periphery of the liver. The curved-tip metal introducer sheath tip had been advanced down the wire into the periphery of the liver (*arrow*). A 20-gauge Trucut needle is advanced coaxially through the metal curved-tip introducer sheath (housed within sheath). The sheath directs the needle to the desired location (hepatic periphery) without injuring the structures it passes (cava, right atrium, hepatic veins). As can be seen the needle is tip-to-tip with the sheath.

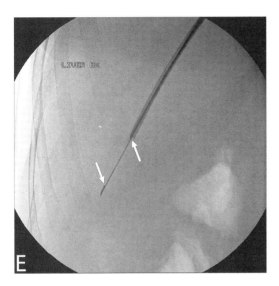
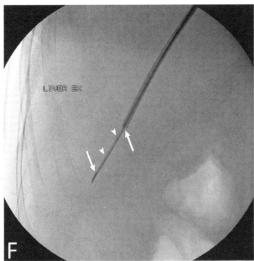

Fig. 1.1 *(Continued)* **(E)** Single fluoroscopic image that is a magnified view of the periphery of the liver. The 20-gauge Trucut needle is advanced coaxially through the metal sheath. The Trucut needle has a groove along its side *(between arrows)*. The hepatic parenchyma falls into it. **(F)** Single fluoroscopic image that is a magnified view of the periphery of the liver. The 20-gauge Trucut needle has been "fired." The outer metal covering *(arrowheads)* quickly passes over the needle groove and "shaves" off the hepatic parenchyma, which had fallen into the groove *(between arrows)*. The shaved hepatic parenchyma now housed in the needle groove is the 20-gauge core sample.

Contraindications

Absolute Contraindications

- Uncorrected coagulopathy (see **Table 1.1** for suggested thresholds)

Relative Contraindications

- Ascites (can be drained just prior to biopsy procedure)
- Liver transplantation within one month of the transplantation
- Concerns for seeding of hepatocellular carcinoma in a patient with a high α-fetoprotein without dissemination and a candidate for liver transplantation

Preprocedural Evaluation

Evaluate Prior Cross-sectional Imaging

- Look for ascites
  - When there is no ascites, bleeding can seize due to the tamponade effect of adjacent organs and particularly the chest wall (rib cage).
  - Due to this, some operators consider ascites an increased risk for bleeding (controversial).
  - Many operators would drain ascites prior to the liver biopsy.

- Evaluate the size of the hepatic lobes and their location (**Fig. 1.2**)
  - For random liver biopsies, some operators prefer to biopsy the left hepatic lobe.
    - Evaluate whether the left hepatic lobe is accessible; it may be positioned behind the anterior aspect of the rib cage.
    - The left hepatic lobe may be small and inaccessible from the epigastric region.
  - If evaluating for a random liver biopsy for the right hepatic lobe:
    - Make sure the right hepatic lobe is accessible and that the right hemicolon does not stand in the way (**Fig. 1.2**).
    - For history of hepatic lobectomies, evaluate prior operative notes and prior computed tomography (CT) examinations to see which lobe was resected and how the remaining liver has hypertrophied to decide which ultrasound approach is best for a random liver biopsy sample (**Fig. 1.2**).
- Look for adjacent organs that can be traversed (**Figs. 1.2, 1.3**)
  - This helps plan the needle trajectory (biopsy approach).
  - This can help reduce transgression of adjacent organs with subsequent potential major complication.
  - Particular organs that may be traversed include the colon, gallbladder, lung, and, less likely, the small bowel.

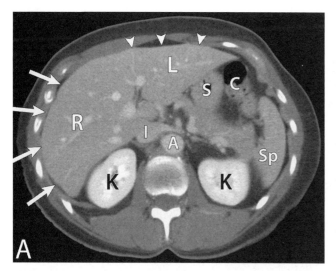

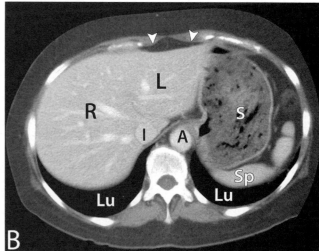

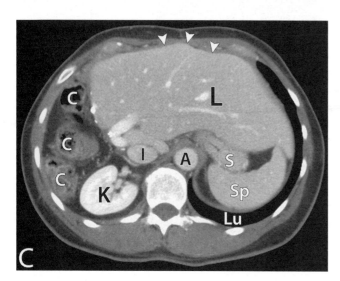

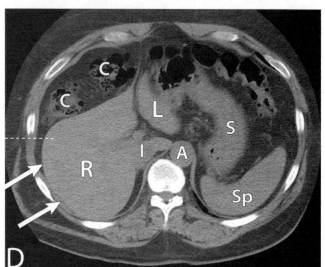

Fig. 1.2 Planning ultrasound-guided biopsy approach based on computed tomography (CT) findings. **(A)** Contrast-enhanced axial CT image at the level of the porta hepatis. The image demonstrates an easily accessible right hepatic lobe from intercostal approaches (*arrows*) and an easily accessible left hepatic lobe from a subxyphoid (epigastric) approach (*arrowheads*). **(B)** Contrast-enhanced axial CT image at the level of the aortic hiatus. The image demonstrates a small left hepatic lobe, which is still accessible from a subxyphoid (epigastric) approach (*arrowheads*). The purpose of this image is to compare with the prior image (**Fig. 1.2A**) the different sizes and configurations of left hepatic lobes. **(C)** Contrast-enhanced axial CT image at the level of the aortic hiatus. The patient is status post right hepatic lobectomy with resultant left hepatic compensatory hypertrophy. The image demonstrates a large left hepatic lobe (L), which is still accessible from a subxyphoid (epigastric) approach (*arrowheads*). An intercostal approach is not feasible. There is no right hepatic lobe. The place of the right hepatic lobe is occupied by the right hemicolon (C). **(D)** Unenhanced axial CT image at the level of the aortic hiatus. The patient has not had any liver surgery. The right hemicolon (C), however, rides high and occupies the right upper quadrant anteriorly. The image demonstrates that an intercostal approach is feasible (*arrows*) only posterior to the midaxillary line (*dashed line*). A focused ultrasound posterior to the midaxillary line should be performed to find the target liver. **(E)** Unenhanced axial CT image at the level of the porta hepatis. The patient has not had any liver surgery. The right

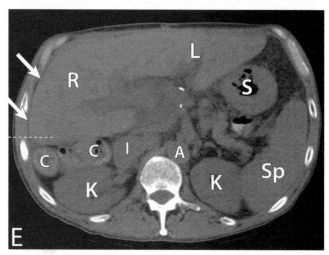

hemicolon (C), however, rides high and occupies the right upper quadrant posteriorly between the kidney and the right hepatic lobe. The image demonstrates that an intercostal approach is feasible (*arrows*) only anterior to the midaxillary line (*dashed line*). (K, kidney; R, right hepatic lobe; L, left hepatic lobe; Sp, spleen; C, colon; S, stomach; A, aorta; I, inferior vena cava; Lu, lung)

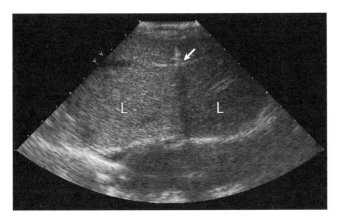
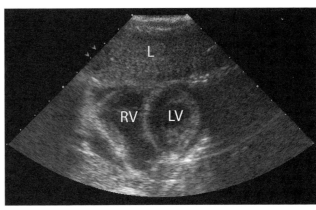

A   B

Fig. 1.3 **(A)** Preliver biopsy examination gray-scale ultrasound exam (transverse to the abdomen in the epigastric region) as a 21-gauge lidocaine needle is advanced to locally anesthetize the subcutaneous tissue and Glisson's capsule. The lidocaine needle tip (*arrow*) is at the liver (Glisson's) capsule. **(B)** Gray-scale ultrasound exam (transverse to the abdomen in the epigastric region). The operator has just "panned" the transducer cephalad. Right above the left liver lobe (L) sits the base of the heart. The image shows the left hepatic lobe between the transducer and the heart, which is seen in its short axis. (L, liver; RV, right ventricle; LV, left ventricle)

- For hepatic lesion biopsy, look for normal hepatic parenchymal segments for peripherally located subcapsular lesions.
  - This helps plan the biopsy needle trajectory to traverse normal hepatic parenchyma by the needle prior to entering the target lesion.
  - Traversing normal hepatic parenchyma may reduce the risk of bleeding.
  - Traversing normal hepatic parenchyma may reduce the risk of tumor seeding.

Evaluate Prebiopsy Laboratory Values

Laboratory value evaluation mostly revolves around ruling out coagulopathy.

- Suggested coagulopathy thresholds are presented in **Table 1.1**.
- Serum creatinine may be considered for transjugular liver biopsies, although the use of contrast can be minimal and certain operators can argue that a transjugular liver biopsy can be obtained without venography (contrast utilization).

Obtain Informed Consent

- Indications
  - To evaluate for diffuse liver disease versus focal liver lesion
  - The expected diagnostic pathology yield from a random renal biopsy is 97–100%.

- Alternatives
  - To refuse the biopsy
  - Percutaneous versus transjugular liver biopsy
  - Surgical wedge biopsy
- Procedural risks
  - Infection
    - This is a rare complication (<1%).
    - It is most common (up to 1.8% of cases) in liver transplant recipients in the form of postbiopsy fevers and rigors (presumed to be postbiopsy cholangitis).
  - Bleeding
    - This is the most common major complication.
    - It may present as pain and/or hypotension.
    - Bleeding may be transient with or without blood transfusion.
    - In rare cases, bleeding may require intervention such as transcatheter hepatic arterial embolization or exploratory surgery.
  - Injury to surrounding organs and/or structures
    - Pleura (pneumo- and hemothorax)
    - Gallbladder (pain and/or biloma)
    - Kidney and bowel
  - Others

Equipment

Ultrasound Guidance

- Ultrasound machine with Doppler capability
- Multiarray 4–5 MHz ultrasound transducer
- Transducer guide bracket
- Sterile transducer cover

Standard Surgical Preparation and Draping

- Chlorhexidine skin preparation/cleansing fluid
- Fenestrated drape

Local Infiltrative Analgesia Administration

- 21-gauge infiltration needle
- 10–20 mL 1% lidocaine syringe

Sharp Access and Biopsy

- 11-blade incision scalpel
- Coaxial access needle (see below); 17- and 19-gauge coaxial needles for delivery of core biopsy needles (18-gauge and 20-gauge core biopsy needles, respectively)
- Coaxial access needle (see below); 20-gauge coaxial needles for delivery of fine-needle aspiration 22-gauge needles

Technique

Intravenous Access

- The necessity of moderate sedation (administered intravenously) for liver biopsies varies from one institution to another. My institution prefers moderate sedation for liver biopsies.
- If moderate sedation is not routinely administered, intravenous (IV) access is still reasonable as a standby for any complication (including pain related complications), or if the need arises to administer sedation.

Prebiopsy Ultrasound Examination

- Determine easiest visibility of lesion in cases of target lesion biopsy
- Determine access (intercostal, subcostal, subxyphoid) (**Fig. 1.2**)
- For random liver biopsies, determine a region of hepatic parenchyma with paucity of larger intrahepatic vessels.
- Look for ascites
- Evaluate the size of the left hepatic lobe and its location/accessibility (**Fig. 1.2**)
- Look for adjacent organs that can be traversed (**Figs. 1.2 and 1.3**)
- For hepatic lesion biopsy, look for normal hepatic parenchymal segments for peripherally located subcapsular lesions.

Standard Surgical Preparation and Draping

- Prepare/cleanse skin in the region chosen as an ultrasound imaging portal and a needle access portal
- Place a fenestrated drape at the prepared skin region

Local Infiltrative Analgesia Administration

- Utilizing a 21-gauge (by at least a 3.7 cm long) infiltration needle, 1% lidocaine infiltration is performed. The infiltration should not be limited to the skin and subcutaneous tissue, but should include infiltration of the very sensitive hepatic capsule (Glisson's capsule) (**Fig. 1.3**).

Sharp Access

- An incision is made utilizing an 11-blade scalpel, usually by a 3-mm-depth stab.
- A coaxial access needle (17- or 19-gauge coaxial needles for core biopsies) can be passed across the hepatic capsule in the direction of the chosen parenchyma (for a random biopsy) or the hepatic lesion (for target lesion biopsy).
- When utilizing a midaxillary intercostal approach, the coaxial needle (or biopsy needle itself) should be passed over (cephalad) the ribs to avoid injury to the intercostal neurovascular bundle (intercostal vessels and nerve).
- The coaxial access needle allows multiple coaxial passes of the actual biopsy needle (pathology-sample acquisition needle), while only inflicting a single puncture of the hepatic capsule. This theoretically may reduce bleeding risk and possibly tract seeding (**Fig. 1.4**).
- The coaxial access needle also allows for the embolization of the transhepatic tract with Gelfoam (Pfizer Pharmaceuticals, New York, NY) or coils after the biopsy has been performed (**Fig. 1.4**).

Pathology Sample Acquisition (Biopsy)

- An automated spring-loaded core-biopsy needle is passed to the end of a coaxial needle, "fired" (automatically deployed), and withdrawn.
- Without the use of coaxial needle access, the core-biopsy needle is passed to the edge of the intended region (specific target lesion or the intended parenchyma for the random biopsy). It is then "fired" or deployed (**Figs. 1.5, 1.6, 1.7**).
- When it comes to lesion biopsy, at least one biopsy sample should be obtained by having the core biopsy needle be deployed from outside the lesion (from a position falling short of the lesion border) so as to obtain "normal" hepatic parenchyma and sample the pathologic junction/margin of the lesion.
- Usually one to five core (20-gauge, 18-gauge, or, by some operators, larger caliber) biopsy needle passes/deployments are made.

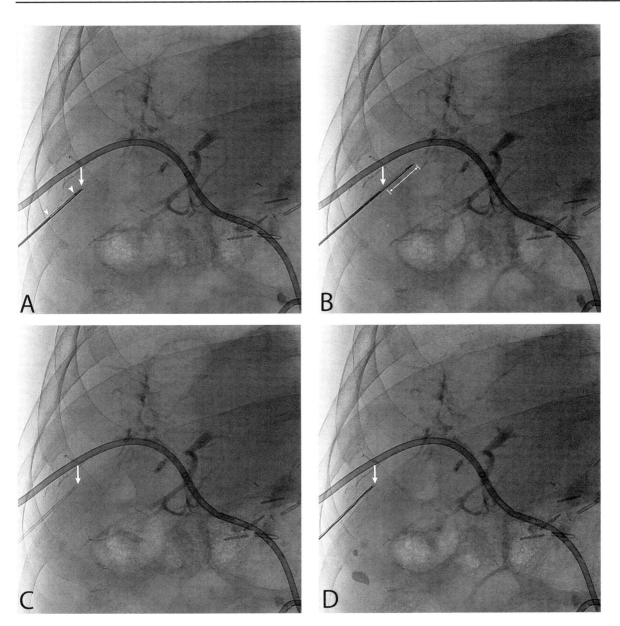

Fig. 1.4 Fluoroscopic step-by-step liver biopsy and coil embolization through a coaxial needle. **(A)** Fluoroscopic image demonstrates an 18-gauge Trucut needle positioned within a 17-gauge coaxial needle. The 18- and 17-gauge needles are tip-to-tip (*arrow*). The 18-gauge Trucut needle is "cocked" and ready to be "fired." The Trucut needle has a side groove (between the *arrowheads*). Incidentally, this random liver biopsy is subsequent to a transhepatic biliary drain placement; despite that, this is a fluoroscopic liver biopsy. The fluoroscopic images allow the readers to see the step-by-step sample acquisition and transhepatic liver biopsy. **(B)** Fluoroscopic image following **Fig. 1.4A**. The 18-gauge Trucut needle has been "fired" from the 17-gauge coaxial needle. This particular 18-gauge Trucut needle (Bard Manopty needle; BARD, Covington, GA) protrudes 2.2 cm (*bi-way arrow*) outside the 17-gauge needle (17-gauge coaxial needle tip at *arrow*). The outer Trucut needle metal cover has shaved the liver parenchyma thus acquiring the 18-gauge core sample (please see **Figs. 1.1D, 1.1E, 1.1F**). In fact, this needle fires automatically and does the three steps described from **Fig. 1.1D** to **Fig. 1.1F** in one button push (fully automated; the needle in **Fig. 1.1** is semiautomated). **(C)** Fluoroscopic image following **Fig. 1.4B**. The 18-gauge Trucut needle has been removed from the 17-gauge coaxial needle. The core sample has been obtained. The 17-gauge coaxial needle tip (*arrow*) is still in place. **(D)** Fluoroscopic image following **Fig. 1.4C**. A 0.035-inch stainless steel fibered coil (Cook Medical, Bloomington, IN) is being pushed up the 17-gauge needle. The coil once pushed out will form a 9-mm diameter helical coil. At this moment, the coil tip is at the tip of the 17-gauge coaxial needle tip (*arrow*). *(Continued on page 10)*

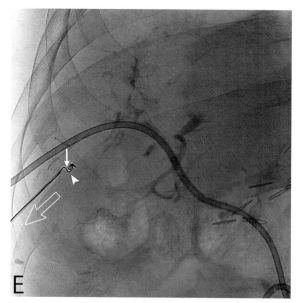

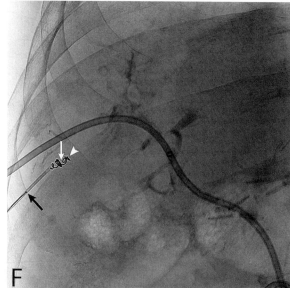

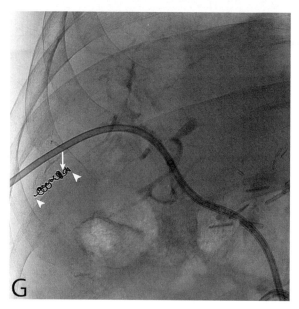

Fig. 1.4 *(Continued)* **(E)** Fluoroscopic image following **Fig. 1.4D**. The 0.035-inch stainless steel fibered coil (*arrowhead*) has been pushed beyond the tip of the 17-gauge needle (*arrow*). From this point, the 17-gauge coaxial needle is pulled back (*directional hollow arrow*), thus unsheathing the coil. **(F)** Fluoroscopic image following **Fig. 1.4E**. The 0.035-inch stainless steel fibered coil (*arrowhead*) has been deployed completely. The arrow points to where the tip of the 17-gauge needle used to be positioned before it was pulled back (*arrow*). A second stainless steel coil is being advanced up the 17-gauge coaxial needle (*black arrow*). **(G)** Fluoroscopic image following **Fig. 1.4F**. This is the final (completion) image. The two 0.035-inch stainless steel fibered coils (*between arrowheads*) have been deployed completely. Their coil diameters are 9 mm. The arrow points to where the tip of the 17-gauge needle used to be positioned before it was pulled back (*arrow*). Typically, this is the ideal transhepatic coil deployment: part of the first coil is beyond the coaxial needle in the vicinity of the hepatic parenchyma that has been biopsied (sampled) and the remainder of the coils is along the transhepatic tract as the needle has been pulled back.

Transhepatic Tract Embolization

- This is not routinely performed.
- It may be performed in significantly coagulopathic patients after a core biopsy or if there is inadvertent active bleeding.
- Transhepatic needle tract embolization requires a coaxial access needle technique (**Figs. 1.4, 1.8**).
- Gelfoam pledgets, Gelfoam slurry, or metal coils can be blindly deployed through the coaxial needle as it is slowly withdrawn along the transhepatic tract (**Figs. 1.4, 1.8**).
- If fluoroscopy is available, the coils can be deployed under fluoroscopy. Deploying Gelfoam pledgets under fluoroscopy guidance requires the Gelfoam pledgets to be soaked in contrast for them to be visualized.

Immediate Postbiopsy Ultrasound Imaging

- Immediate postbiopsy ultrasound imaging is for documentation and obtaining an image baseline for capsular or subcapsular hematomas.
- Visualizing a hepatic capsular hematoma does not alter postprocedural care or management.
- Visualizing active bleeding in the presence of ascites (**Fig. 1.9**). The ascites allows the visualization of the active bleeding and not necessarily increases the risk of active bleeding. This last statement is controversial; some would argue that ascites increases the risk for bleeding.

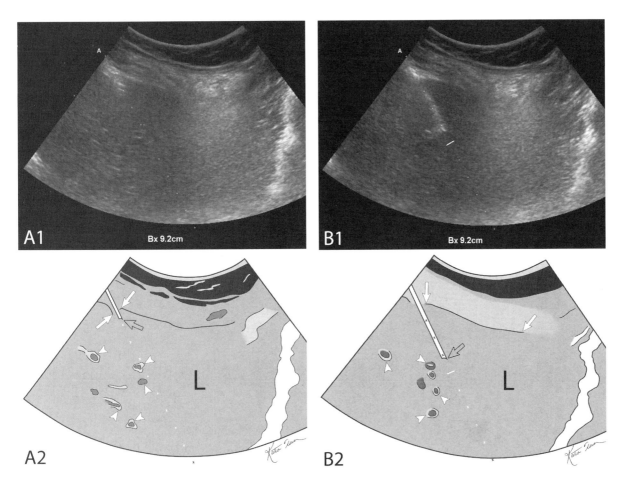

Fig. 1.5 **(A)** Ultrasound-guided random left liver biopsy gray-scale ultrasound image of the upper abdomen (*top*) and schematic sketch of it (*bottom*). The liver parenchyma seen is the left hepatic lobe (L). An 18-gauge needle is seen indenting and just passing through the hepatic capsule (*between arrows*). The operator attempts to direct the needle away from the majority of visualized blood vessels and bile ducts (*arrowheads*). **(B)** Gray-scale ultrasound image of the upper abdomen (*top*) and schematic sketch of it (*bottom*). The 18-gauge Trucut biopsy needle has been "fired" and the liver sample has been obtained. The operator has avoided the majority of visualized blood vessels and bile ducts (*arrowheads*). The arrows point to the hepatic capsule.

Endpoints

The overall endpoint is to obtain a tissue sample that is representative of the liver lesion or of the hepatic parenchyma and that is adequate enough to obtain a pathologic diagnosis of the disease process in question. The operator in this instance evaluates the gross tissue sample by the naked eye to determine if he or she has obtained enough core samples. This is a personal evaluation, however, and not an exact quantitative science.

Random Nontarget Liver Biopsy

- Usually one to three 18-gauge needle passes are required to obtain an adequate pathology sample.
- An adequate pathology sample is obtained by real-time ultrasound guidance in 97–100% of the time.

- Smaller caliber needles (20-gauge core biopsy needles) and larger caliber needles (16-gauge core biopsy needles) may require more needle passes or fewer needle passes, respectively.
- The operator grossly evaluates the core sample and determines when to stop making core biopsy needle passes (after the first, second, or third needle pass).
- For a virology evaluation or an electron microscopy evaluation, or the case of metal deposition disease (hemachromatosis or Wilson's disease), additional samples are required. Samples should be placed in reagents and containers that are appropriate for the desired tests. Consultation with your institution's pathologist is recommended.
- Advanced cirrhosis may cause the core samples to fragment. As a result, more than the usual number of needle passes may be required in cases of friable/fragmented samples.

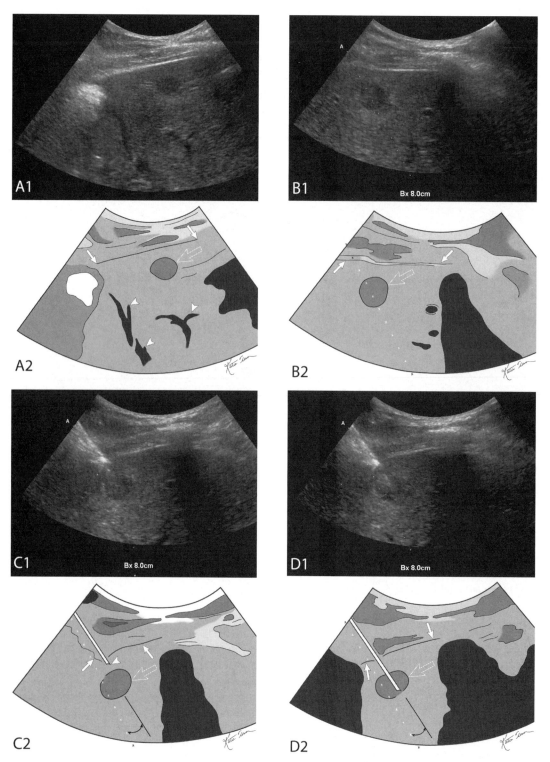

Fig. 1.6 Ultrasound-guided target lesion liver biopsy. **(A)** Gray-scale ultrasound image of the upper abdomen (*top*) and schematic sketch of it (*bottom*). A hypoechoic lesion (*hollow arrow*) is seen in a subcapsular location. The arrows point to the hepatic capsule. Deep to this lesion are hepatic blood vessels (*arrowheads*). **(B)** Gray-scale ultrasound image of the upper abdomen (*top*) and schematic sketch of it (*bottom*). The operator puts on the ultrasound guidance sites through the hypoechoic lesion (*hollow arrow*) is seen in a subcapsular location. The arrows point to the hepatic capsule. **(C)** Gray-scale ultrasound image of the upper abdomen (*top*) and schematic sketch of it (*bottom*). The image is acquired after **Fig. 1.6B**. The operator advances an 18-gauge biopsy needle toward the hypoechoic lesion (*hollow arrow*). The hepatic capsule (*arrows*) is seen being indented by the needle tip (*arrowhead*). Note that the needle passes along a trajectory that is off (*curved bi-arrow*) the ultrasound-guidance sites (*dotted line*). In this situation, the operator should correct for the offset needle trajectory so that the target lesion is sampled. **(D)** Gray-scale ultrasound image of the upper abdomen (*top*) and schematic sketch of it (*bottom*). The image is acquired after **Fig. 1.6C**. The operator has "fired" the18-gauge Trucut biopsy needle into the hypoechoic lesion (*hollow arrow*). The arrows point to the hepatic capsule. Note that the operator has corrected for the discrepancy between the ultrasound-guidance site and the actual needle trajectory (*curved bi-arrow*).

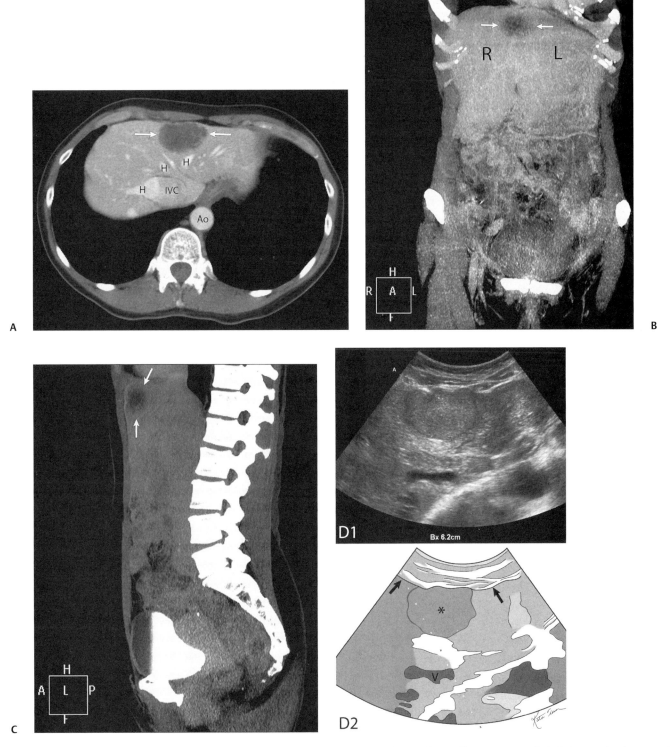

Fig. 1.7 Ultrasound-guided target lesion liver biopsy. **(A)** Axial image of a contrast-enhanced computed tomography (CT) scan of the upper abdomen at the level of convergence of the hepatic veins (H) around the inferior vena cava (IVC). A low-density lesion is seen (*between arrows*). **(B)** Coronal reconstruction of the contrast enhanced CT of **Fig. 1.7A**. Noted is the low-density lesion (*between arrows*). **(C)** Sagittal reconstruction of the contrast-enhanced CT of **Fig. 1.7A**. Noted is the low-density lesion (*between arrows*). **(D)** Gray-scale ultrasound image of the upper abdomen (*top*) and schematic sketch of it (*bottom*) of the same patient with the same lesion as in **Figs. 1.7A, 1.7B, and 1.7C**. An isoechoic lesion (*asterisk in center of lesion*) is seen in an immediate subcapsular location. The arrows point to the hepatic capsule. Deep to this lesion is hepatic vein (V). *(Continued on page 14)*

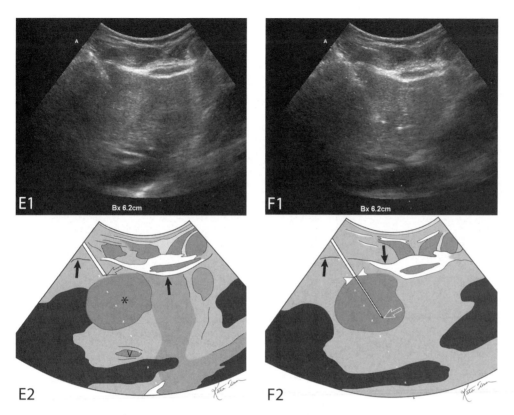

Fig. 1.7 *(Continued)* **(E)** Gray-scale ultrasound image of the upper abdomen *(top)* and schematic sketch of it *(bottom)*. The isoechoic lesion *(asterisk in center of lesion)* is again seen in an immediate subcapsular location. Deep to this lesion is hepatic vein (V). A 17-gauge coaxial needle has been passed through the hepatic capsule *(arrows)*. Its tip *(hollow arrow)* is just short of the target lesion edge. **(F)** Gray-scale ultrasound image of the upper abdomen *(top)* and schematic sketch of it *(bottom)*. The isoechoic lesion is again seen in an immediate subcapsular location. An 18-gauge Trucut biopsy needle has been passed through the 17-gauge coaxial needle and has been "fired" or deployed into the target lesion. The tip of the 17-gauge coaxial needle sits at the edge of the target lesion *(arrowheads)*. The hollow arrow points to the 18-gauge biopsy needle tip. (Ao, aorta; R, right hepatic lobe; L, left hepatic lobe.)

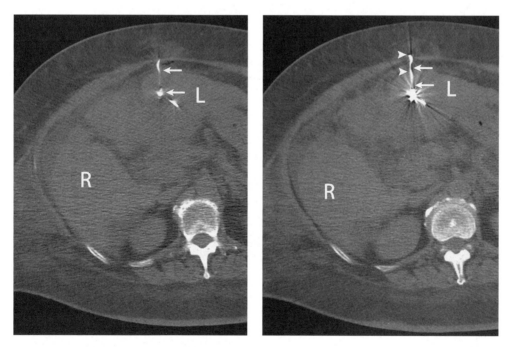

Fig. 1.8 Transhepatic coil placement after a liver biopsy. **(A)** Axial image of a noncontrast-enhanced computed tomography (CT) scan of the upper abdomen. Transhepatic coils are seen traversing the transhepatic tract *(between arrows)*. **(B)** Axial image of a noncontrast-enhanced CT of the upper abdomen. Transhepatic coils are seen traversing the transhepatic tract *(between arrows)*. The coils are seen extending outside the liver in the soft tissue tract *(arrowheads)*. (R, right hepatic lobe; L, left hepatic lobe.)

14

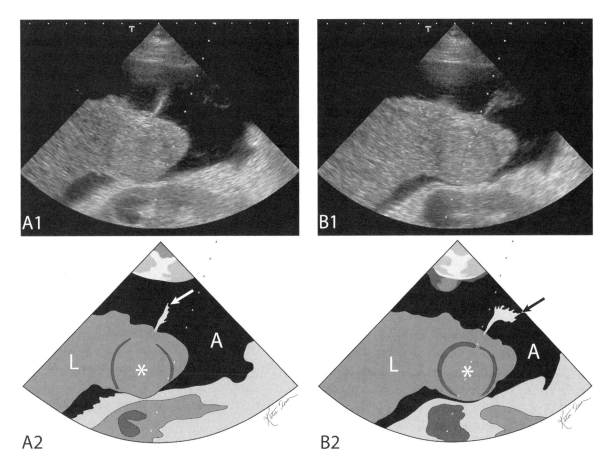

Fig. 1.9 Active bleeding into ascetic fluid after a liver lesion biopsy. **(A)** Gray-scale ultrasound image of the upper abdomen (*top*) and schematic sketch of it (*bottom*) of a patient with a large liver lesion (*asterisk in center of lesion*). An isoechoic lesion (*asterisk in center of lesion*) is seen in an immediate subcapsular location. Ascites (A) is seen surrounding the liver (L). There is a fountain of blood spurting (*arrow*) out of the liver after a core biopsy was obtained. The ascites allows us to see the spurting fountain of bleeding. **(B)** Gray-scale ultrasound image of the upper abdomen (*top*) and schematic sketch of it (*bottom*). An isoechoic lesion (*asterisk in center of lesion*) is seen in an immediate subcapsular location. Ascites (A) is seen surrounding the liver (L). There is a fountain of blood spurting (*arrow*) out of the liver after a core biopsy was obtained. Despite the alarming appearance of the bleeding, the patient was always stable and did well. Treat the patient and not the images. (Courtesy of Dean Nakamoto, MD of Case Western University)

Lesion-specific Target Liver Biopsy

- Usually one to three 18-gauge needle passes are required to obtain an adequate pathology sample.
- Smaller caliber needles (20-gauge core biopsy needles) and larger caliber needles (16-gauge core biopsy needles) may require more needle passes or fewer needle passes, respectively.
- The operator grossly evaluates the core sample and determines when to stop making core biopsy needle passes (after the first, second, or third needle pass). This decision is not based on evidence-based research.
- In cases of suspicion of lymphoma, fine needle aspirates (22-gauge needle passes) should be obtained prior to the core biopsy sample for flow-cytometry evaluation.

Postprocedural Evaluation and Management

There is no clear set standard for outpatient postbiopsy care. The following are suggestions with some variations mentioned for discussion and flexibility to accommodate particular institutional and practice settings.

Outpatient Ambulatory Stay/Observation Period

- Postprocedural stay varies from one institution to another.
- It should be noted that almost all complications (bleeding is the foremost concern) present within the first 3 hours after the liver biopsy.
- At my institution, postliver biopsy outpatients are kept under observation for 3–4 hours after the liver biopsy.

Intravenous Fluid and Diet

- IV access should be kept until just prior to discharge.
- Institutions that practice moderate sedation start with a clear liquid diet and advance it as tolerated. This helps to offset patients' nausea and vomiting.
- Other institutions/operators commence a clear liquid diet after a period of abstinence of oral intake. This period could be one hour, for example.
- Give IV fluid until oral intake is adequate

Activity

- Bed rest for the observation period prior to discharge
- Some institutions/operators would keep the patient in a right-side-down position in cases where a right midaxillary intercostal approach was sought for the live biopsy. The idea is that this would tamponade the right hepatic lobe capsular puncture and prevent/stop bleeding. There is no evidence-based research to support this practice; however, it is practiced at some institutions including my own.
- Patients, on discharge, are instructed not to engage in strenuous activity for 24–48 hours postbiopsy.

Pain Management

- Narcotics are usually not required during the postbiopsy stay of the patient prior to discharge. Occasionally, some patients require oral narcotic analgesics such as acetaminophen and hydrocodone combination medication. Rarely does a patient require IV narcotics such as fentanyl.
- Pain radiating to the left shoulder would further support chemical/irritant peritonitis. However, if coupled with shortness of breath and desaturation (not splinting) one should suspect a significant pneumothorax. A chest x-ray is warranted.
- On discharge, patients usually tolerate the procedure well and do not require more potent analgesics than over-the-counter medications.

Monitoring Vital Signs

- Vital sign monitoring includes blood pressure and heart rate. Occasionally, oxygen saturation monitoring is required in cases of shortness of breath and/or chest pain.
- Institutions/operators that practice conscious sedation may record a softer blood pressure than a patient's baseline blood pressure after the biopsy. This is most likely due to sedation with or without dehydration. The patient usually responds in time with hydration, particularly as the sedatives wear off.

- Continued hypotension and, more importantly, a rise in heart rate are concerning for hypovolemia (bleeding). If signs of hypovolemia occur, an IV volume bolus is given and a noncontrast CT exam is performed to confirm the clinical suspicion of bleeding.
- Prior to discharge, some operators/institutions measure orthostatic pressures. At my institution, they are considered unnecessary and are not specific, particularly when we keep the postliver biopsy patients for 4 hours. Obviously, patients who on standing erect become light-headed are not discharged.

Complications and Their Management

At the postliver biopsy evaluation and during the management period, the main concerns revolve around the most common complication – pain and pain-related morbidity – and the most serious complication, bleeding (**Fig. 1.9**). Please see **Table 1.2** for the list of types of complications and their incidence following liver biopsies. Most complications, particularly life-threatening complications, are clinically unmasked within 3 hours of the liver biopsy.

Management of Pain and Pain-related Morbidity

- Continued pain requires further clinical and possibly imaging evaluation. Signs of peritonitis may denote chemical peritonitis from intraperitoneal bleeding or bile leak. The degree of pain does not correlate with the degree of bleeding. However, changes in vital signs do signify a significant bleed.
- Occasionally, operators respond to continued pain by performing a diagnostic imaging exam.
  - A limited ultrasound examination at the site to evaluate for a capsular hematoma
  - Or a more global exam such as a noncontrast abdominal CT exam. Ultimately, the decisive factor for determining significant bleeding is the patient's stability (vitals) – not what is seen on the images.
- If there is no bleeding and the patient is stable but requires narcotic analgesics for pain, the patient can be admitted for pain management. Hospital admission for pain management is rare; however, it has been reported in up to 2–3% of cases.

Management of Bleeding Complications

- IV access should be kept until just after discharge in case fluid resuscitation is required.
- Bleeding can take several forms and have different sources.
  - Skin bleeding (external)
  - Intercostal bleeding (hemothorax, external skin bleeding, or hemoperitoneum)

Table 1.2 Complications of Ultrasound-guided Liver Biopsies

Complication	Incidence
Abdominal and/or shoulder pain	36–37%*
Pain-associated morbidity (increased outpatient stay, hospitalization, or the use of narcotic analgesics)	1.8%*
Postbiopsy hospitalization (usually due to pain)	0.5–3.0%*
Mortality	Rare†
Pericapsular hematoma	0.5%
Hemobilia	Rare†
Hemo- and/or pneumothorax	0.0–0.4%
Arterioportal fistulae	Rare†
Vasovagal reaction	0.4–3.6%
Puncture to adjacent organs	0.0–1.8%
Bleeding/hypotension	1.5%

Source: Data from Lindor KD, Bru C, Jorgensen RA, et al. The role of ultrasonography and automatic-needle biopsy in outpatient percutaneous liver biopsy. Hepatology 1996;23(5):1079–1083; Little AF, Ferris JV, Dodd GD III, Baron RL. Image-guided percutaneous hepatic biopsy: effect of ascites on the complication rate. Radiology 1996;199(1):79–83; Nazarian LN, Feld RI, Herrine SK, et al. Safety and efficacy of sonographically guided random core biopsy for diffuse liver disease. J Ultrasound Med 2000;19(8): 537–541; Nobili V, Comparcola D, Sartorelli MR, et al. Blind and ultrasound-guided percutaneous liver biopsy in children. Pediatr Radiol 2003;33(11):772–775; Saad WEA, Ryan CK, Davies MG, et al. Safety and efficacy of fluoroscopic versus ultrasound guidance for core liver biopsies in potential living related liver transplant donors: preliminary results. J Vasc Interv Radiol 2006;17(8): 1307–1312; Sheets PW, Brumbaugh CJ, Kopecky KK, Pound DC, Filo RS. Safety and efficacy of a spring-propelled 18-gauge needle for US-guided liver biopsy. J Vasc Interv Radiol 1991; 2(1):147–149.

Note. Complications are mentioned when they constitute a percentage. Not all studies mention all complications.

*Due to varying definitions among prior studies, there is an overlap between criteria.

†This is not mentioned in the ultrasound-guided biopsy literature; however, it is mentioned in the blind liver biopsy literature.

○ Hepatic parenchyma/capsule (hemoperitoneum if not contained, capsular hematoma if contained) (**Fig. 1.9**).
○ Hemobilia (gastrointestinal bleeding)
• Significant bleeding affecting vital signs and patient stability should be managed by
○ Fluid resuscitation starting with crystalloid fluid bolus
○ Type and cross
○ Repeat hematocrit to compare with baseline

○ Blood transfusion to maintain hematocrit at or above 30%
○ Surgical consult/interventional radiology consult
• Interventional radiology offers
○ Hepatic arteriography with super-selective arterial embolization if bleeding or a pseudoaneurysm is seen
○ Hepatic arteriography with global arterial Gelfoam embolization to reduce arterial perfusion in the liver if bleeding or a pseudoaneurysm is not seen. One should be cautious about globally embolizing the hepatic artery in a patient who has had a liver biopsy. There is a good chance that he or she may be cirrhotic. Cirrhotic patients may have a higher incidence of hepatic infarction after global arterial embolization.
• In cases of severe uncontrolled bleeding, surgical consultation may offer open surgery, exploration, and local hemostasis of surface bleeding.

Management of Pleural/Thoracic Complications

• One must be able to differentiate clinically:
○ Referred shoulder pain from irritant peritonitis versus pleurisy from a hemo- and/or pneumothorax
○ Reduced oxygen saturation from poor inspiratory effort secondary to pain-related respiratory splinting versus reduced oxygenation due to hemo- and/or pneumothorax
• If chest pain with or without reduced oxygen saturation is encountered, a chest x-ray should be obtained to rule out pneumothorax or hemothorax. This is particularly true of liver biopsies using an intercostals-approach.
• Clinically significant hemo- and/or pneumothorax require chest tube placement, increased nasal cannula oxygenation, and fluid resuscitation/bleeding management in case of the former (see above).

Management of Puncture of Adjacent Organs

• With image guidance, this is a rare complication (up to 1.8% of cases).
• When it occurs, it is usually detected during the procedure by imaging or from the pathology report (renal glomeruli in a liver biopsy sample).
• When transgression of adjacent organs occurs, the result is clinically inconsequential. The problem is incidental and does not rise to the level of a minor clinical complication, let alone a major complication.
• Bile leak from inadvertent puncture of the gallbladder (rare) would require percutaneous drainage of the resultant biloma and perhaps cholecystectomy.

Further Reading

Cardella JF, Bakal CW, Bertino RE, et al; Society of Interventional Radiology Standards of Practice Committee. Quality improvement guidelines for image-guided percutaneous biopsy in adults. J Vasc Interv Radiol 2003;14(9 Pt 2):S227–S230

Lindor KD, Bru C, Jorgensen RA, et al. The role of ultrasonography and automatic-needle biopsy in outpatient percutaneous liver biopsy. Hepatology 1996;23(5):1079–1083

Little AF, Ferris JV, Dodd GD III, Baron RL. Image-guided percutaneous hepatic biopsy: effect of ascites on the complication rate. Radiology 1996;199(1):79–83

Nazarian LN, Feld RI, Herrine SK, et al. Safety and efficacy of sonographically guided random core biopsy for diffuse liver disease. J Ultrasound Med 2000;19(8):537–541

Nobili V, Comparcola D, Sartorelli MR, et al. Blind and ultrasound-guided percutaneous liver biopsy in children. Pediatr Radiol 2003;33(11): 772–775

Saad WEA, Ryan CK, Davies MG, et al. Safety and efficacy of fluoroscopic versus ultrasound guidance for core liver biopsies in potential living related liver transplant donors: preliminary results. J Vasc Interv Radiol 2006;17(8):1307–1312

Sheets PW, Brumbaugh CJ, Kopecky KK, Pound DC, Filo RS. Safety and efficacy of a spring-propelled 18-gauge needle for US-guided liver biopsy. J Vasc Interv Radiol 1991;2(1):147–149

2 Renal Biopsy
Wael E.A. Saad

Classification

Kidney biopsies are classified into random renal biopsies and target-specific renal lesion biopsies.

Random Renal Biopsy

A random renal biopsy is a kidney tissue sample that is obtained to evaluate diffuse kidney disease (medicorenal disease) such as

- Proteinuria (nephrotic syndrome)
- Microscopic hematuria
- Urologically unexplained macroscopic hematuria
- Renal manifestation of systemic disease
  ○ Systemic lupus erythematosus (SLE)
  ○ Scleroderma
  ○ Systemic vasculitis
  ○ Antiphospholipid
  ○ Multiple myeloma
  ○ Monoclonal gammopathy of uncertain significance
- Unexplained renal failure
- Renal transplant rejection
- Renal transplant ischemia/drug-induced toxicity
- Renal transplant chronic allograft nephropathy

There are two types of random renal biopsies (**Table 2.1**):

- Transjugular random renal biopsies (native kidney) (**Fig. 2.1**)

Table 2.1 Comparison of Transjugular Renal Biopsy and Percutaneous Renal Biopsy

	Transjugular Renal Biopsy	Percutaneous Renal Biopsy
Indications	Second-line biopsy when percutaneous renal biopsy is contraindicated or difficult: Patient unable to lie prone Morbidly obese Borderline coagulopathy (see below) Can be performed in conjunction with transjugular hepatic and/or cardiac biopsies	First-line biopsy (see general indications in text)
Skill Set Required	Requires a specialized skill set: Vascular access Transcatheter skills	Requires a less specialized skill set However, requires good command of ultrasound guidance
Diagnostic Yield	Generally less pathologic diagnostic yield due to (a study has shown no difference in yield compared with percutaneous renal biopsy): Little parenchymal imaging/image guidance Needle caliber smaller than 18-gauge (20-gauge)	Generally higher pathologic diagnostic yield due to: Parenchymal imaging/image guidance Needle caliber can be 18-gauge or higher
Additional Diagnostic Yield	Usually no additional information on the renal disease being evaluated	Can characterize superadded focal renal disease Can identify medicorenal disease findings, however, these findings are nonspecific
Coagulopathy Thresholds*	Higher threshold for coagulopathy Suggested thresholds: INR: ≤1.7 PLT: ≥50,000 aPTT: ≤60 s	Lower threshold for coagulopathy Suggested thresholds: INR: ≤1.4–1.5 PLT: ≥50,000–70,000 aPTT: ≤45–50 s

*Coagulopathy thresholds are suggestions. Variations of set thresholds among institutions and individual operators are typical. Safe thresholds are difficult to set (prove based on evidence-based science) due to numerous clinical variables.

Abbreviations: INR, international normalized ration; PLT, platelets; aPTT, active prothrombin time.

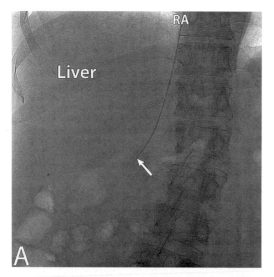

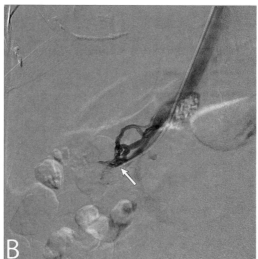

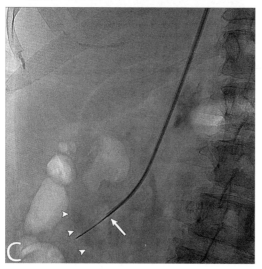

Fig. 2.1 **(A)** Fluoroscopic image during a transjugular renal biopsy. The catheter tip (*arrow*) is in the right renal vein. The hepatic (Liver) shadow is seen above it. The catheter has been passed down (in order): the right jugular vein, the superior vena cava, the right atrium (RA), the inferior vena cava, and the right renal vein. **(B)** Image from a digital subtraction venogram of the right renal vein. The catheter tip (*arrow*) is in the renal vein. The venogram is for documentation that the catheter is actually in the renal vein and not another vein such as a right hepatic vein. An accessory right hepatic vein is more cephalad than the main right hepatic vein and may be thought to be a renal vein especially if venography is not performed. **(C)** Fluoroscopic image during a transjugular renal biopsy. The 20-gauge needle has been passed down its metal introducer sheath (so not to injure adjacent structures). The arrow is at the tip of the metal-coated introducer sheath. The semiautomatic needle has been passed and then "fired" from the metal introducer sheath tip (*arrow*) toward and reaching the renal capsule (*arrowheads*). Remember that the cortex needs to be sampled and so the needle should be passed to the capsule.

- Percutaneous random renal biopsies
  - Transretroperitoneal (through the back) random renal biopsy for native kidney (right or left) (**Figs. 2.2, 2.3, 2.4, and 2.5**)
  - Transabdominal (through the anterior abdominal wall) random renal biopsy for:
    - Transplanted kidney (most common) (**Fig. 2.6**)
    - Anatomically disoriented native kidney (not common)
    - Ptosed native kidney that has undergone nephropexy procedure to fixate it (not common)

Target-selected Renal Biopsy/Renal Lesion Biopsy

A renal lesion biopsy is a kidney tissue sample that is obtained to evaluate a specific focal kidney lesion such as (**Fig. 2.7**):

- Renal cell carcinoma (RCC)
- Oncocytoma

- Papillary adenoma
- Renal lymphoma
- Renal leiomyoma (capsuloma)
- Angiomyolipoma

Conventional management of focal renal masses is based on the assumption that they are almost all RCC; thus, they are removed surgically. In cases of small renal masses (<3 cm in diameter) in nonsurgical candidates follow-up imaging is advocated. In both these scenarios and their corresponding treatment strategies, percutaneous renal biopsy has not played a role. However, Wood et al reported a series of 73 renal lesion biopsies; 40% of patients had disease management changed by the results of the percutaneous biopsy. These patients had preexisting malignancy where focal renal metastasis disease was found and not primary RCC. Furthermore, the incidence of renal masses detected by imaging has risen over the past years due to improvements in imaging including the use of thin slice computed tomography (CT). When it comes

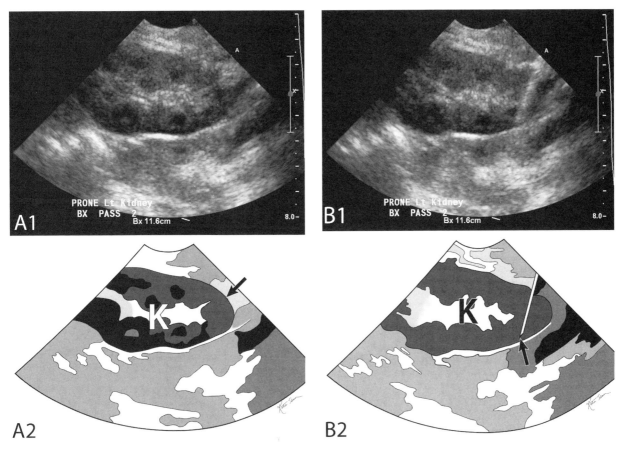

Fig. 2.2 Common setup/layout for random parenchymal renal biopsy. **(A)** Gray-scale ultrasound image of the left kidney (K) (*top*) and schematic sketch of it (*bottom*). The transducer is long on the left kidney and is clearly visualizing the lower pole of the kidney (*arrow*). The needle is to be guided to sample the lower pole of the kidney and slanted toward the renal sinus. This is a common layout for a random renal biopsy. **(B)** Ultrasound image of the left kidney (K) (*top*) and sketch of same (*bottom*). The transducer is long on the left kidney and is clearly visualizing the lower pole of the kidney. An 18-gauge biopsy needle has been passed through the lower pole of the kidney (*arrow at needle tip*).

to small renal masses (<3 cm in diameter) the incidence of benign lesions actually rises:

- Overall incidence of benignity in renal masses is 12.8%.
- The incidence of benignity in renal masses <3 cm is 25%.
- The incidence of benignity in renal masses <2 cm is 30%.
- The incidence of benignity in renal masses <1 cm is 44%.

An additional potential problem with percutaneous renal mass biopsies is the potential for tract seeding and converting a locally confined tumor to a locally disseminated tumor. Needle tract seeding after renal biopsies most likely occurs at a rate similar to other types of tumor biopsies, which is estimated at 0.01% of cases (1/1000 biopsies). There is no evidence that renal malignancies have a higher incidence of seeding than any other malignancy in the body.

Indications

The indications for focal renal mass percutaneous biopsies are limited, but growing as the old doctrine is gradually changing. Currently, the established indications for focal renal lesion biopsy are

- Biopsy of renal mass with prior history of nonrenal malignancy or concomitant/synchronous extrarenal primary tumor
- Unresectable retroperitoneal mass involving the kidney (Is it RCC invading extracapsular or is it a retroperitoneal sarcoma invading the kidney?)
- Suspicion of lymphoma or atypical radiologic appearance of RCC
- Focal pyelonephritis to identify the causing organism

The emerging indications for focal renal lesion biopsy are

- Immediately (intraprocedurally) prepercutaneous ablation

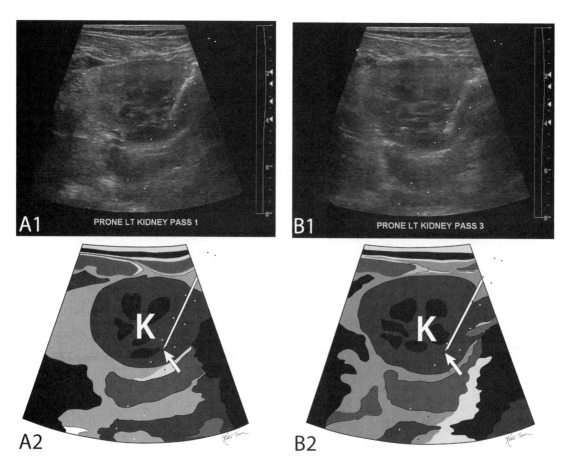

Fig. 2.3 Obliqued random parenchymal renal biopsy. **(A)** Ultrasound image of the left kidney (*top*) and sketch of same (*bottom*). The transducer is obliqued (midway between long and transverse) on the lower pole of the left kidney. An 18-gauge biopsy needle has been passed through the lower pole of the kidney (*arrow at needle tip*).

(B) Gray-scale ultrasound image of the left kidney (K) (*top*) and schematic sketch of it (*bottom*). The transducer is obliqued (midway between long and transverse) on the lower pole of the left kidney. Another 18-gauge biopsy needle has been passed through the lower pole of the kidney (*arrow at needle tip*).

- Patients with <3 cm solid hyperattenuating enhancing renal masses
- Indeterminate cystic renal mass

Contraindications

Absolute Contraindications

- Uncorrected coagulopathy (see **Table 2.1** for suggested thresholds)
- Uncontrolled severe hypertension (increased risk of bleeding)

Relative Contraindications

- Solitary native kidney
- Pregnancy
- Concerns for seeding of RCC and spreading tumor locally outside the Gerota's fascia

- Hydronephrosis
  - The cause of the hydronephrosis should be investigated first. This may be the cause of the renal disease and the biopsy is not necessary.
  - Hydronephrosis increases risk of hematuria.
- Upper urinary tract infection (concerns for spread of infection)
- Horseshoe kidney. This condition was labeled a contraindication prior to the advent of cross-sectional imaging and image-guided biopsies (biopsy can be performed after careful examination of anatomy, which can be provided by magnetic resonance imaging [MRI] and/or a dedicated gray-scale and Doppler ultrasound exam).

Relative Contraindications with Indication

- Patient unable to lie prone
- Morbidly obese (poor ultrasound visual of kidney + difficulty lying prone)
- Borderline coagulopathy

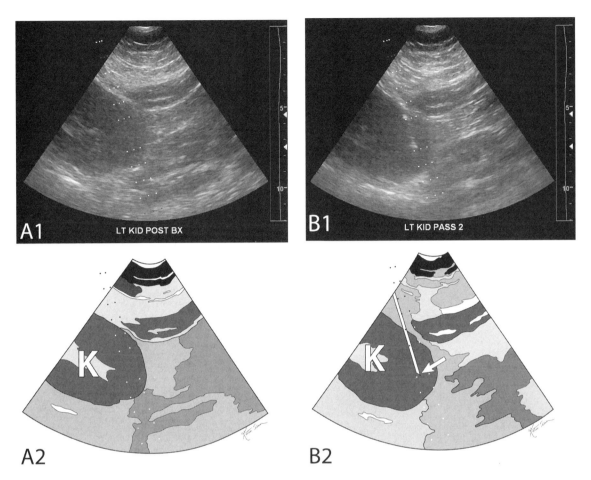

Fig. 2.4 Random parenchymal renal biopsy with needle directed away from the renal sinus. **(A)** Ultrasound image of the left kidney (K) (*top*) and sketch of same (*bottom*). The transducer is long on the left kidney and is clearly visualizing the lower pole of the kidney. The needle is to be guided to sample the lower pole of the kidney and slanted away from the renal sinus. The operators who use this technique (needle directed away from the renal sinus) feel that this is safer as the needle is directed away from the larger vessels in the center of the kidney. **(B)** Ultrasound image of the left kidney (K) (*top*) and sketch of same (*bottom*). The transducer is long on the left kidney and is clearly visualizing the lower pole of the kidney. An 18-gauge biopsy needle has been passed through the lower pole of the kidney (*arrow at needle tip*) directed away from the renal sinus.

Preprocedural Evaluation

Evaluate Prior Cross-sectional Imaging

- Look for anatomic abnormalities
  - Kidney malrotation/malposition
  - Horseshoe kidneys as well as other kidney fusions
  - Solitary kidney (considered a contraindication by some, however, a transplanted kidney is a solitary functioning kidney and they are not infrequently biopsied)
- Look for pathologic/morphologic abnormalities
  - Hydronephrosis
  - Polycystic kidney
- Look for adjacent organs that can be traversed
  - This helps plan the needle trajectory (biopsy approach).
  - This can help reduce transgression of adjacent organs with subsequent potential major complications.

  - Particular organs that may be traversed include colon, spleen, and liver for native kidneys and small bowel, urinary bladder, and iliac vessels for transplanted kidneys.
- Look for the safest renal pole to biopsy
  - In native kidneys the choice is right versus left. The room setting and operator preference may make the decision as to which side is chosen over the other.
  - Avoid the side that is away from vessels or local parenchymal cysts
  - The lower pole is chosen because it is away from adjacent organs that are closer to the upper poles (lung, adrenal, liver, and spleen).
  - In transplant kidneys, the choice is usually medial versus lateral pole. The safest and most accessible pole should be chosen with the planned needle trajectory away from iliac vessels and small bowel.

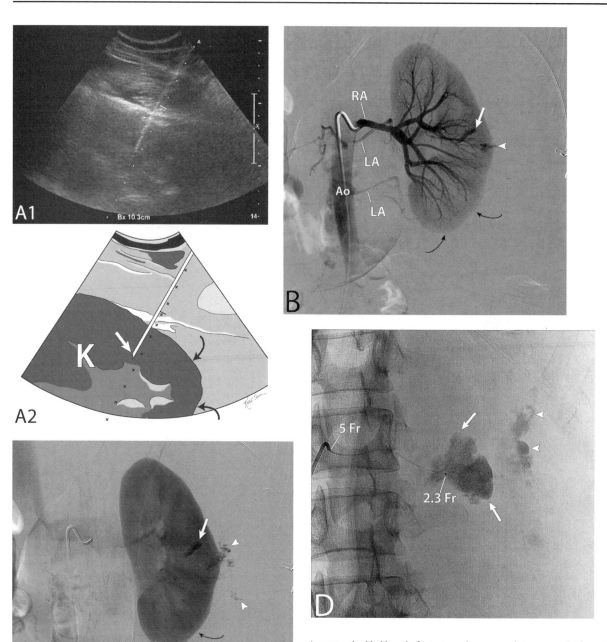

Fig. 2.5 Random parenchymal renal biopsy complicated by bleeding. **(A)** Ultrasound image of the left kidney (K) (*top*) and sketch of same (*bottom*). An 18-gauge biopsy needle has been passed through the midportion of the kidney (*arrow at needle tip*) directed at the renal sinus. The needle is not passing through the lower pole of the kidney (*between curved arrows*). Needle passage directed at the midportion of the kidney reduces the likelihood of obtaining a cortex dominant sample (which is required) due to a relatively thinner cortex in the midportion of the kidney. In addition, inadvertent deep passage of the needle in the midportion of the kidney may increase the likelihood of injuring a larger renal sinus vessel. The patient bled after the renal biopsy, dropping hematocrit and having a subcapsular hematoma. The patient was taken to the angiography suite to evaluate for the source of bleeding with possible embolization of the vessels. **(B)** Digitally subtracted arteriogram of the left kidney through a 5-French SOS catheter during the late arterial phase. The arteriogram demonstrates extravasation of contrast (bleeding) where the biopsy was taken (*arrowhead*). In addition, a stagnant linear collection of contrast is seen signifying a second site of bleeding (*arrow*). The two curved black arrows point to the lower pole where the biopsy should have been taken (RA, renal artery; LA, lumbar artery(ies); Ao, aorta). **(C)** Digitally subtracted arteriogram of the left kidney during the nephrogram phase. Again noted is the extravasation of contrast (bleeding) where the biopsy was taken (*arrowheads*). In addition, the stagnant linear collection of contrast is seen signifying the second site of bleeding (*arrow*). The two curved black arrows point to the lower pole where the biopsy should have been taken. **(D)** Super-selective arteriogram of the left kidney segment in the midportion of the left kidney utilizing a 2.3-French (2.3Fr) microcatheter passed coaxially through the 5-French SOS catheter (5 Fr). The renal segment stains with contrast (*between arrows*) and the pooling of contrast (bleeding) is again seen (*arrowheads*).

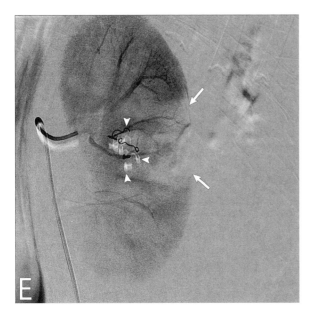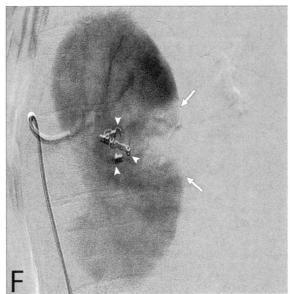

Fig. 2.5 *(Continued)* **(E)** Digitally subtracted arteriogram of the left kidney during the late arterial phase after embolization utilizing microcoils (*arrowheads*). There is a wedge-shaped segmental infarct (*between coils and arrows*) correlating with the wedge-shaped super-selective angiogram in **Fig. 2.5D**. No bleeding is identified. **(F)** Digitally subtracted arteriogram of the left kidney during the nephrogram phase after embolization utilizing microcoils (*arrowheads*). There is a wedge-shaped segmental infarct (*between coils and arrows*) correlating with the wedge-shaped super-selective angiogram in **Fig. 2.5D**. No bleeding is identified.

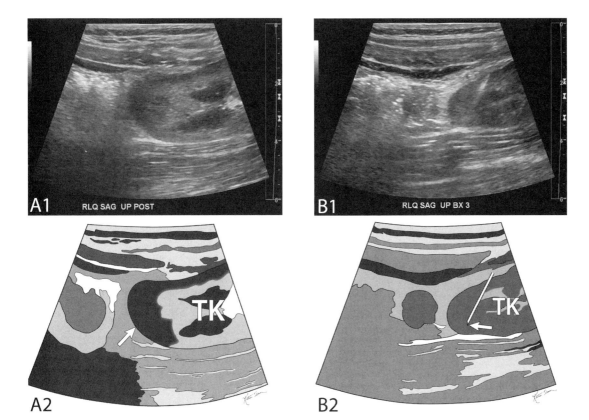

Fig. 2.6 Random parenchymal renal biopsy of a transplanted kidney in the right lower quadrant. **(A)** Ultrasound image of the transplanted right lower quadrant kidney (TK) (*top*) and sketch of same (*bottom*). The transducer is long on the transplanted kidney and is clearly visualizing the lateral pole of the kidney (*arrow*). In transplanted kidneys that usually lie across (transversely) in the abdomen, the poles are usually referred to medial and lateral. Avoiding the small bowel and the iliac vessels are the major concerns for this biopsy. **(B)** Ultrasound image of the transplanted right lower quadrant kidney (TK) (*top*) and sketch of same (*bottom*). The transducer is long on the transplanted kidney and is clearly visualizing the lateral pole of the kidney (*arrow*). An 18-gauge biopsy needle has been passed through the lateral pole of the kidney (*arrow at needle tip*) directed away from the renal sinus. *(Continued on page 26)*

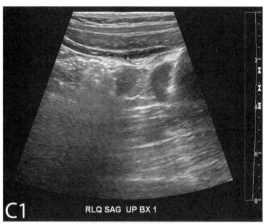

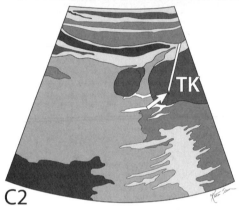

Fig. 2.6 *(Continued)* **(C)** Ultrasound image of the transplanted right lower quadrant kidney (TK) *(top)* and sketch of same *(bottom)*. The transducer is long on the transplanted kidney and is clearly visualizing the lateral pole of the kidney *(arrow)*. Another 18-gauge biopsy needle has been passed through the lateral pole of the kidney *(arrow at needle tip)* directed away from the renal sinus.

- For renal lesion biopsy, look for target lesion and its characteristics.
  - This helps plan biopsy needle trajectory leading to the target lesion.
  - Traversing normal renal parenchyma may reduce the risk tumor seeding.
  - Avoid needle trajectories that are close to the renal pelvicalyceal collecting system or avoid obtaining specimens from the mass that is close to the collecting system.

Evaluate Prebiopsy Laboratory Values

- Laboratory value evaluation mostly revolves around ruling out coagulopathy.
  - Suggested coagulopathy thresholds are presented in **Table 2.1**.
  - Serum creatinine may be considered for transjugular renal biopsies although the use of contrast can be minimal.

Obtain Informed Consent

- Indications
  - To evaluate for parenchymal renal disease (medicorenal disease) versus evaluate nature of focal renal/retroperitoneal lesion

- Alternatives
  - To refuse the biopsy
  - Percutaneous versus transjugular renal biopsy
  - Surgical wedge biopsy (mostly historical)
- Procedural risks
  - Infection
    - This is a rare complication.
    - It may occur at higher frequency with upper urinary tract infection (not proven).
  - Bleeding
    - This is the most common major complication.
    - It may present as hematuria, pain, and/or hypotension.
    - Clinically, the most common presentation of bleeding is hematuria.
    - Bleeding may be transient with or without blood transfusion.
    - In rare cases, bleeding may require intervention such as transcatheter renal arterial embolization or exploratory surgery.
  - Injury to surrounding organs and/or structures
    - Pleura (pneumo- and hemothorax)
    - Spleen, liver, and large bowel

Equipment

Ultrasound Guidance

- Ultrasound machine with Doppler capability
- Multiarray 4–5 MHz ultrasound transducer
- Transducer guide bracket
- Sterile transducer cover

Standard Surgical Preparation and Draping

- Chlorhexidine skin preparation/cleansing fluid
- Fenestrated drape

Local Infiltrative Analgesia Administration

- 21-gauge infiltration needle
- 10–20 mL 1% lidocaine syringe

Sharp Access and Biopsy

- 11-blade incision scalpel
- Coaxial access needle (see below); 17-gauge coaxial needle for delivery of 18-gauge core biopsy needle
- Coaxial access needle (see below); 20-gauge coaxial needles for delivery of fine-needle aspiration 22-gauge needles

Technique

Intravenous Access

- The necessity of moderate sedation (administered intravenously) for renal biopsies varies from one institution to another. My institution performs moderate sedation for renal biopsies.
- If moderate sedation is not routinely administered, intravenous (IV) access is still reasonable as a standby for any complication (including pain-related complications), or if the need arises to administer sedation.

Prebiopsy Ultrasound Examination

- Determine the easiest visibility of the lesion in cases of target lesion biopsy.
- Determine the easiest and safest lower renal pole (right versus left) in native kidneys or medial versus lateral pole in transplanted kidney.
- Look for adjacent organs that can be traversed (spleen, colon). Avoid too lateral a trajectory; this increases the risk of colon transgression.
- For a renal lesion biopsy, avoid sampling mass close to the collecting system or traversing close to the collecting system.

Standard Surgical Preparation and Draping

- Skin preparation/cleansing in the region that was chosen as an ultrasound imaging portal and a needle access needle portal
- Place a fenestrated drape at the prepared skin region

Local Infiltrative Analgesia Administration

- Utilizing a 21-gauge (by at least a 3.7 cm long) infiltration needle and 1% lidocaine, infiltration is performed.

Sharp Access

- An incision is made utilizing an 11-blade scalpel usually by a 3- to 5-mm-depth stab of the 11-blade.
- A 19-gauge coaxial access needle can be passed across the retroperitoneum in the direction of the chosen parenchyma (for a random biopsy) or the renal lesion (for target lesion biopsy) (**Fig. 2.7**).
- The coaxial access needle also allows for the embolization of the transretroperitoneal tract with Gelfoam (Pfizer Pharmaceuticals, New York, NY) or coils after the biopsy has been performed (**Fig. 2.7**).
- A coaxial needle is not necessary in renal biopsies.

Pathology Sample Acquisition (Biopsy)

- An automated spring-loaded core biopsy needle is passed to the end of a coaxial needle, "fired" (automatically deployed), and withdrawn (**Fig. 2.7**).
- Without the use of coaxial needle access, the core biopsy needle is passed to the edge of the intended region (specific target lesion or the intended parenchyma for the random biopsy). It is then "fired" or deployed (**Fig. 2.7**).
- Regarding lesion biopsy, at least one biopsy sample should be obtained by having the core biopsy needle be deployed from outside the lesion (from a position falling short of the lesion border) so as to obtain "normal" renal parenchyma/retroperitoneum and sample the pathologic junction/margin of the lesion.
- Regarding random renal biopsies:
  - Usually, one to five core (18-gauge or by some operators, larger caliber such as 14-gauge) biopsy needle passes/deployments are made.
  - With 18-gauge biopsy needles, at least three passes are required (some authors recommend more than three passes as a minimum) for sample adequacy. This is moot if an experienced renal pathology technician evaluates the samples under microscopy.
  - The target renal parenchyma is classically the lower pole.

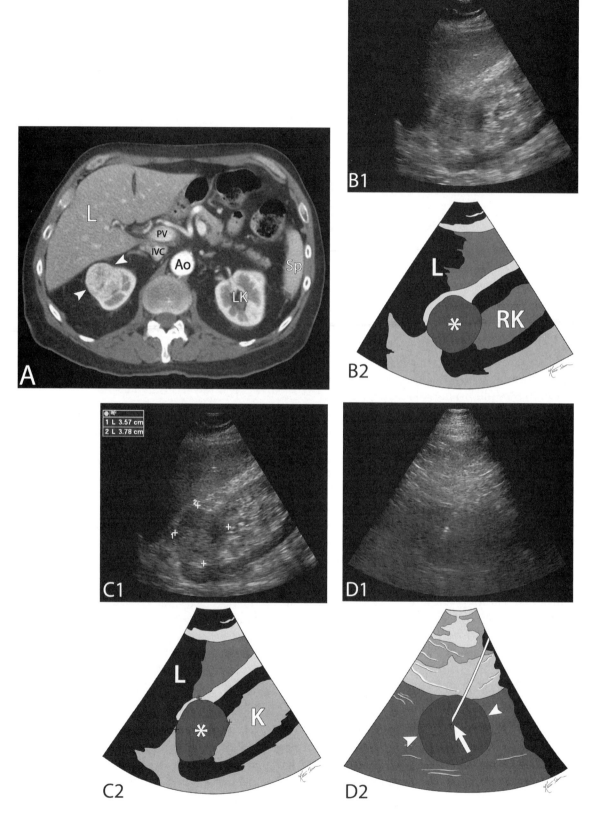

Fig. 2.7 (Continued)

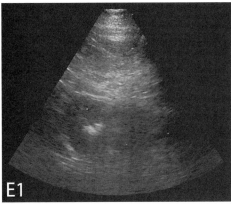

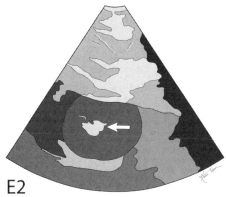

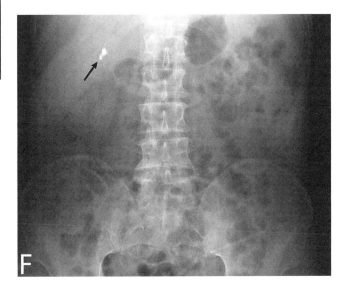

Fig. 2.7 Upper pole right renal mass biopsy. **(A)** Contrast-enhanced computed tomography (CT) scan of the abdomen demonstrating an enhancing heterogeneous mass (*between arrowheads*) in the upper pole of the right kidney. (L, liver; LK, left kidney; Ao, aorta; IVC, inferior vena cava; PV, portal vein; Sp, spleen) **(B)** Ultrasound image of the right kidney (RK) (*top*) and sketch of same (*bottom*). The transducer is long on the right kidney and visualizes the upper pole mass (*asterisk in center of mass*). The sonographer is utilizing the liver (L) as an acoustic window. This explains the clarity of the image. When actually performing the procedure/biopsy the use of the liver as a sonographic window is usually not feasible and thus the images during the biopsy may be less clear (**Figs. 2.7D and 2.7E**). **(C)** Ultrasound image of the right kidney (*top*) and sketch of same (*bottom*). The transducer is long on the right kidney and visualizes the upper pole mass (*asterisk in center of mass*). The sonographer is utilizing the liver (L) as an acoustic window. This explains the clarity of the image. When actually performing the procedure/biopsy the use of the liver as a sonographic window is usually not feasible and thus the images during the biopsy may be less clear (**Figs. 2.7D and 2.7E**). **(D)** Ultrasound image of the right kidney mass (*top*) and sketch of same (*bottom*). A coaxial 17-gauge needle (*arrow at needle tip*) has been passed into the lesion (*between arrowheads*). Several 18-gauge coaxial biopsy needles can be passed through the 17-gauge needle at this point. **(E)** Ultrasound image of the right kidney mass (*top*) and sketch of same (*bottom*). The 18-gauge samples have been obtained. Coils have been passed coaxially through the 17-gauge needle and the coaxial 17-gauge needle has been removed. The coils, with air trapped in them, are seen to be an echogenic focus in the middle of the mass (*arrow*). **(F)** Flat-plate plain film of the abdomen (KUB) demonstrating the radiopaque coils (*arrow*) in the right upper quadrant projecting over the upper pole of the right kidney.

- Lower pole is away from the spleen, liver, and lung.
- Usually has more renal parenchyma/cortex (fewer passes, more safe; away from interlobar arteries)
  ○ Any position to visualize the lower pole and to biopsy it will do. This includes
    - The classic longitudinal view of the kidney and deploying the biopsy needle toward the renal sinus (**Fig. 2.2**)
    - Transverse or oblique views of the lower pole of the kidney (**Fig. 2.3**)

- Longitudinal view of the kidney and deploying the biopsy needle away from the renal sinus (presumed safer by some operators) (**Fig. 2.4**)
- The midportion should be avoided (**Fig. 2.5**) unless certain circumstances dictate to biopsy the midportion of the kidney.
- Regarding transplanted kidneys, there is usually no clear upper or lower pole (usually medial and lateral) (**Fig. 2.6**). The end of the kidney chosen depends on the thickness of the cortex and the distance the pole is from surrounding structures such as iliac vessels and/or small bowel.

Transretroperitoneal Tract Embolization

- This is not routinely performed.
- It may be performed in significantly coagulopathic patients after a core biopsy or if there is inadvertent active bleeding.
- Transretroperitoneal needle tract embolization requires a coaxial access needle technique (**Fig. 2.7**).
- Gelfoam pledgets, Gelfoam slurry, or metal coils can be blindly deployed through the coaxial needle as it is slowly withdrawn along the transhepatic tract.
- If fluoroscopy is available, the coils can be deployed under fluoroscopy. Deploying Gelfoam pledgets under fluoroscopy guidance requires the Gelfoam pledgets to be soaked in contrast for them to be visualized.

Immediate Postbiopsy Ultrasound Imaging

- Immediate postbiopsy ultrasound imaging is for documentation and obtaining imaging baseline for capsular or subcapsular hematomas, if any (**Fig. 2.8**).
- Visualizing a renal capsular hematoma does not alter postprocedural care or management. Treat the patient and not the images.

Endpoints

Random Nontarget Liver Biopsy

- Usually three or four 18-gauge needle passes are required to obtain an adequate random renal parenchymal pathology sample.
- Smaller caliber needles (20-gauge core biopsy needles) and larger caliber needles (14-gauge core biopsy needles) may require more needle passes or fewer needle passes, respectively.
- The operator grossly evaluates the core sample and determines when to stop making core biopsy needle passes (after the first, second, or third needle pass).

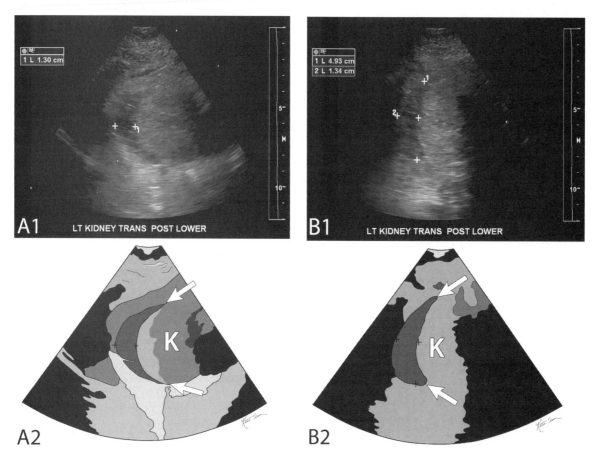

Fig. 2.8 Postrandom biopsy image. **(A)** Ultrasound image of the lower pole of a left kidney (K) (*top*) and sketch of same (*bottom*). The transducer is transverse on the lower pole. A random parenchymal biopsy has been obtained. A postbiopsy subcapsular crescent-shaped hematoma is seen (*between arrows and crosshairs*). **(B)** Ultrasound image of the lower pole of a left kidney (K) (*top*) and sketch of same (*bottom*). The transducer is transverse on the lower pole. A random parenchymal biopsy has been obtained. A postbiopsy subcapsular crescent-shaped hematoma is seen (*between arrows and crosshairs*).

Lesion-specific Target Liver Biopsy

- Usually one to three 18-gauge needle passes are required to obtain an adequate pathology sample.
- Smaller caliber needles (20-gauge core biopsy needles) and larger caliber needles (16-gauge core biopsy needles) may require more needle passes or fewer needle passes, respectively.
- The operator grossly evaluates the core sample and determines when to stop making core biopsy needle passes (after the first, second, or third needle pass).
- In cases of suspect of lymphoma, fine needle aspirates (22-gauge needle passes) should be obtained prior to the core biopsy sample for flow-cytometry evaluation.

Postprocedural Evaluation and Management

There is no clear set standard for postbiopsy outpatient care. Some institutions do not perform outpatient renal biopsies and admit patients for a 23-hour stay. The following are suggestions with some variations mentioned for discussion and flexibility to accommodate particular institutional and practice settings.

Outpatient Ambulatory Stay/Observation Period

- Postprocedural stay varies from one institution to another.
- Some institutions admit patients overnight (23-hour admission).
- It should be noted that
  - 40–50% of complications present <4 hours from the biopsy
  - 67–80% of complications present <8 hours from the biopsy
  - 80–100% of complications present <12 hours from the biopsy
- Keep patients who have undergone renal biopsy in the hospital for at least 8–12 hours.

Intravenous Fluid and Diet

- IV access should be kept until just prior to discharge.
- Institutions that practice moderate sedation start with a clear liquid diet and advance it as tolerated. This helps to offset patients' nausea and vomiting.
- Other institutions/operators commence a clear liquid diet after a period of abstinence of oral intake. This period could be one hour, for example.
- Give IV fluid until oral intake is adequate

Activity

- Bed rest for approximately 4 hours is recommended.
- Patients, on discharge, are instructed to not engage in strenuous activity for 24–48 hours postbiopsy.

Pain Management

- Narcotics are usually not required during the postbiopsy stay of the patient prior to discharge. Occasionally, some patients require oral narcotic analgesics such as acetaminophen and hydrocodone combination medication. Rarely does a patient require IV narcotics such as fentanyl.
- On discharge, patients usually tolerate the procedure well and do not require analgesics more potent than over-the-counter medications.

Monitoring Vital Signs

- Vital sign monitoring includes blood pressure and heart rate. Occasionally, oxygen saturation monitoring is required in cases of shortness of breath and/or chest pain.
- Institutions/operators that practice conscious sedation may record a softer blood pressure than a patient's baseline blood pressure after the biopsy. This is most likely due to sedation with or without dehydration. The patient usually responds in time with hydration, particularly as the sedatives wear off.
- Continued hypotension and, more importantly, a rise in heart rate are concerning for hypovolemia (bleeding). If signs of hypovolemia occur, an IV volume bolus is given and a noncontrast CT exam is performed to confirm the clinical suspicion of bleeding.
- Prior to discharge, some operators/institutions measure orthostatic pressures.

Complications and Their Management

Most complications (67–100%), particularly life-threatening complications, are clinically unmasked within 8–12 hours for the renal biopsy (**Table 2.2**).

Management of Pain and Pain-related Morbidity

- Continued pain requires further clinical and possibly imaging evaluation. An expanding retroperitoneal hematoma can cause pain. The degree of pain does not correlate with the degree of bleeding. However, changes in vital signs do signify a significant bleed.
- Occasionally, operators respond to continued pain by performing a diagnostic imaging exam.

Table 2.2   Complications of Ultrasound-guided Renal Biopsies

Complication	Incidence
Pain	<17%*
Mortality	0.0–0.05%
Nephrectomy	0.0–0.06%
Paged kidney	Rare†
Arteriovenous fistulae	0.3–19.0‡
Puncture to adjacent organs	0.0–1.0%
Gross hematuria	0.5–12.0%
Bleeding/hematomas	2.7–5.6%
Pericapsular hematoma causing increased morbidity including increased hospital stay	0.3%
Bleeding/hypotension	1.5%
Tract seeding in renal cell carcinoma	0.01%

Note. Complications are mentioned when they constitute a percentage. Not all studies mention all complications.

*May vary widely due to varying definitions and methodology among studies.

†Rarely mentioned in the ultrasound-guided biopsy literature without an incidence.

‡Higher risk (up to 3–4-fold increase) in transplanted kidneys compared with native kidneys.

○ A limited ultrasound examination at the site to evaluate for a capsular hematoma
○ Or a more global exam such as a noncontrast abdominal CT exam. Ultimately, the decisive factor for determining significant bleeding is the patient's stability (vitals) – not what is seen on the images.
• If there is no bleeding and the patient is stable but requires narcotic analgesics for pain, the patient can be admitted for pain management.

Management of Bleeding Complications

• IV access should be kept until just after discharge in case fluid resuscitation is required.
• Bleeding can take several forms and have different sources.
  ○ Skin bleeding (external)
  ○ Musculoskeletal bleeding

○ Renal parenchyma/capsule (retroperitoneal hematoma if not contained, capsular hematoma if contained) (**Fig. 2.2**)
○ Hematuria (this is the most common clinically apparent type of bleeding)
• Significant bleeding affecting vital signs and patient stability should be managed by
  ○ Fluid resuscitation starting with crystalloid fluid bolus
  ○ Type and cross
  ○ Repeat hematocrit to compare with baseline
  ○ Blood transfusion to maintain hematocrit at or above 30%
  ○ Urology consult/interventional radiology consult
• Interventional radiology offers
  ○ Renal/lumbar arteriography with super-selective arterial embolization if bleeding or a pseudoaneurysm is seen.
• Urology consultation may offer, in the cases of severe uncontrolled bleeding, open surgery, exploration, and local hemostasis of surface bleeding.

Management of Pleural/Thoracic Complications

• This complication is not common particularly when the lower poles are used as a target region.
• If chest pain with or without reduced oxygen saturation is encountered, a chest x-ray should be obtained to rule out pneumothorax or hemothorax.
• Clinically significant hemo- and/or pneumothorax require chest tube placement, increased nasal cannula oxygenation, and fluid resuscitation.

Management of Puncture of Adjacent Organs

• With image guidance, this is a rare complication (up to 1.0% of cases).
• When it occurs, it is usually detected during the procedure by imaging or from the pathology report.
• When transgression of adjacent organs occurs, the result is clinically inconsequential. The problem is incidental and does not rise to the level of a minor clinical complication, let alone a major complication.
• Splenic injury is the only adjacent organ injury that should be taken more seriously due to the risk of increased hemorrhage or even delayed splenic rupture. These patients should be observed closely.

Further Reading

Cardella JF, Bakal CW, Bertino RE, et al; Society of Interventional Radiology Standards of Practice Committee. Quality improvement guidelines for image-guided percutaneous biopsy in adults. J Vasc Interv Radiol 2003;14(9 Pt 2):S227–S230

Cluzel P, Martinez F, Bellin MF, et al. Transjugular versus percutaneous renal biopsy for the diagnosis of parenchymal disease: comparison of sampling effectiveness and complications. Radiology 2000;215(3):689–693

Gervais DA. Percutaneous image-guided biopsy: review of and emphasis on special approaches. In: Ray CE Jr., Hicks ME, Patel NH, eds. SIR Syllabus. Fairfax, VA: Society of Interventional Radiology; 2003:63–72

Silverman SG, Gan YU, Mortele KJ, Tuncali K, Cibas ES. Renal masses in the adult patient: the role of percutaneous biopsy. Radiology 2006;240(1):6–22

Stiles KP, Yuan CM, Chung EM, Lyon RD, Lane JD, Abbott KC. Renal biopsy in high-risk patients with medical diseases of the kidney. Am J Kidney Dis 2000;36(2):419–433

Wood BJ, Khan MA, McGovern F, Harisinghani M, Hahn PF, Mueller PR. Imaging guided biopsy of renal masses: indications, accuracy and impact on clinical management. J Urol 1999;161(5):1470–1474

3 Extravisceral Abdominal Mass Biopsy

Wael E.A. Saad

Classification

Extravisceral abdominal masses can be classified into extravisceral retroperitoneal masses and extravisceral intraperitoneal masses.

Retroperitoneal Extravisceral Masses

- Musculoskeletal masses/tumors
- Retroperitoneal sarcomas
- Retroperitoneal lymph node enlargement (**Fig. 3.1**)
  - Hyperplastic
  - Infectious
  - Malignant
- Lymphoma
- Retroperitoneal splenosis

Intraabdominal Extravisceral Masses

- Primary mesenteric tumors/sarcomas
- Mesenteric infectious/inflammatory masses (tuberculosis, panniculitis)
- Infected or dysplastic mesenteric cysts
- Peritoneal seeding/caking/metastasis (**Fig. 3.2**)
- Mesenteric lymph node enlargement
  - Malignant
  - Hyperplastic (lymphadenitis)
  - Infectious
    - Nonspecific lymphadenitis
    - Tuberculosis
    - Yersinia
    - Actinomycosis
    - Sarcoidosis (granulomatous inflammatory, not infectious)
    - Lymphoma/leukemia
    - Intraperitoneal splenosis
    - Gastrointestinal duplication cysts
    - Desmoplastic small round cell tumors
    - Endometrioma (4% of endometriosis patients)
    - Misdiagnosed visceral masses (not truly extravisceral masses)

Indications

Extravisceral abdominal lesions/masses biopsies can be sampled utilizing ultrasound or computed tomography (CT) guidance. The choice of CT versus ultrasound guidance depends on operator preference, experience, and the availability of adequate ultrasound and/or CT imaging. The size of the target lesion/mass, its location, and its proximity to important organs and/or structures, as well as the proximity of structures and/or viscera in the needle path all contribute to the choice of imaging modality. Certainly, ultrasound guidance can be used for large lesions; however, small lesions/masses adjacent to important abdominal structures usually require CT guidance for precision biopsy. Generally, at my institution the majority of retroperitoneal masses are biopsied utilizing CT guidance. Intraperitoneal masses are biopsied by either ultrasound guidance (superficial lesions with a wide window for the needle trajectory) or by CT (deeper lesions with a narrow window of needle trajectory).

Contraindications

Absolute Contraindications

- Uncorrected coagulopathy – suggested thresholds are
  - International normalized ration (INR): 1.7
  - Active prothrombin time (aPTT): 65 seconds
  - Platelet count of 50,000
- Vascular masses (aneurysms and pseudoaneurysms)

Relative Contraindications

- Certain masses that can cause acute systemic effects when biopsied such as pheochromocytomas (controversial)

Preprocedural Evaluation

Evaluate Prior Cross-sectional Imaging

- Exclude visceral involvement (truly extravisceral mass)
  - Mass adherent to adjacent organ
  - Adjacent organ creating a claw sign with the target mass
  - The enhancement pattern of the target mass mimics the enhancement pattern of an adjacent organ.

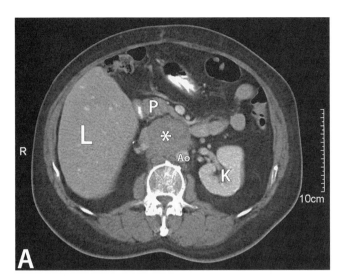

Fig. 3.1 Retroperitoneal mass biopsy (fine-needle aspirate [FNA]). **(A)** Contrast-enhanced axial computed tomography (CT) image of the abdomen. The image demonstrates a large retroperitoneal mass (*asterisk*) most likely the result of amalgamated paraaortic retroperitoneal lymph nodes. **(B)** Doppler ultrasound image of the retroperitoneal mass seen in **Fig. 3.1A** (*top*) and sketch of same (*bottom*). The retroperitoneal mass is again seen (*asterisk at epicenter*). It is avascular and the aorta is seen to its left. The needle trajectory guide (*dotted line*) is seen going through the mass. **(C)** Ultrasound image of the retroperitoneal mass (*asterisk in center of mass*) seen in **Figs. 3.1A and 3.1B** (*top*) and sketch of same (*bottom*). A 19-gauge coaxial needle has been passed into the mass (*arrow at coaxial needle tip*). The operator now is ready to pass the 22-gauge FNA needle sequentially. (K, left kidney; L, liver; Ao, aorta; P, pancreas; LT, left; RT, right)

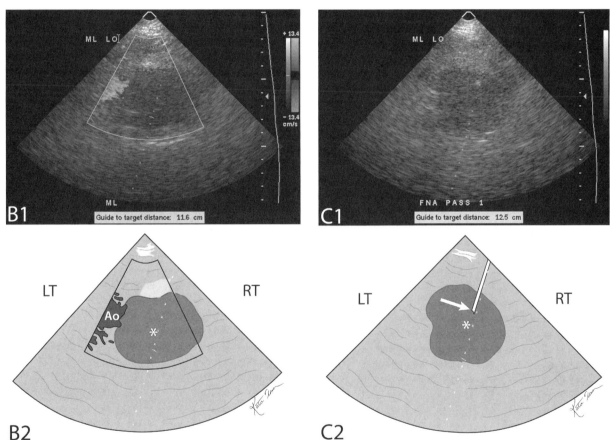

- Look for anatomic hints for the diagnosis
  - Retroperitoneal versus intraperitoneal?
  - If retroperitoneal, is it inside or outside the Gerota's fascia?
  - Lesion completely surrounded by small bowel and mesentery (mesenteric lesion)
  - Mass in the perivascular retroperitoneum and associated with multiple adjacent enlarged lymph nodes (aggregated/amalgamated lymph nodes)
- Exclude that the mass/target lesion is vascular
  - Must review contrast-enhanced CT or magnetic resonance (MR) images to exclude that the mass is not an aneurysm or a pseudoaneurysm

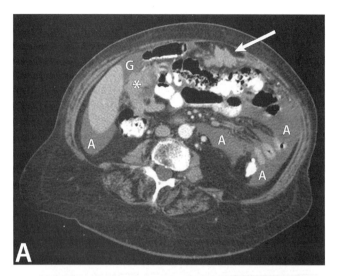

Fig. 3.2 Omental mass biopsy. **(A)** Contrast-enhanced axial computed tomography (CT) image of the abdomen. The image demonstrates peritoneal fluid (A, ascites) and omental masses (*asterisk and arrow*). Peritoneal fluid is also seen at the gallbladder fundus (G). The omental mass deep to the gallbladder (*asterisk*) is difficult to access. The operator decided to biopsy the more superficial left-sided mass (*arrow*), which is more accessible. Hypothetically, if the right-sided omental mass was the only mass (no left-sided mass), a transhepatic approach utilizing a coaxial needle would be reasonable to entertain. Strictly speaking, when trying to determine the diagnosis (which is most likely malignant in this setting) from the least risky to the more risky, the following (in order) should be performed: (1) Cytology evaluation of ascetic fluid aspirate; (2) direct percutaneous left-sided-mass aspiration/biopsy, and (3) transhepatic fine-needle aspiration of the right-sided mass. **(B)** Ultrasound image of the left-sided mass seen in **Fig. 3.2A** (*top*) and sketch of same (*bottom*). An insert is placed in the bottom left-hand corner, which is a cropped CT image from **Fig. 3.2A**. Again seen is the mesenteric mass (*arrow*), which has a superficial "double-humped" component (*asterisk*)

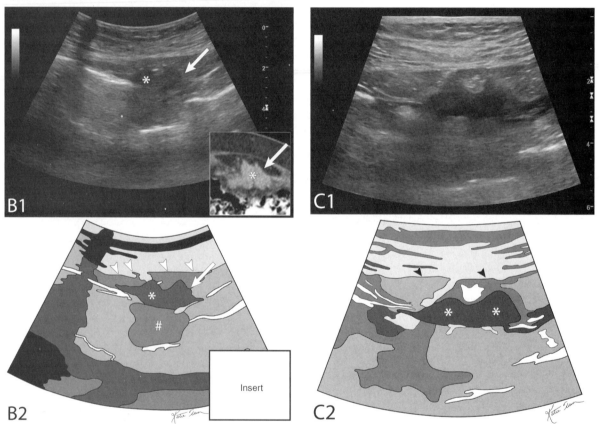

and a deeper component (#) which is relatively more echogenic than the more superficial double-humped component. The *arrowheads* point to the sonographic plain of the deep fascia. **(C)** Ultrasound image utilizing a linear transducer of the same mass seen in **Figs. 3.2A and 3.2B** (*top*) and sketch of same (*bottom*). The more superficial double-humped component (*asterisks*) is more closely seen. The *arrowheads* point to the sonographic plain of the deep fascia. **(D)** Ultrasound image utilizing a linear transducer of the same mass (*top*) and sketch of same (*bottom*). The operator has switched on the needle trajectory guide (*sites: diverging dotted lines*), which traject through the more superficial double-humped component (*asterisk*). The *arrowheads* point to the

sonographic plain of the deep fascia. **(E)** Ultrasound image utilizing a linear transducer of the same mass (*top*) and sketch of same (*bottom*). The operator has passed an 18-gauge Trucut biopsy needle, which is indenting the tissue plain superficial to the mass (*asterisks*). **(F)** Ultrasound image utilizing a linear transducer of the same mass (*top*) and sketch of same (*bottom*). The operator has "fired" or deployed the 18-gauge Trucut biopsy needle (*arrow*), which has penetrated the mass (*asterisks*). **(G)** Ultrasound image utilizing a linear transducer of the same mass (*top*) and sketch of same (*bottom*). The operator has made a second 18-gauge Trucut biopsy needle (*arrow*) pass, which has again penetrated the mass (*asterisks*).

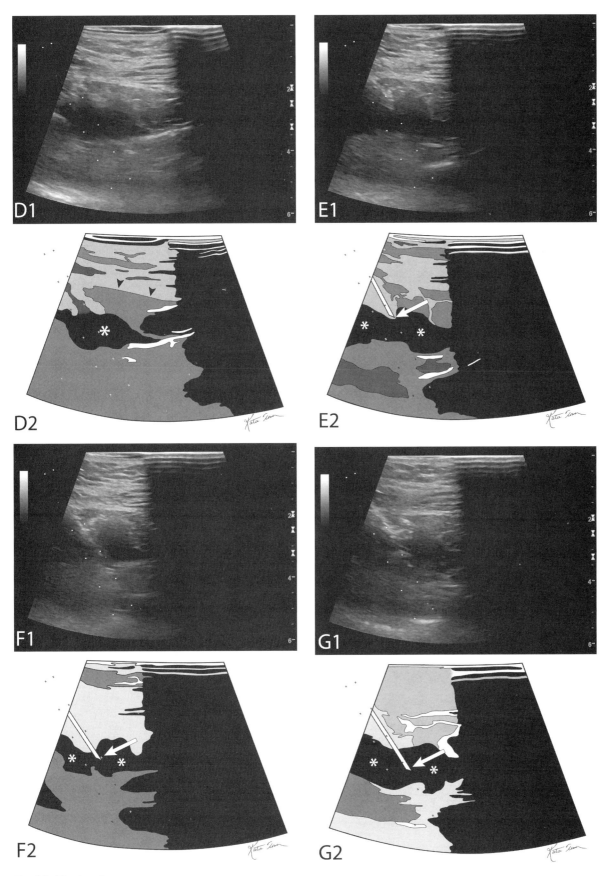

Fig. 3.2 *(Continued)*

○ If there are no prior contrast-enhanced studies, Doppler ultrasound evaluation of the mass should be performed just prior to the biopsy (intraprocedurally) to exclude pseudoaneurysm/aneurysm.

○ If a pseudoaneurysm or aneurysm is inadvertently accessed using a coaxial needle, keep the needle in its location, and call an interventionalist immediately.

• Look for adjacent organs that can be traversed

○ This helps plan the needle trajectory (biopsy approach).

○ This can help reduce transgression of adjacent organs with subsequent potential major complications.

○ When choosing amid multiple lesions, choose the least risky lesion that is farthest from adjacent organs that might be injured (**Fig. 3.2**).

○ Particular organs that may be intentionally traversed by a coaxial fine-needle aspiration (FNA) kit (outer 19-gauge/inner 22-gauge needle) include liver, stomach, colon, and even the inferior vena cava (IVC). However, these intended visceral transgressions are usually planned and performed utilizing CT guidance. The two exceptions are the liver and possibly the stomach (see below).

○ The liver can be used as an acoustic window as well as a traversal organ.

○ The stomach can also be used as an acoustic window as well as a traversal organ if it is filled with water. However, the patient in this case is not NPO (nothing by mouth) and cannot be sedated fully.

Evaluate Prebiopsy Laboratory Values

• Laboratory value evaluation mostly revolves around ruling out coagulopathy.

○ Suggested coagulopathy thresholds for core biopsy are as follows:

• aPTT: ≤45–50 seconds
• INR: ≤1.4–1.5
• Platelet count: >70,000

○ Suggested coagulopathy thresholds for FNA are as follows:

• aPTT: ≤60 seconds
• INR: ≤1.7
• Platelet count: >50,000

• In cases of borderline coagulopathy, FNA can be utilized to potentially reduce the risk of bleeding. To counter the risk of reduced sample adequacy with FNA, collaborating with the cytology department for feedback on adequacy prior to terminating the procedure is recommended.

Obtain Informed Consent

• Indications

○ To evaluate the true nature of the mass:

• Evaluate for benign versus malignant disease
• Evaluate if this is an infectious process
• Evaluate the type of malignancy

• Alternatives

• To refuse the biopsy
• Surgical excision biopsy

• Procedural risks

○ There are no data in the literature discussing the incidence of complications regarding the biopsy of nonvisceral abdominal masses. The incidence of complications should be extrapolated from the liver biopsy literature (see Chapter 1) for intraperitoneal mass biopsy and renal biopsy literature (see Chapter 2) for retroperitoneal mass biopsy.

○ Infection

• This is a rare complication.
• It may occur at higher frequency with traversal of bowel (not proven).

○ Bleeding

• This is the most common major complication.
• Bleeding may be transient with or without blood transfusion.
• In rare cases, bleeding may require intervention such as transcatheter renal arterial embolization or exploratory surgery.

○ Injury to surrounding organs and/or structures

• Vessels (bleeding)
• Spleen, liver, and bowel

Equipment

Ultrasound Guidance

• Ultrasound machine with Doppler capability
• Multiarray 4–5 MHz ultrasound transducer
• Transducer guide bracket (unless free-hand is being attempted)
• Sterile transducer cover

Standard Surgical Preparation and Draping

• Chlorhexidine skin preparation/cleansing fluid
• Fenestrated drape

Local Infiltrative Analgesia Administration

• 21-gauge infiltration needle
• 10–20 mL 1% lidocaine syringe

Sharp Access and Biopsy

- 11-blade incision scalpel
- Coaxial access needle (see below); 17-gauge coaxial needle for delivery of 18-gauge core biopsy needle
- Coaxial access needle (see below); 20-gauge coaxial needles for delivery of FNA 22-gauge needles

Technique

Intravenous Access

- The necessity of moderate sedation (administered intravenously) for renal biopsies varies from one institution to another. My institution performs moderate sedation for nonvisceral abdominal mass biopsies.
- If moderate sedation is not routinely administered, intravenous (IV) access is still reasonable as a standby for any complication (including pain-related complications) or if the need arises to administer sedation.

Prebiopsy Ultrasound Examination

- Determine easiest visibility of lesion in cases of target lesion biopsy
- Look for adjacent organs that can be inadvertently traversed (spleen, colon)
- For mesenteric lesion biopsy, avoid traversing areas of the mesentery that show numerous vessels by contrast-enhanced CT if possible.

Standard Surgical Preparation and Draping

- Skin preparation/cleansing in the region that was chosen as an ultrasound imaging portal and a needle access needle portal
- Place a fenestrated drape at the prepared skin region

Local Infiltrative Analgesia Administration

- Utilizing a 21-gauge (by at least a 3.7 cm long) infiltration needle, 1% lidocaine infiltration is performed.

Sharp Access

- An incision is made utilizing an 11-blade scalpel usually by a 3- to 5-mm-depth stab of the 11-blade.
- A 17- to 19-gauge coaxial access needle can be passed across and into the target lesion.
- The coaxial access needle also allows for the embolization of the biopsy tract with Gelfoam (Pfizer Pharmaceuticals, New York, NY) or coils after the biopsy has been performed.

Pathology Sample Acquisition (Biopsy)

- It is advisable to obtain a fine needle aspirate for flow cytometry evaluation for diagnosing lymphoma prior to any core biopsy sample.
  - Evaluate for lymphoma in any extravisceral abdominal mass biopsy because lymphoma is not uncommon in this setting.
  - The FNA flow cytometry sample is obtained prior to the core biopsy because bleeding from the core biopsy may give a false reading on subsequent flow cytometry evaluation.
- An automated spring-loaded core biopsy needle is passed to the end of a coaxial needle, "fired" (automatically deployed), and withdrawn (**Fig. 3.2**).
- Without the use of coaxial needle access, the core biopsy needle (or fine needle) is passed to the edge of the intended target lesion. The biopsy needle is then "fired" or deployed (**Figs. 3.1 and 3.2**).
- In cases of lesion heterogeneity, sampling different areas of the lesion to obtain representing samples of all the acoustic characteristic areas is advisable. Heterogeneity commonly, but not necessarily, represents areas of degeneration or necrosis of the mass.

Immediate Postbiopsy Ultrasound Imaging

- To evaluate if there is associated bleeding/hematoma

Endpoints

Lesion-specific Target Liver Biopsy

- Usually one to three 18-gauge needle passes are required to obtain an adequate pathology sample. More needle samples are required in heterogeneous/necrotic masses.
- The operator grossly evaluates the core sample and determines when to stop making core biopsy needle passes.
- White/pale-appearing samples usually correlate with malignancy.

Postprocedural Evaluation and Management

There is no clear set standard for patient care following biopsy of a miscellaneous abdominal mass (extravisceral abdominal mass). At my institution, these patients are treated like liver biopsy patients and are observed postbiopsy for 3–4 hours.

Outpatient Ambulatory Stay/Observation Period

- Postprocedural stay varies from one institution to another.
- At my institution, these patients are treated similar to liver biopsy patients and are observed postbiopsy for 3–4 hours.

Intravenous Fluid and Diet

- IV access should be kept until just prior to discharge.
- Institutions that practice moderate sedation start with a clear liquid diet and advance it as tolerated. This helps to offset patients' nausea and vomiting.
- Other institutions/operators commence a clear liquid diet after a period of abstinence of oral intake. This period could be one hour, for example.
- Give IV fluid until oral intake is adequate

Activity

- Bed rest for approximately 4 hours is recommended.
- Patients, on discharge, are instructed to not engage in strenuous activity for 24–48 hours postbiopsy.

Pain Management

- Narcotics are usually not required during the postbiopsy stay of the patient prior to discharge. Occasionally some patients require oral narcotic analgesics such as acetaminophen and hydrocodone combination medication. Rarely does a patient require IV narcotics such as fentanyl.
- On discharge, patients usually tolerate the procedure well and do not require analgesics more potent than over-the-counter medications.

Monitoring Vital Signs

- Vital sign monitoring includes blood pressure and heart rate. Occasionally, oxygen saturation monitoring is required in cases of shortness of breath and/or chest pain.
- Institutions/operators that practice conscious sedation may record a softer blood pressure than a patient's baseline blood pressure after the biopsy. This is most likely due to sedation with or without dehydration. The patient usually responds in time with hydration, particularly as the sedatives wear off.
- Continued hypotension and, more importantly, rise in heart rate are concerning for hypovolemia (bleeding).

If signs of hypovolemia occur, an IV volume bolus is given and a noncontrast CT exam is performed to confirm the clinical suspicion of bleeding.

Complications and Their Management

Management of Pain and Pain-related Morbidity

- Continued pain requires further clinical and possibly imaging evaluation. An expanding retroperitoneal hematoma can cause pain. The degree of pain does not correlate with the degree of bleeding. However, changes in vital signs do signify a significant bleed.
- Occasionally, operators respond to continued pain by performing a diagnostic imaging exam.
  - A limited ultrasound examination at the site to evaluate for a capsular hematoma
  - Or a more global exam such as a noncontrast abdominal CT exam. Ultimately, the decisive factor for determining significant bleeding is the patient's stability (vitals) – not what is seen on the images.
- If there is no bleeding and the patient is stable but requires narcotic analgesics for pain, the patient can be admitted for pain management.

Management of Bleeding Complications

- IV access should be kept until just after discharge in case fluid resuscitation is required.
- Significant bleeding affecting vital signs and patient stability should be managed by
  - Adequate IV access (two 18-gauge IV access or central venous catheters)
  - Fluid resuscitation starting with crystalloid fluid bolus
  - Type and cross
  - Repeat hematocrit to compare with baseline
  - Blood transfusion to maintain hematocrit at or above 30%
  - Surgical consult/interventional radiology consult
- Interventional radiology offers
  - Arteriography with super-selective arterial embolization if bleeding or a pseudoaneurysm is seen
- Surgical consultation may offer, in the cases of severe uncontrolled bleeding, open surgery, exploration, local hemostasis of surface bleeding, or excision of the mass.

Management of Puncture of Adjacent Organs

- With image guidance, this is a rare complication.
- When it occurs, it is usually detected during the procedure by imaging or from the pathology report.
- When transgression of adjacent organs occurs the result is clinically inconsequential. The problem is incidental and does not rise to the level of a minor clinical complication, let alone a major complication.

Special Issues

Splenic Mass Biopsy

Splenic mass biopsies are rarely done. They should be approached with caution; splenic rupture and bleeding are primary concerns. The approach and technique used are similar to those for an intraperitoneal mass biopsy. Unlike a liver biopsy where it is advisable to cross normal liver parenchyma to reduce bleeding, the needle path should not cross normal spleen and should enter the mass directly to avoid splenic rupture. This, of course, can only be achieved in peripheral lesions. Lesions deeper than the splenic capsule require the needle to pass the capsule.

Pancreatic Mass Biopsy

Pancreatic biopsies are routinely performed. Trans-retroperitoneal, transhepatic, and transgastric routes can be used to mention common needle paths that require visceral/organ transgression. Intentional visceral/organ transgression is not necessary but is common. The method utilized is usually FNA, similar to those methods described above. The key issue with pancreatic biopsies is to make sure that the mass is not a pseudoaneurysm. Careful examination of contrast-enhanced CT and/or MR images is required, as well as Doppler ultrasound evaluation, before performing a pancreatic biopsy. In addition, pancreatitis (although not common postbiopsy) should be included in the risks for the formal consent.

Further Reading

Cardella JF, Bakal CW, Bertino RE, et al; Society of Interventional Radiology Standards of Practice Committee. Quality improvement guidelines for image-guided percutaneous biopsy in adults. J Vasc Interv Radiol 2003;14(9 Pt 2):S227–S230

Gervais DA. Percutaneous image-guided biopsy: review of and emphasis on special approaches. In: Ray CE Jr., Hicks ME, Patel NH, eds. SIR Syllabus. Fairfax, VA: Society of Interventional Radiology; 2003:63–72

Silverman SG, Deuson TE, Kane N, et al. Percutaneous abdominal biopsy: cost-identification analysis. Radiology 1998;206(2): 429–435

4 Chest Mass Biopsy

Sudhir Vinayak

The first percutaneous transthoracic needle biopsy was reported in 1883; a century later, ultrasound guidance was used to biopsy a lung nodule. It is now common practice and has become an invaluable diagnostic procedure to determine the etiology of masses arising from the lung, pleura, mediastinum, and the chest wall. As image resolution improves, this technique is becoming more accurate, safer, and more widely accepted.

Ultrasound has several strengths as a biopsy guidance system. It is readily available, relatively inexpensive, and portable. In addition, it uses no ionizing radiation and can provide guidance in multiple transverse, longitudinal, or oblique planes. The greatest advantage, however, is that it allows real-time visualization of the needle tip as it passes through tissues into the target. This allows precise needle placement and avoidance of important intervening structures. In addition, color flow Doppler imaging can help prevent complications of needle placement by identifying the vascular nature of a mass and by allowing the clinician to avoid vascular structures lying within the needle path.

Air in the lungs intervening between the transducer and the lesion prevents its use in the majority of pulmonary lesions. However, when a pulmonary process abuts the pleura or has arisen within the pleura, the chest wall, or a portion of the mediastinum contiguous with the chest wall, ultrasound may be the method of choice for localizing the lesion and guiding the biopsy needle. This may be especially true for apical pulmonary and extrapulmonary lesions for which computed tomography (CT) and fluoroscopy cannot demonstrate an easy access route.

Ultrasound-guided biopsy is significantly faster than CT-guided biopsy with average procedure times of 31.4 minutes and 45.2 minutes, respectively. The diagnostic yield with ultrasound guidance is also superior to CT with accuracies of 91% and 71%, respectively. The overall accuracy of ultrasound-guided biopsy ranges between 91 and 98%.

Classification

Ultrasound-guided needle biopsy can be classified by the preferred method of approach and anatomical location of the lesion.

- Mediastinum – extrapleural access: suprasternal, parasternal, transsternal, and paravertebral approaches

- Apical – apical lesions of the lung and pleura, as well as supraclavicular lymph nodes
- Peripheral – lesions abutting the anterior, lateral, and posterior pleural linings of the chest
- Others
  - Transpulmonary – lesions in the mediastinum and perihilar regions may have to be approached in this manner to avoid injury to major vessels.
  - Endoscopic ultrasound – lower paratracheal, subcarinal, aortopulmonary, and paraesophageal regions. Main indication is for posterior mediastinal lesions especially in the case of preoperative staging of nonsmall cell lung cancer.

Indications

- Evaluation of a focal pulmonary process (solid nodule or infective) abutting the pleura. This may be primary or secondary (metastatic).
- Evaluation of hilar and mediastinal lesions
- Staging of tumors (lung cancer or extrathoracic malignancies)
- Evaluation of a pleural mass or pleural thickening (focal or diffuse)
- Evaluation of chest wall masses arising from or extending into the chest cavity

Contraindications

Absolute Contraindications

There are no absolute contraindications to percutaneous chest biopsy.

Relative Contraindications

- An uncooperative patient
- Patient on positive pressure ventilation
- Abnormal coagulation – international normalized ratio (INR) of more than 1.3 or platelet count of less than 50,000/mm^3
- Pulmonary arterial hypertension – if projected needle path involves transgression of lung tissue
- Other severe underlying pulmonary disease such as severe chronic obstructive airway disease (COAD)

- Severely limited function of contralateral lung or contralateral pneumonectomy
- Intractable cough
- Suspicion of hydatid cyst
- Lack of a safe biopsy route – inaccessible location of lesion such as adjacent to large blood vessels that cannot be circumnavigated

In some patients, the platelet count may be normal, but platelet function is decreased in uremia, liver disease, hematologic neoplasms, and in patients taking acetylsalicylic acid.

Preprocedural Evaluation and Preparation of the Patient

Prior to the procedure, the following should be rechecked:

- Written consent, if required; obtain informed or written consent as prescribed by hospital policies
- Correction of any abnormal coagulation discovered during preexamination
- Confirmation that patient's general health has not changed since preevaluation, for example, fever, dyspnea, etc.

Hospitals have their own policies for obtaining verbal or written informed consents. Regardless of the policy, the procedure, its inherent risks, alternatives, and benefits should be explained in a manner that the patient understands. The physician must be empathetic of patient apprehension regarding pain, and reassurance helps gain patient cooperation during the procedure. An apprehensive patient will not follow breathing instructions and will cause unnecessary delays with poor biopsy results.

The patient need not be fasting and no blood is required for transfusion. Therefore, the procedure can be performed on an outpatient basis. Premedication is only advised for percutaneous biopsies of mediastinal lesions. Conscious sedation is induced using midazolam and fentanyl citrate in addition to administration of local anesthesia. For mediastinal biopsies, it is also advised to have noninvasive blood pressure monitoring with continuous pulse oxymetry.

- Coagulation screen – The prothrombin time, partial thromboplastin time, and platelet count are obtained to exclude any bleeding disorder before the biopsy. INR of <1.3 and platelet count of >50,000/mm^3 are generally acceptable. However, a higher platelet count of >100,000/mm^3 is desirable. Bleeding disorders should be corrected with fresh frozen plasma, platelets, or vitamin K.

- Discontinue aspirin 5 days before biopsy and other antiinflammatory agents 2 days prior. Patients on oral anticoagulants should be switched to heparin 2–3 days prior to the procedure, and it should be discontinued several hours before the procedure.
- Check pulmonary function tests in compromised patients

Equipment

The choice of transducer for biopsy is important. A 2–5 MHz convex probe allows visualization of deeper structures; a sector probe with a small footprint allows a wider field of view and is also convenient to place in the intercostal space and suprasternal notch. For superficial lesions a higher frequency linear probe of 5–10 MHz will improve resolution and depict relationship of the lesion to the pleura.

When necessary, color Doppler is used to detect potential blood vessels in the needle path. Doppler sensitivity should be set to a low velocity (typically 0.25 m/s) and the wall filter is adjusted to minimize rejection of small frequency shifts to avoid interference from respiratory and cardiac movements.

The patient is positioned depending upon the chosen needle entry site. For a parasternal, transsternal, and anterior wall approach, the patient should lie supine. For supraclavicular and suprasternal approach, a pillow is placed under the shoulders and the neck hyperextended. If the approach is lateral, the patient can be positioned in supine, oblique, or lateral decubitus position.

The posterior chest is best imaged with the patient sitting upright. Raising the arm above the patient's head increases the rib space on the ipsilateral side thereby facilitating scanning and allowing for a larger window for needle entry.

Percutaneous Needle Biopsy

Percutaneous needle biopsy (PNB) can be performed by the patient's bedside or in the department. It is useful to have the following three probes at hand:

- 2–5 MHz multifrequency convex transducer with needle guide – useful for deeper lesions
- 3.5 MHz sector transducer – small footprint allows intercostal scanning
- 5–10 MHz linear transducer for superficial lesions

As with other ultrasound-guided biopsies, there are two methods for acquiring tissue, fine-needle aspiration biopsy (FNAB) and core needle biopsy (CNB).

Fine-Needle Aspiration Biopsy

FNA can be used for sampling both solid (soft tissue) and fluid. A fine needle is defined as one with an outside diameter of <1 mm and is generally 20–25 gauge in size. FNAB causes less pleural and pulmonary trauma than cutting needles used for CNB. Aspiration produces a highly diagnostic sample for cytologic analysis and is particularly useful for small mediastinal lesions that make the placement and activation of cutting needles (CNB) a daunting prospect. However, the cell aspirate from FNAB may not be sufficient for a definitive diagnosis, thereby necessitating a CNB.

Core Needle Biopsy

CNBs are performed using larger caliber cutting needles of 14–19 gauges to obtain greater amounts of material thereby preserving the histologic integrity of the tissue. The structural relationships of cellular elements and the preserve as well as distribution of noncellular matrix provide useful information thereby improving the certainty of a diagnosis. Both types of needles should be available during the procedure and a cytopathologist or a cytotechnologist should be present if FNAB is planned.

Technique

Most patients are referred for biopsy after a previous CT or ultrasound examination, and these images should be viewed prior to starting the procedure. Once the lesion is identified, the ideal probe for biopsy is chosen. The desirable needle path is planned and skin entry is marked. The needle path should be the shortest possible, making sure that large blood vessels are avoided by using color Doppler to chart the path. Lesions lying posterior to a rib can be targeted by angling the probe and using an oblique approach.

If the needle entry is through the intercostal space, it should be superior to the rib so as to avoid the neurovascular bundle just inferior to the rib, because entry at this level can cause discomfort to the patient and result in bleeding (**Fig. 4.1**).

Ultrasound guidance can be performed using a needle guide or free hand. Inexperienced physicians are advised to use the needle guide prior to trying the free-hand technique so as to familiarize themselves with applying the needle with one hand while controlling the transducer with the other. For difficult target lesions, the needle guide is a necessity even in experienced hands.

A needle guide is a dedicated device made to fit a specific transducer in a way that produces an electronically

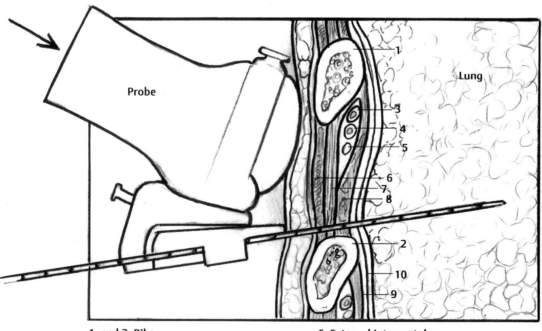

1. and 2. Ribs
3. Posterior intercostal a.
4. Posterior intercostal v.
5. Intercostal nerve.

6. External intercostal m.
7. Internal intercostal m.
8. Internal intimi m.
9. Subserous fascia
10. Parietal pleura

Fig. 4.1 Probe with needle guide attached. Needle placement is just superior to rib 2, thereby avoiding the neurovascular bundle that is inferior to the adjacent rib 1.

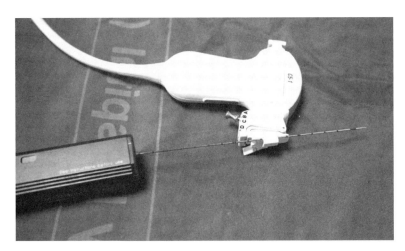

Fig. 4.2 Convex probe with attached needle guide, Trucut needle, and spring-loaded trigger device.

displayed puncture line on the monitor corresponding to the needle canal on the guide. Though it provides safer control of the needle during insertion, there is less flexibility of needle manipulation and limited degree of freedom regarding direction of puncture. Most needle guides have three adjustable needle angles, which help to align the electronic puncture line through the target (**Fig. 4.2**).

With the free-hand technique, there is no physical connection between needle and probe giving greater flexibility for needle entry. By inserting the needle from the end of the transducer parallel to the scanning plane, the entire length of the needle can be seen on the monitor, but no electronic puncture line is seen with the free-hand technique. If the needle entry is perpendicular to the scanning plane, it will appear as a single or double dot.

For sterility, the ultrasound transducer can be covered with a sterile plastic sheath containing sterile gel. However, many physicians prefer to clean the probe with povidone–iodine (Betadine; Purdue Pharma, Stamford, CT) and place it directly on the skin using sterile gel as an acoustic coupling agent. After the procedure, the transducer is soaked for 10 minutes in a bactericidal dialdehyde solution. Caturelli et al reviewed their experience with a similar degree of antisepsis and found no increase in postbiopsy infection.

Biopsy Methods

After the lesion has been identified and skin marked, the skin site is prepped and draped in a sterile fashion. The skin and subcutaneous tissues are anesthetized using a 1% solution of lidocaine down to, but not traversing, the parietal pleura. It is imperative to anesthetize well the vicinities of the periosteum and parietal pleura (which is very sensitive) to minimize patient discomfort during biopsy. A small skin incision may be required for core

biopsy needles. There are two methods for acquiring tissue at biopsy:

- Aspiration, which produces a cellular slurry for cytology examination
- CNB, which produces a piece of tissue with histologic integrity

Fine-Needle Aspiration Biopsy

Having a cytopathologist or cytotechnologist present during the procedure is beneficial because they can determine that a sufficient diagnostic sample has been obtained before the procedure is terminated. A wide range of FNAB needles are available, ranging from 20–25 gauges. Twenty-gauge needles harvest more cells due to the larger size. A useful technique for biopsy, used by many physicians, aims to prevent a continuous needle tract following withdrawal of the needle after biopsy. Prior to placing the needle, the overlying skin is pulled or pushed and the biopsy is performed in the normal manner (**Fig. 4.3**). The needle is then withdrawn and the skin tension is relieved. This helps to avoid a continuous needle tract, thereby decreasing the chances of fistula formation.

FNAB can be performed by simply attaching a syringe to the needle and aspirating cells by pulling on the plunger. However, by attaching the syringe to a vacuum device, there is firmer control of the needle and suction is greatly improved (**Fig. 4.4**).

To aspirate cells from a lesion, the needle (with stylet) is advanced along the planned trajectory, in suspended respiration, until the tip lies within the target lesion. The patient is allowed to take a few shallow breaths and then again is instructed to suspend respiration while the stylet is withdrawn and syringe attached to the needle with vacuum device in place.

1. Skin
2. Subcutaneous or
   intrathoracic tissues
3. Nodule

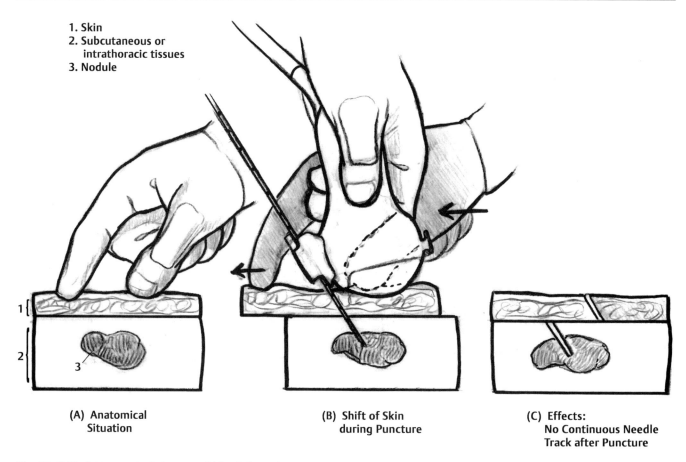

(A) Anatomical
Situation

(B) Shift of Skin
during Puncture

(C) Effects:
No Continuous Needle
Track after Puncture

Fig. 4.3 Shift of skin over the lesion to avoid fistula formation.

The vacuum syringe plunger is then pulled back to generate suction and the needle passed in and out of the lesion several times in a gentle fashion to free material from the lesion and draw it into the needle's lumen. The suction is then relieved as the needle and attached syringe are withdrawn. The patient can then resume breathing.

Cellular material in the needle is placed on a slide for staining and cytology and extrusion of the material from the needle onto the slide may require passing the stylet through the needle's lumen. The cytopathologist is asked to confirm that an adequate number of cells have been harvested before terminating the procedure.

Core Needle Biopsy

Numerous kinds of CNB devices are commercially available based either on the Trucut principle (more common) whereby a tissue core is cut by an outer needle overriding

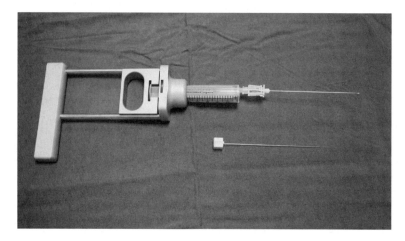

Fig. 4.4 Vacuum device attached to the syringe improves suction and provides firmer control of the needle during aspiration.

an inner needle with a slot for retrieval or the Menghini principle whereby the tissue core is cut loose by a rotating maneuver and sampled into the needle by suction. Most devices are spring loaded with automatic triggers that produce a sharp sound (**Fig. 4.2**). As with FNAB, the patient is prepped and a local anesthetic administered. CNBs can be performed with a needle guide or by the free-hand technique. The needle is advanced to a point just short of the nodule and, depending on the setting, triggering the gun will advance the needle by a preset distance through the nodule (usually 15 or 22 mm). The needle is then withdrawn and the cylindrical tissue sample revealed by pulling back the outer needle. The specimen is placed in formalin and sent for histopathology.

Key Points Pertaining to FNA and CNB

- Coaxial technique is sometimes used whereby, a larger needle is placed into the mass, the stylet is removed, and a longer, smaller caliber needle is placed through the lumen of the first needle, which serves as a guide. Multiple samples can then be obtained with the smaller needle without the need to reposition the large needle. In this way, the pleura need only be punctured once by the large needle. The coaxial technique is more commonly used for aspiration biopsies, but may also be used for CNBs.
- Having identified the needle entry point, color Doppler is used to confirm that there are no blood vessels in the trajectory path.
- In tumors exhibiting central necrosis, ultrasound-guided biopsy of the solid viable portions of the tumor improves sensitivity.
- The choice of biopsy mode (FNA versus CNB) is important. In patients with no known primary tumor, CNB specimens are preferred because immunohistochemical studies are often required to determine a more specific primary tumor. CNBs are also preferred in histologic tumor types such as thymoma, germ cell tumors, neurogenic tumors, and benign tumors. FNAB is useful in documenting metastatic disease in a patient with a known primary malignancy. It is also used in complex cases where the needle path involves transgression of lung tissue, when lesions are located adjacent to great vessels, or when highly vascular lesions are suspected. In patients with suspected lymphoma, both CNB and FNAB samples are obtained for histology and flow cytometry.

Endpoints

- Mediastinal masses can be approached in the following manner:
  - Parasternal approach – for biopsy of anterior mediastinal lesions that extend to the anterior parasternal chest wall (**Figs. 4.5, 4.6, and 4.7**)
  - Paravertebral approach – Patient is placed in prone or oblique prone position. However, it is rarely used for ultrasound-guided biopsies.
  - Suprasternal approach – This is best performed using a 5 MHz sector probe and the free-hand technique. FNAB is performed using a 22-gauge needle inserted through the suprasternal fossa. This is a safe and effective method to biopsy lesions in the pretracheal, right paratracheal, and prevascular compartments of the superior mediastinum. CNB is seldom performed. FNAB of superior mediastinal lesions using the suprasternal approach has a yield of 86.8%.
- Apical lesions and supraclavicular lymph nodes are biopsied using the supraclavicular route. Bronchogenic carcinoma is the most common cause of supraclavicular nodal metastasis, but other primary tumors also spread to these nodes. In patients with lung cancer, metastatic supraclavicular nodes must reach a size of at least 22 mm to have a 50% chance of being palpable. Most supraclavicular nodal metastases can be detected with ultrasound and it is considered the gold standard in identifying suspicious nodes. The FNAB technique is commonly used and a CNB is usually reserved for larger apical lobe lesions. When the arms are positioned at the patient's side in a sitting position, the clavicles drop and apical lung lesions are more clearly visible on ultrasound.

  In a series of 12 sonographically guided supraclavicular FNA biopsies reported by Yang et al, the needle had to pass through the jugular vein in four patients and no complication occurred. The authors believed that penetration of neck veins by thin (22-gauge) needles is acceptable if the vessels are unavoidable.

Postprocedural Management

- An immediate postprocedure upright expiratory chest radiograph is taken to detect a pneumothorax. This may be repeated after 4 hours.
- Outpatients should be observed in the recovery area for 2–4 hours and vital signs (including oxygen saturation) monitored every 20 minutes. Stable inpatients can be returned to the ward.
- The patient is placed with puncture site dependent (if tolerated). This prevents the occurrence of pneumothorax and can facilitate the resorption of a small pneumothorax.
- Pneumothoraces that are small, asymptomatic and stable do not require treatment unless:
  - Patient is dyspneic or has acute onset of chest pain.
  - Size of pneumothorax exceeds 30% of chest volume.
  - Pneumothorax continues to increase in volume.

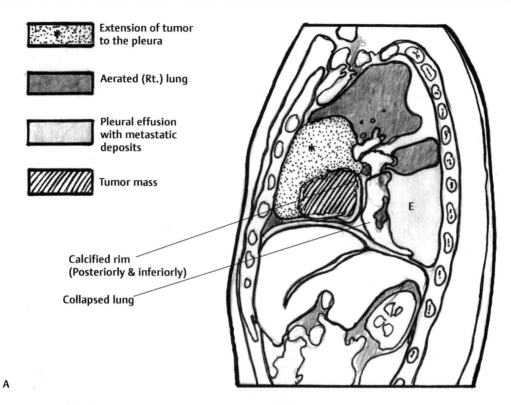

Extension of tumor
to the pleura

Aerated (Rt.) lung

Pleural effusion
with metastatic
deposits

Tumor mass

Calcified rim
(Posteriorly & inferiorly)

Collapsed lung

A

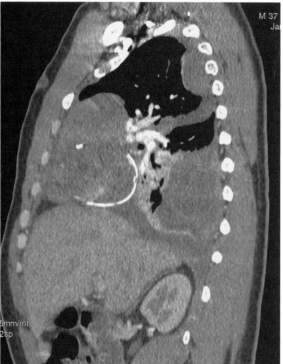

B

Fig. 4.5 (A) Sketch of **(B)** sagittal image of parasternal lesion with calcified rim. Core needle biopsy was positive for thymoma.

- Two general approaches can be undertaken in the treatment of post biopsy pneumothorax.
  - Aspiration of pneumothorax by insertion of an 18-gauge intravenous catheter into the pleural space and suction using a 50 mL syringe. The catheter is withdrawn and patient observed.
  - Place a chest drain for larger pneumothorax and admit patient for observation.
- Stable outpatients can be discharged after 4 hours and instructed not to exert themselves for the rest of the day.

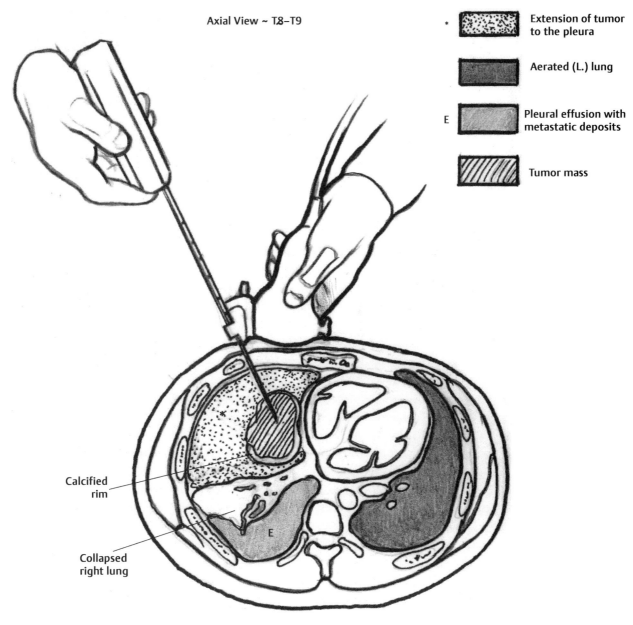

Axial View ~ T8–T9

* Extension of tumor to the pleura

Aerated (L.) lung

E Pleural effusion with metastatic deposits

Tumor mass

Calcified rim

Collapsed right lung

A

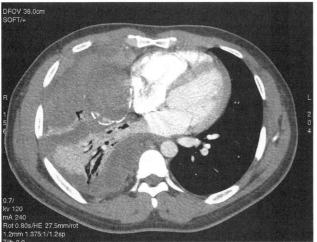

B

Fig. 4.6 (A) Sketch and **(B)** axial image of chest. Diagram shows position of probe with needle guide and needle placement. Core needle biopsy was positive for thymoma.

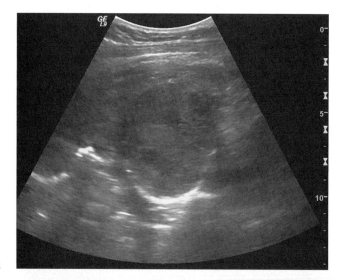

A

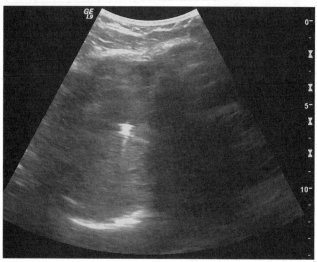

B

Fig. 4.7 **(A)** Ultrasound images showing parasternal thymoma before biopsy and **(B)** during biopsy with hyperechoic needle tip within the lesion.

Complications and Their Management

Ultrasound-guided percutaneous lung biopsy is extremely safe and has an overall complication rate of <6%. In these series, none of the complications was serious, mainly self-resolving pneumothoraces and hemoptysis that resolved spontaneously.

Pneumothorax

This is the most common complication and is easily diagnosed on an upright expiratory chest radiograph. If it occurs during the procedure (sudden onset of dyspnea), the biopsy should be discontinued. Factors that increase the occurrence of pneumothorax include

- Increasing the number of needle passes
- Duration of the procedure
- Concomitant lung disease such as COAD
- CNB as opposed to FNAB (gauge of needle)
- Increased depth of lesion (length of needle pass)
- Size of the lesion
- Patient compliance
- Inability to place the patient with biopsy site in the dependent position following the procedure

Hemorrhage and Hemoptysis

Hemoptysis is uncommon and generally resolves spontaneously. Incidence ranges between 2 and 6%. The occurrence of hemorrhage complications depends on the presence of a bleeding diathesis, vascularity of the lesion, intake of medication that induces bleeding tendency, and underlying uremia or liver disease. If hemoptysis occurs, the patient should be reassured and observed; massive, life-threatening hemorrhage is rare. Placing the biopsy side in a dependent position prevents transbronchial aspiration into the contralateral lung.

Pleural Pain

This is commonly associated with complications such as pneumothorax and hemoptysis. It can be managed with mild doses of codeine, which as an antitussive agent is also useful for hemoptysis.

Other Complications

Infrequent and rare complications are

- Hemothorax and chest wall hematoma
- Vasovagal reaction
- Air embolism
- Bronchopleural fistula
- Tumor seeding
- Massive hemoptysis

Further Reading

Caturelli E, Giacobbe A, Facciorusso D, et al. Free-hand technique with ordinary antisepsis in abdominal US-guided fine-needle punctures: three-year experience. Radiology 1996;199(3): 721–723

Gupta S, Gulati M, Rajwanshi A, Gupta D, Suri S. Sonographically guided fine-needle aspiration biopsy of superior mediastinal lesions by the suprasternal route. AJR Am J Roentgenol 1998; 171(5):1303–1306

Gupta S, Seaberg K, Wallace MJ, et al. Imaging-guided percutaneous biopsy of mediastinal lesions: different approaches and anatomic considerations. Radiographics 2005;25(3):763–786, discussion 786–788

Koh DM, Burke S, Davies N, Padley SP. Transthoracic US of the chest: clinical uses and applications. Radiographics 2002;22(1):e1

Liao W-Y, Chen M-Z, Chang Y-L, et al. US-guided transthoracic cutting biopsy for peripheral thoracic lesions less than 3 cm in diameter. Radiology 2000;217(3):685–691

Morvay Z, Szabó E, Tiszlavicz L, Furák J, Troján I, Palkó A. Thoracic core needle biopsy using ultrasound guidance. Ultrasound Q 2001; 17(2):113–121

Middleton WD, Teefey SA, Dahiya N. Ultrasound-guided chest biopsies. Ultrasound Q 2006;22(4):241–252

van Overhagen H, Brakel K, Heijenbrok MW, et al. Metastases in supraclavicular lymph nodes in lung cancer: assessment with palpation, US, and CT. Radiology 2004;232(1):75–80

Pan JF, Yang PC, Chang DB, Lee YC, Kuo SH, Luh KT. Needle aspiration biopsy of malignant lung masses with necrotic centers. Improved sensitivity with ultrasonic guidance. Chest 1993;103(5): 1452–1456

Sheth S, Hamper UM, Stanley DB, Wheeler JH, Smith PA. US guidance for thoracic biopsy: a valuable alternative to CT. Radiology 1999; 210(3):721–726

Yang PC, Chang DB, Lee YC, Yu CJ, Kuo SH, Luh KT. Mediastinal malignancy: ultrasound guided biopsy through the supraclavicular approach. Thorax 1992;47(5):377–380

5   Breast Biopsy

Jennifer A. Harvey

Classification

Percutaneous image-guided breast biopsy is less invasive, less expensive, and more efficient than diagnostic surgical biopsy.

- Sensitivity of ultrasound-guided breast core needle biopsy (CNB): 97–99%
- Fine-needle aspiration biopsy (FNAB) is less sensitive, but can be very useful in evaluating additional lesions or abnormal lymph nodes in the setting of a known primary breast cancer.
- Most breast masses are amenable to ultrasound-guided biopsy.

Initial Training

American College of Radiology (ACR) Practice Guidelines for performance of ultrasound-guided breast biopsy recommends that radiologists who are beginning to perform these procedures meet practice guidelines for performing breast ultrasound and obtain

- At least 3 hours of continuing professional education hours in breast ultrasound intervention, and perform at least three procedures under direct supervision. These training suggestions can be met in residency or fellowship training programs.
- In addition, the ACR recommends that radiologists perform at least 12 ultrasound-guided procedures annually to maintain skills.

Advantages of image-guided preoperative diagnosis of breast cancer over diagnostic surgical biopsy:

- Reduces the number of women undergoing surgical procedures
- Allows the patient and surgeon to discuss therapeutic options in advance of surgery
- Once a breast cancer has been diagnosed, the extent of disease can be evaluated by ultrasound or magnetic resonance imaging (MRI). Ultrasound-guided biopsy documenting multifocal or multicentric disease may alter surgical management.
  - Percutaneous biopsy of nonpalpable cancer results in a single therapeutic surgical operation in 81% of

women. Receptor status as determined by CNB samples can also guide neoadjuvant chemotherapy if needed.

Other advantages of ultrasound guidance for breast CNB over stereotactic guidance include

- The lack of ionizing radiation is particularly important for pregnant women with a breast mass.
- Real-time visualization of the needle during biopsy improves confidence that a small lesion has been accurately sampled.
- The supine position of the patient for an ultrasound-guided procedure is often more comfortable than the prone or sitting position used for stereotactic procedures.
- Stereotactic biopsy is also limited by compressed breast thickness of at least 2.5 cm, whereas small breast thickness rarely affects the ability to perform ultrasound-guided breast biopsy.
- Ultrasound-guided breast biopsies (in experienced hands) are often more efficient than stereotactic biopsy.

Indications

Percutaneous image-guided biopsy has largely replaced diagnostic surgical biopsy in the evaluation of breast lesions in many practices. Most breast lesions that are visible on ultrasound that are suspicious (Breast Imaging Reporting and Data System [BI-RADS] assessment category 4) or malignant (BI-RADS 5) are amenable to ultrasound-guided core needle biopsy. Image-guided biopsy is not typically performed for

- Lesions with BI-RADS assessment category 3: Probably benign, unless there is undue patient anxiety or the reliability of the patient for return visit is uncertain, for example a homeless woman with limited healthcare resources.
- In the setting of a palpable finding, diagnostic ultrasound-guided biopsy can be an alternative to excision.

Some lesions will not be amenable to percutaneous biopsy. Of 630 breast cancers diagnosed over a 3-year period at Yale University, 17% were not diagnosed by percutaneous biopsy. The most commonly cited reasons were

- Lesion was difficult to visualize for image-guided biopsy.
- Patient preference
- Lesion was superficial or very small.

Although most masses identified on mammography can be identified on ultrasound for biopsy, lesions presenting as architectural distortion or calcifications on mammography may be more difficult to identify on ultrasound. If a lesion is much better visualized on mammography than ultrasound, then stereotactic-guidance may be the better choice to improve confidence that the correct area was sampled (**Fig. 5.1**).

Microcalcifications

Should typically undergo sampling using stereotactic guidance, but can be identified and undergo biopsy using ultrasound in some cases. In a prospective study, Soo et al identified 23% of 111 lesions on ultrasound that presented as microcalcifications without a mass on mammography, and subsequently performed successful CNB using ultrasound. When calcifications were identified on ultrasound, lesions were more likely to be larger, malignant (69% versus 21%), and invasive when malignancy

was diagnosed (72% versus 28%) than lesions not identified on ultrasound. Ultrasound-guidance can be a useful option when percutaneous biopsy using stereotactic guidance is not feasible (**Fig. 5.2**).

Ultrasound-Guided Biopsy of Abnormal Axillary Lymph Nodes

- Can reduce the number of women undergoing sentinel lymph node biopsy.
- Women with a newly diagnosed invasive breast cancer undergo sentinel lymph node biopsy at the time of lumpectomy or mastectomy (unless there is palpable adenopathy).
- If FNA of an axillary lymph node in a woman with diagnosed breast cancer shows metastatic breast cancer, she can undergo axillary dissection at the first surgical procedure.
- If ultrasound shows normal axillary lymph nodes or the ultrasound-guided FNA or CNB is negative, sentinel node biopsy can be performed.

Axillary Adenopathy of Unknown Cause

- Can also undergo diagnostic percutaneous biopsy using ultrasound guidance
- In the setting of a known malignancy, FNA of an abnormal lymph node is typically adequate.

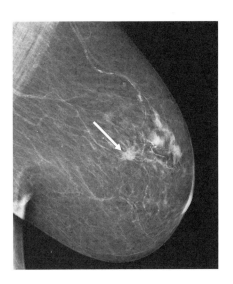

A

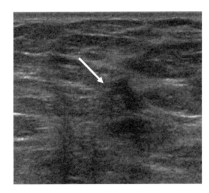

B

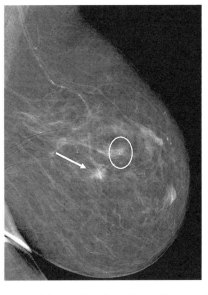

C

Fig. 5.1 A 67-year-old woman with abnormal right mammogram. **(A)** Right mediolateral (ML) view shows an 8-mm mass with spiculated margins (*arrow*). **(B)** Ultrasound shows a corresponding subtle hypoechoic solid mass in the right breast at 10 o'clock (*arrow*). **(C)** Postprocedure ML view shows that the clip (circle) is located ~2 cm from the lesion (*arrow*). Core biopsy was immediately repeated using stereotactic guidance. Histology from ultrasound-guided core needle biopsy (CNB) showed only stromal fibrosis, whereas the stereotactic-guided CNB showed ductal carcinoma in situ. In retrospect, stereotactic-guided CNB would likely have been a better choice initially because the finding was subtle on ultrasound.

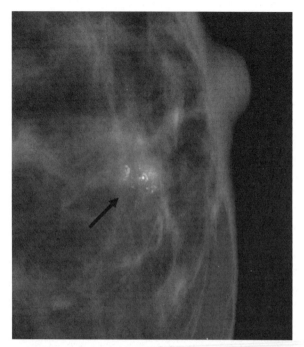

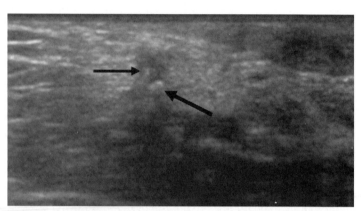

Fig. 5.2 A 68-year-old woman with suspicious microcalcifications on mammography who underwent diagnostic ultrasound-guided core needle biopsy. Stereotactic-guided biopsy could not be performed due to small compressed breast thickness. **(A)** Craniocaudal magnification view of the left breast shows grouped heterogeneous calcifications (*arrow*). **(B)** The calcifications were visualized on ultrasound (*arrows*).

A

B

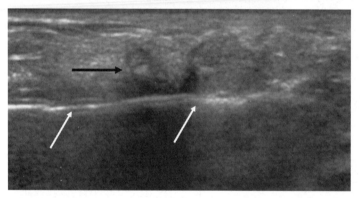

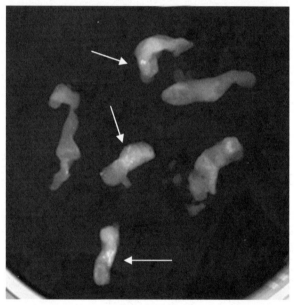

C

D

(C) Ultrasound-guided vacuum-assisted biopsy was performed by placing the needle (*white arrows*) posterior to the calcifications (*black arrow*). **(D)** Specimen radiograph contains numerous calcifications (*arrows*). Histology revealed invasive ductal carcinoma and ductal carcinoma in situ.

- When there is no known malignancy, CNB may be needed to exclude lymphoma.

Contraindications

Contraindications to ultrasound-guided breast biopsy:

- Uncooperative patient during the procedure
  - Mild sedation using fast-acting oral agents can be helpful if necessary.
- An uncorrectable known bleeding disorder
  - For these women, FNA or surgical biopsy may be reasonable alternatives.

Women who are not good candidates for stereotactic biopsy due to stroke or small breast size can usually undergo ultrasound-guided breast biopsy if the lesion is identified. The presence of a breast implant can increase the complexity of the approach, but is not necessarily a contraindication.

Preprocedural Evaluation

- A complete diagnostic imaging workup should be performed prior to scheduling a procedure. This improves efficiency of the procedure schedule, as no additional diagnostic imaging need be obtained that would result in delay or canceling of the procedure.

- Communication regarding the need for biopsy, procedural information, and an appointment can be given to the patient by the radiologist and an onsite nurse or technologist at the time of diagnostic imaging.
- A list of the patient's medications should be reviewed prior to scheduling the biopsy appointment. Management of anticoagulant medication is coordinated with the prescribing physician. We request that patients discontinue use of aspirin and nonsteroidal antiinflammatory medications for 5 days prior to the procedure if possible, though it is not mandatory.
- On the day of the procedure, informed consent can be obtained by the radiologist or a nurse.
- During the consent process, women are queried regarding known vascular disease or diabetes to avoid the use of lidocaine with epinephrine to reduce the risk of skin injury.
- Discuss possibility of surgery after a benign CNB that shows a high-risk lesion (i.e., atypical ductal hyperplasia or radial scar). If the biopsy does indeed show a high-risk lesion, the patient will have been forewarned that surgery was a possible recommendation even if the CNB did not show cancer.

Equipment

High-Frequency Linear Array Transducers

- Use of 10 MHz or higher linear transducer is highly recommended.
- Focal zones should be adjustable rather than fixed in position.

Needle Selection (Core versus Vacuum)

Either automated throw needle (CNB) or vacuum-assisted (VAB) biopsy devices may be used for ultrasound-guided breast biopsy.

Core Needle Biopsy

- 14-gauge needles are most commonly used for ultrasound-guided CNB, but range in size from 12–18 gauge.
- Higher diagnostic yields have been demonstrated for 14-gauge needles compared with 16- or 18-gauge core biopsy needles.

Vacuum-assisted Biopsy

- Needle size ranges from 8–14 gauge.
- VAB devices may collect single samples that must be retrieved after each pass (similar to CNB devices) or may collect multiple samples with a single needle insertion.
- VAB is more advantageous for calcified lesions. Bleeding complications may be slightly higher with VAB devices than CNB devices.

VAB can be useful for selective cases:

- A small lesion that may be difficult to visualize after the first one or two samples. In these cases, the needle can be placed posterior to the lesion and kept stationary during the biopsy. The lesion can be observed for resolution during sampling under real-time.
- VAB is also useful for the uncommon case when calcifications are sampled by ultrasound rather than stereotactic-guidance as VAB devices that require only one needle insertion often result in less introduction of air that may obscure calcifications.

Fine-Needle Aspiration Biopsy

- The Radiologic Diagnostic Oncology Group V found the sensitivity and specificity of FNAB of nonpalpable breast lesions to be 85–88% and 56–90%, respectively, which is considerably lower than CNB.
- FNAB has lower sensitivity for invasive lobular carcinoma compared with invasive ductal carcinoma.
- CNB should be performed instead of FNAB for most breast lesions.

FNAB can be very useful in

- The evaluation of cystic lesions of the breast
- A complicated cyst or complex mass may initially undergo FNAB. If a residual solid component remains, CNB can then be performed.
- FNAB of suspicious axillary lymph nodes can circumvent the need for sentinel node biopsy in the setting of known breast cancer.

Room Setup

Prior to beginning the procedure, diagnostic breast imaging including any mammograms, ultrasound, and MR images should be reviewed.

- An examination table that is adjustable in height is convenient to accommodate for radiologist stature.
- A table that rotates is useful for radiologists who prefer to use their dominant hand to manage the biopsy device.
- Lights should be dim enough to visualize the lesion well on the ultrasound screen.

Preparation for Procedure

- The patient lies supine on the examination table.
  - If the breast is large, an oblique position using wedge supports under the ipsilateral shoulder and back can improve access to lateral lesions.
  - The ipsilateral arm is placed above the head.
  - The breast is scanned to localize the lesion of interest.
- In planning the biopsy, the natural curvature of the breast can be used to advantage.
  - Visualization of the needle will be optimal when perpendicular to the ultrasound beam, which occurs when the needle is parallel to the surface of the transducer.
  - If the surface of the ultrasound transducer is placed parallel to the chest wall, needle entry from the periphery of the breast yields a path that is both parallel to the pectoral muscle, reducing risk of chest wall injury, and perpendicular to the ultrasound beam (**Fig. 5.3**).
  - Once the approach is decided, a "T" mark is placed on the breast marking the edge of the transducer and the anticipated entry site (**Fig. 5.4A**).
  - Skin is cleansed with an iodine solution. The use of a sterile eye-drape with an adhesive back (Steri-drape; 3M, St. Paul, MN) can be helpful to ensure a clean field without the drape changing position during the procedure (**Fig. 5.4B**).

  - The transducer can likewise be covered with a sterile cover (IsoSilk; Microtech, Columbus, MS) or cleansed with an antiseptic solution.

Technique

Core Needle Biopsy

Before beginning the procedure, the patient's identity and willingness to proceed should be verbally confirmed, as well as the laterality and location of the lesion that is to undergo sampling. Free-hand technique is used for ultrasound-guided breast procedures.

- The transducer is held in one hand and the biopsy device in the other (**Figs. 5.4A-F**).
- Using the dominant hand for either function is a useful skill to develop.
- If the radiologist does not feel comfortable using his or her nondominant hand with the biopsy device, the patient's head may be placed at the opposite end of the examination table to change the position of access without losing the ability to view the ultrasound screen.
- Lining up the long axis of the transducer along the lesion and the skin nick defines the planned path of the biopsy needle (**Figs. 5.3, 5.4D**). Keeping the lesion under constant visualization from the time of lidocaine

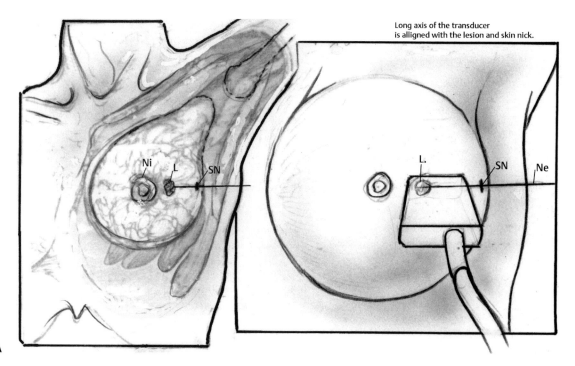

Fig. 5.3 Positioning of the transducer and biopsy needle. **(A)** The skin nick is made at the side of the breast in the same plane as the transducer.

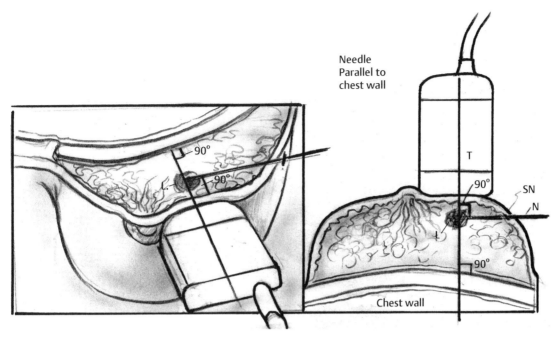

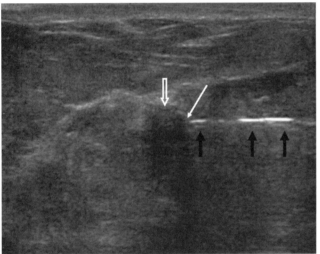

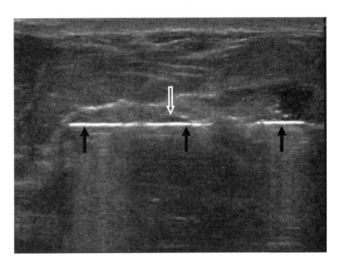

Fig. 5.3 *(Continued)* **(B)** Using this approach, the needle will be parallel to the chest wall and perpendicular to the ultrasound beam, which optimizes needle visualization. **(C)** Prefire ultrasound image with the needle tip (*white arrow*) positioned at the edge of the lesion (*open arrow*).

Note that the needle (*black arrows*) is parallel to the surface of the transducer and chest wall. **(D)** Postfire ultrasound image confirming that the needle (*black arrows*) has traversed the lesion (*open arrow*).

injection until the biopsy marker is placed is very important. Small lesions may be difficult to localize after injection of lidocaine or after the first sample is obtained. The transducer must therefore remain in a steady, stable position.

- Hold the transducer near the breast between the thumb and index fingers while using the fanned out fourth and fifth fingers to stabilize the position of the transducer (**Fig. 5.4C**).
- Lidocaine (2%) is injected in the skin, along the anticipated needle path, as well as in and at the far side of the lesion for anesthesia.

- Buffering of the lidocaine by adding sodium bicarbonate (8.4%) in a volume ratio of 10:1 (5 cc of lidocaine with 0.5 cc of bicarbonate) may reduce pain associated with injection because lidocaine is an acidic compound.
- Lidocaine with epinephrine (1:100,000) can be used to reduce bleeding during the procedure.
  - An injection of lidocaine with epinephrine in the skin may result in focal necrosis.
  - Avoid using lidocaine with epinephrine in women who may have compromised vasculature, such as diabetes or known vascular disease, or if the lesion is close to the skin

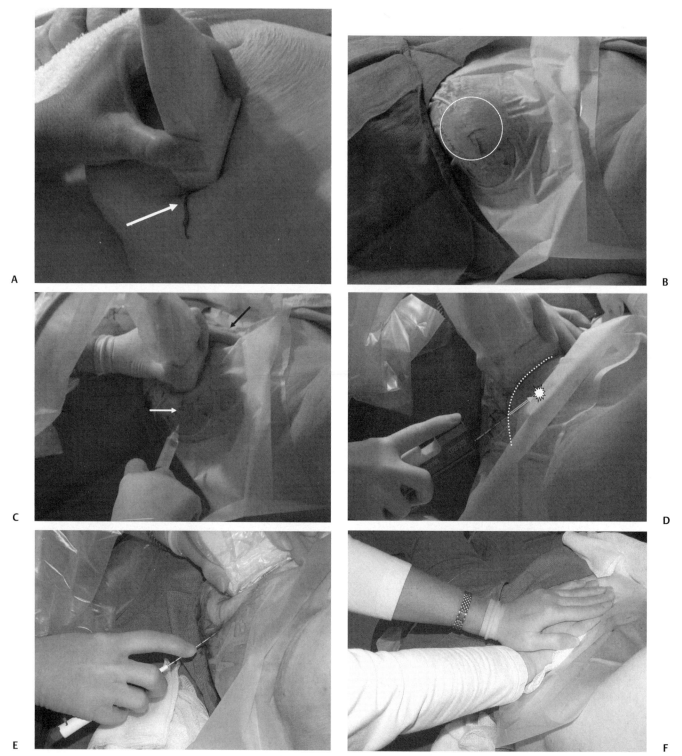

Fig. 5.4 Ultrasound-guided core-needle biopsy method. **(A)** Typically, a lateral approach is easiest. Once the lesion is located and an approach is decided, a "T" is marked on the breast (*arrow*) with the top of the "T" at the side of the transducer and the vertical portion of the "T" marking the plane of the transducer. The base of the "T" is made at the approximate depth of the lesion. **(B)** The skin is cleansed. A sterile drape is placed with the aperture over the area of the lesion to the bottom of the "T." **(C)** The lesion is again localized using the "T" mark. Note the index finger and thumb are located at the base of the transducer, while the remaining fingers anchor the transducer position (*black arrow*). Local anesthetic is injected by entering at the base of the "T" (*white arrow*). **(D)** After a skin nick is made, the biopsy needle is placed in the breast, also entering at the base of the "T." Entry at the lateral curvature of the breast (*dashed line*) results in the needle (*gray arrow*) being parallel to the face of the transducer as it approaches the lesion (*drawn white mass*). Further throw of the needle when fired to obtain a sample will not result in injury to the chest wall using this position. **(E)** A marker is placed after the samples are obtained using the same path as the biopsy needle. Note the positioning of the transducer has remained stable and unchanged during the entire procedure. **(F)** Following the procedure, manual pressure is placed over the entire needle path, which includes the skin nick and area of the lesion.

- Be aware that the terms "gun" and "fire" can increase patient anxiety. Substituting the terms "biopsy device" and "sample" may help patients stay more relaxed during the procedure. The biopsy needle is placed a short distance into the breast, but deep enough to identify the leading edge.
- If the transducer is aligned with the skin nick and the lesion, a small sweeping motion of the needle should bring it into the plane of the transducer resulting in visualization of the shaft of the needle (**Fig. 5.5**).

- Once the needle is identified, adjustments to the depth or angle can be made prior to advancing toward the lesion.
- The needle is then advanced to the proximal edge of the lesion. Continuous observation of the needle is important.
- Before taking a sample, ensure that the 2.2-cm excursion of the biopsy needle will not result in injury to the chest wall.
- After the sample is obtained, scan and take images to document that the needle traversed the lesion.

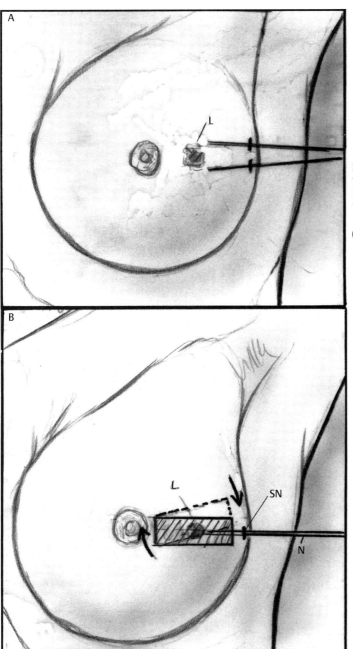

Sweeping motion to bring needle into plane of the transducer

(Keep transducer fixed)

Realign lesion and nick along long axis of transducer

SN- Skin nick
N- Needle
L- Lesion

Fig. 5.5 Visualizing the needle. **(A)** If the transducer is lined up with the lesion and skin nick, a small sweeping motion of the needle will bring the needle into the plane of the transducer. **(B)** If the needle is not visualized using this technique, realign the lesion with the skin nick by rotating the transducer.

If there is difficulty identifying the needle during the procedure, it is usually due to lack of alignment of the needle and transducer. Looking down at the relationship between the skin nick, needle, and transducer facilitates correction. The needle position can be adjusted or the transducer can be rotated to improve visualization of the needle (**Fig. 5.5**).

- At least four samples should be obtained if using a 14-gauge throw needle.
- More samples may be useful if the samples appear fragmented or do not sink when placed in fixative. (More samples are useful in the case of large cancers due to tumor heterogeneity. It is helpful in patients managed with neoadjuvant chemotherapy where receptor status from the core biopsy samples may be used to guide therapy.)

Placement of a Radiopaque Marker

Placement of a radiopaque marker (Ultraclip; Inrad, Kentwood, MI) is helpful for several reasons after the samples have been taken (**Fig. 5.4E**).

- A postprocedure mammogram with a biopsy marker can confirm concordance between a sonographic and mammographic finding.
- Even when a mass is highly suspicious and large, marker placement is often useful. The patient may ultimately be managed with neoadjuvant chemotherapy

and the marker will remain as the tumor shrinks in response to treatment.

- When a biopsy is performed for a small or potentially cystic mass, the marker can be placed just posterior to the lesion prior to sampling. This helps subsequent localization.
- Titanium markers have minimal interference with breast MRI. When more than one lesion undergoes sampling in the same breast, the use of different shaped markers can help distinguish the location of the lesion in different mammographic views.

Fine-Needle Aspiration Biopsy

For FNAB, the shortest approach to the lesion is used.

- Needle enters the skin at the edge of the transducer, approaching the lesion at a 30–45 degree angle (**Fig. 5.6**).
- Lidocaine without epinephrine is injected locally for anesthesia; 22-gauge spinal needles are used.
- The needle is placed within the lesion, the inner stylet removed, and the needle is moved rapidly back and forth in the lesion. In this technique, cells are removed from the lesion using capillary action.
- Typically, two or three passes are made.
- Slides can be made immediately by a cytopathology technologist or the needles can be rinsed in a preservative solution (Cytolyte; Cytyc Corp., Marlborough, MA) and slides made later.

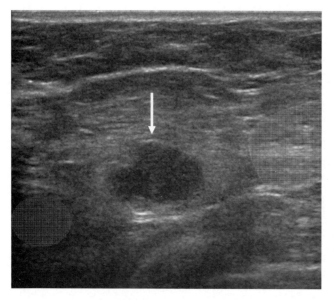
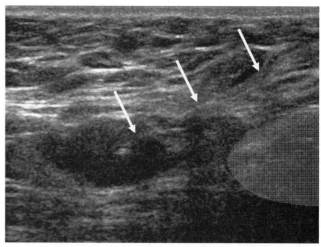

A

B

Fig. 5.6 Ultrasound-guided fine-needle aspiration technique. **(A)** Suspicious lymph node (*arrow*) in the left axilla in a 48-year-old woman with newly diagnosed left invasive breast cancer. Note that the lymph node lies adjacent to the latissimus dorsi muscle (*pink area*) and axillary vessels (*red area*). **(B)** A steep needle angle (*arrows*) is used to avoid the latissimus dorsi muscle (*pink area*). The tip of the needle is within the cortex of the lymph node. Cytology showed metastatic adenocarcinoma in the lymph node.

Challenging Cases

Dense Breast Tissue

- Can make it difficult to advance the needle
- A coaxial system with placement of a 12-gauge trocar (TruGuide; Bard, Covington, GA) provides a path to the lesion that can be altered slightly to sample different areas of the lesion without having to traverse the dense tissue for each sample.

Implants

- Stereotactic biopsy may be an easier approach to an identified lesion from a mammography than ultrasound as the implant can be displaced against the chest wall by the compression paddle.
- However, most lesions can still undergo biopsy using ultrasound guidance (**Fig. 5.7**). The presence of an implant increases the need for carefully planning the approach to the lesion.
- Typically, a more oblique needle path along the edge of the breast will allow the needle path to be parallel to the implant.

Small Lesions

- Ultrasound-guided biopsy of a small lesion can be difficult as lesion visualization can decrease after the first pass or two or even after injection of the lidocaine.
- Hence, keeping a small lesion in view during the entire procedure, from injection of lidocaine until the marker is placed, is key.
- Placement of a VAD directly posterior to a small lesion and direct visualization while sampling can help to ensure that a small lesion underwent adequate sampling.

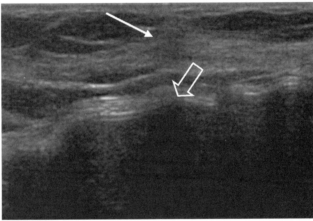

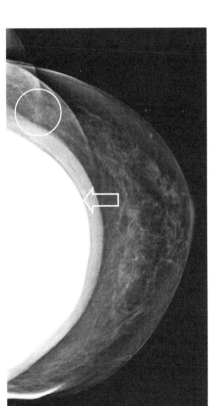

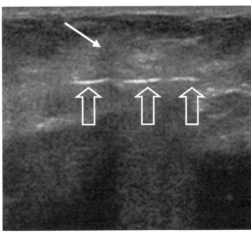

Fig. 5.7 Ultrasound-guided core needle biopsy (CNB) of a suspicious mass in a 52-year-old woman with silicone breast implants. **(A)** Craniocaudal view of the right breast shows a new focal asymmetry in the lateral breast (*circle*). There is a silicone submuscular implant (*open arrow*). **(B)** Ultrasound shows a corresponding irregular hypoechoic mass with an echogenic rim (*arrow*) that is just anterior to the implant (*open arrow*). **(C)** Ultrasound-guided CNB was performed using a needle approach (*open arrows*) that is parallel to the implant. The needle traverses the lesion (*arrow*). Histology showed radial scar.

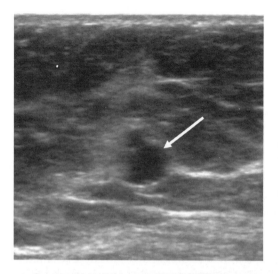

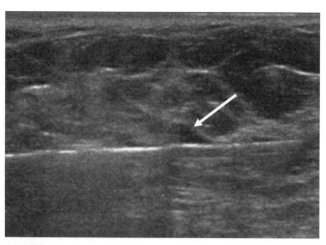

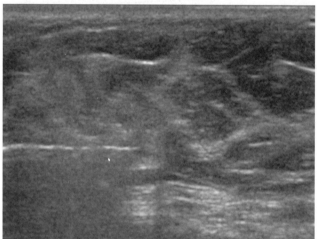

Fig. 5.8 A 60-year-old woman with a new mass on mammography (*not shown*). **(A)** A corresponding very hypoechoic lobular mass with irregular margins is shown on ultrasound (*arrow*). Due to the low echogenicity, a cystic etiology was considered. A biopsy marker was placed prior to the biopsy. **(B)** Postfire image after the first pass shows the needle traversing the lesion (*arrow*). **(C)** Prefire image for the second pass shows near resolution of the mass. Histology showed fibrocystic change.

Potentially Cystic Lesions

- Difficult to discern if it is cystic or solid when a mass when it is very small and very hypoechoic (**Fig. 5.8**). In such cases a clip can be placed posterior to the lesion prior to CNB.
- Placement of a clip will accurately depict the biopsy location in case surgical biopsy is needed based on the CNB results.

Calcifications

Suspicious calcifications are best sampled using stereotactic guidance:

- Calcifications can often be identified on ultrasound; be aware that just a small amount of air can obscure calcifications.
- In cases where stereotactic-guided biopsy is not feasible, calcifications can be sampled using ultrasound guidance (**Fig. 5.2**).

- A VAD may improve retrieval of calcifications.
- Specimen radiograph should be obtained if the lesion primarily presented as calcifications to confirm adequacy of sampling.
- Placement of a radiopaque marker and postprocedure mammogram can also help confirm adequate sampling of the area of mammographic concern.

Lesions in a Large Breast

Entry at the side of the breast is optimal; however,

- Using this approach to biopsy a deep lesion in a large breast may result in traversing a long distance with the needle.
- Alternatively, a shorter and more anterior entry point can be selected.
- To have a needle path that is still parallel to the chest wall, the needle can be used to lift the lesion anterior away from the chest wall (**Fig. 5.9**).

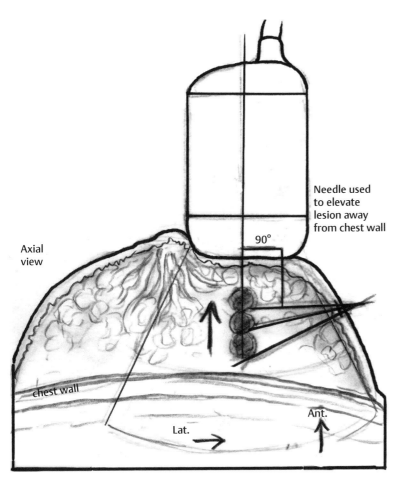

90°

Needle used
to elevate
lesion away
from chest wall

chest wall

Ant.

Lat.

Fig. 5.9 Core needle biopsy of a deep lesion in a large breast. A needle entry site can be made more anterior on the breast. The lesion can be lifted anterior away from the chest wall with the needle to have a path that is still parallel to the chest wall.

Lymph Nodes

Axillary lymph node biopsy is not practical using a parallel approach because

- The axilla is defined at the medial aspect by the pectoral muscles and at the lateral aspect by the latissimus dorsi muscle (**Fig. 5.6**).
- A steep approach must be used, similar to that of FNA.
- Lymph nodes are often just anterior to the axillary artery and vein making the use of long-throw needles difficult.
- Axillary lymph nodes can be sampled using either FNA or a manually controlled core biopsy needle, such as Temno (Cardinel Health, McGaw Park, IL) or Achieve (Cardinal Health, McGaw Park, IL) (**Fig. 5.10**).

If the patient has a known or suspected malignancy, such as a suspicious or malignant-appearing breast mass, then FNA of a lymph node is typically all that is needed. However, if there is no known or suspected malignancy, then core biopsy is useful as the architecture of the lymph node is needed to make a more useful diagnosis. One or

two samples may be sent for evaluation by flow cytometry to assess the likelihood of lymphoma, which can be difficult to diagnose based only on histology of the core biopsy sample.

Postprocedure Evaluation

When the procedure is complete,

- Manual pressure is applied for 5–10 minutes to the entire area of the biopsy to include the region from the skin nick and the entire needle path.
- The skin nick can be closed with either a Steri-Strip (3M, St. Paul, MN) or skin adhesive (Dermabond; Ethicon, Inc., Somerville, NJ).
- A postprocedure mammogram of the sample can confirm that the lesion sampled corresponds to a mammographic finding of concern (**Fig. 5.1**).
- If the biopsy marker placed after ultrasound-guided biopsy is not present in the original lesion of mammographic concern, then stereotactic-guided biopsy of the mammographic finding may be necessary (**Fig. 5.1**).

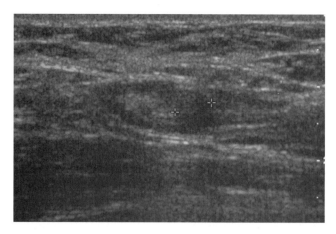
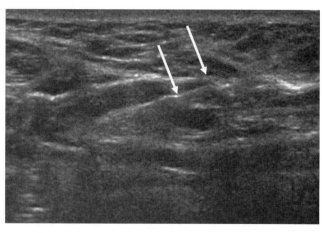

A

B

Fig. 5.10 Ultrasound-guided core needle biopsy (CNB) technique for axillary lymph nodes. **(A)** Ultrasound of the left axilla in a woman with newly diagnosed invasive breast cancer with focal cortical thickening suspicious for metastatic disease (*calipers*). **(B)** Ultrasound-guided CNB of the suspicious area using a manual-throw needle. The needle is in the open position with the notch centered at the lymph node cortex (*arrows*). The tip of the needle is within the lymph node and will not advance when the sample is obtained. Histology showed metastatic invasive ductal carcinoma.

Complications and Their Management

Complications from ultrasound-guided biopsy are few.

- The risk of hematoma for women undergoing ultrasound CNB with a 14-gauge throw needle is ~2%.
- The risk is higher in women using anticoagulants.
- Infection is very uncommon; this occurs in less than 1% of the patients in our practice.
- When there is concern of infection postbiopsy, treatment with a second-generation cephalosporin, such as cephalexin, is usually adequate.
- In a lactating woman, a milk fistula may develop after CNB. Essentially, the core biopsy needle creates a communication between a milk duct and the skin. The fistula will not typically resolve until nursing is finished.

Radiologic–Histologic Correlation

When biopsy results are received,

- All images from that case should be reviewed for correlation.
- The histology should explain the sonographic (and mammographic) finding.
- If the biopsy histology shows malignancy, communication of the results should be given promptly to the patient and her physician.
- If the histology is concordant and benign, ultrasound performed in 6 months is helpful to ensure lesion stability.
- A mammogram can be performed instead of ultrasound if the lesion is well visualized on mammography.

- If the histology is concordant and definitively benign, such as a fibroadenoma, then imaging in one year can be considered.

Discordance occurs resulting in repeat CNB or surgical biopsy in ~3% of cases.

- When the lesion is not explained by the histology, then additional sampling by either surgical biopsy or repeat core biopsy should be recommended (**Fig. 5.1**).
- Cancer is found at repeat sampling in 24–50% of patients. Likewise, if a lesion was assessed as a BI-RADS category 5, surgical biopsy should be considered if a cancer diagnosis is not obtained on CNB histology.
- Certain histologies found on CNB are considered high risk. These include atypical ductal hyperplasia (ADH), lobular carcinoma in situ, atypical lobular hyperplasia, radial sclerosing lesion, and papillary lesions.
- The literature is predominantly based on combined stereotactic (large-gauge) and ultrasound (14-gauge) biopsy, rather than specific to ultrasound biopsy. The upgrade rate to either ductal carcinoma in situ (DCIS) or invasive cancer is best documented for ADH, which is 18–50%.
- Surgical biopsy should be recommended when the core biopsy demonstrates ADH. Management of the remaining lesions is less clear as these are less common and there is a wide range of results in the literature.

Patient Communication

Once the histology is reviewed and a recommendation made, biopsy results can be communicated directly with the patient or to the referring physician who can relay the results to the patient. Discussion of the biopsy results can take place in person or by phone. An addendum to the original report documents recommendations and communication of results.

Quality

An ongoing quality assurance program should be set up to monitor outcome of ultrasound-guided breast biopsy. The program should evaluate

- Positive predictive value
- Benign discordant result
- False-negative outcome

- Complications for the center and by the radiologist
- Available accreditation programs

Summary

The natural curvature of the breast is used to advantage in ultrasound-guided breast core biopsy. Free-hand technique is used. Entry from the periphery of the breast yields a path that is parallel to the chest wall. Contraindications and complications are few. Challenging cases require some planning, but most breast lesions visible on ultrasound are amenable to ultrasound-guided biopsy. Lesions with discordant biopsy results should undergo repeat sampling, either by percutaneous or excisional biopsy. Results of ultrasound-guided biopsy should be monitored for the center and each radiologist for quality assurance.

Further Reading

ACR Breast Imaging and Intervention Practice Guidelines. Available at: http://www.acr.org/SecondaryMainMenuCategories/quality_safety/guidelines/breast.aspx. Accessed

American College of Radiology. Breast imaging reporting and data system (BI-RADS). 4th ed. Reston, VA: American College of Radiology; 2003

Berner A, Davidson B, Sigstad E, Risberg B. Fine-needle aspiration cytology vs. core biopsy in the diagnosis of breast lesions. Diagn Cytopathol 2003;29(6):344–348

Brem RF, Lechner MC, Jackman RJ, et al. Lobular neoplasia at percutaneous breast biopsy: variables associated with carcinoma at surgical excision. AJR Am J Roentgenol 2008;190(3):637–641

Brenner RJ, Jackman RJ, Parker SH, et al. Percutaneous core needle biopsy of radial scars of the breast: when is excision necessary? AJR Am J Roentgenol 2002;179(5):1179–1184

Cavaliere A, Sidoni A, Scheibel M, et al. Biopathologic profile of breast cancer core biopsy: is it always a valid method? Cancer Lett 2005;218(1):117–121

Crystal P, Koretz M, Shcharynsky S, Makarov V, Strano S. Accuracy of sonographically guided 14-gauge core-needle biopsy: results of 715 consecutive breast biopsies with at least two-year follow-up of benign lesions. J Clin Ultrasound 2005;33(2):47–52

Darling MLR, Smith DN, Lester SC, et al. Atypical ductal hyperplasia and ductal carcinoma in situ as revealed by large-core needle breast biopsy: results of surgical excision. AJR Am J Roentgenol 2000;175(5):1341–1346

Deurloo EE, Tanis PJ, Gilhuijs KG, et al. Reduction in the number of sentinel lymph node procedures by preoperative ultrasonography of the axilla in breast cancer. Eur J Cancer 2003;39(8):1068–1073

Deurloo EE, Tanis PJ, Gilhuijs KGA, et al. Reduction in the number of sentinel lymph node procedures by preoperative ultrasonography of the axilla in breast cancer. Eur J Cancer 2003;39(8):1068–1073

Fajardo LL, Pisano ED, Caudry DJ, et al; Radiologist Investigators of the Radiologic Diagnostic Oncology Group V. Stereotactic and sonographic large-core biopsy of nonpalpable breast lesions: results of the Radiologic Diagnostic Oncology Group V study. Acad Radiol 2004;11(3):293–308

Fishman JE, Milikowski C, Ramsinghani R, Velasquez MV, Aviram G. US-guided core-needle biopsy of the breast: how many specimens are necessary? Radiology 2003;226(3):779–782

Foster MC, Helvie MA, Gregory NE, Rebner M, Nees AV, Paramagul C. Lobular carcinoma in situ or atypical lobular hyperplasia at core-needle biopsy: is excisional biopsy necessary? Radiology 2004; 231(3):813–819

Harvey JA, Cohen MA, Brenin DR, Nicholson BT, Adams RB. Breaking bad news: a primer for radiologists in breast imaging. J Am Coll Radiol 2007;4(11):800–808

Jackman RJ, Burbank F, Parker SH, et al. Atypical ductal hyperplasia diagnosed at stereotactic breast biopsy: improved reliability with 14-gauge, directional, vacuum-assisted biopsy. Radiology 1997; 204(2):485–488

Jackman RJ, Nowels KW, Shepard MJ, Finkelstein SI, Marzoni FA Jr. Stereotaxic large-core needle biopsy of 450 nonpalpable breast lesions with surgical correlation in lesions with cancer or atypical hyperplasia. Radiology 1994;193(1):91–95

Lannin DR, Ponn T, Andrejeva L, Philpotts L. Should all breast cancers be diagnosed by needle biopsy? Am J Surg 2006;192(4):450–454

Liberman L, Drotman M, Morris EA, et al. Imaging-histologic discordance at percutaneous breast biopsy. Cancer 2000;89(12): 2538–2546

Liberman L, Ernberg LA, Heerdt A, et al. Palpable breast masses: is there a role for percutaneous imaging-guided core biopsy? AJR Am J Roentgenol 2000;175(3):779–787

Liberman L, Goodstine SL, Dershaw DD, et al. One operation after percutaneous diagnosis of nonpalpable breast cancer: frequency and associated factors. AJR Am J Roentgenol 2002;178(3):673–679

Liberman L. Centennial dissertation. Percutaneous imaging-guided core breast biopsy: state of the art at the millennium. AJR Am J Roentgenol 2000;174:1191–1199

Melotti MK, Berg WA. Core needle breast biopsy in patients undergoing anticoagulation therapy: preliminary results. AJR Am J Roentgenol 2000;174(1):245–249

Nath ME, Robinson TM, Tobon H, Chough DM, Sumkin JH. Automated large-core needle biopsy of surgically removed breast lesions: comparison of samples obtained with 14-, 16-, and 18-gauge needles. Radiology 1995;197(3):739–742

Parker SH, Burbank F, Jackman RJ, et al. Percutaneous large-core breast biopsy: a multi-institutional study. Radiology 1994;193(2): 359–364

Philpotts LE, Hooley RJ, Lee CH. Comparison of automated versus vacuum-assisted biopsy methods for sonographically guided core biopsy of the breast. AJR Am J Roentgenol 2003;180(2):347–351

Pisano ED, Fajardo LL, Caudry DJ, et al. Fine-needle aspiration biopsy of nonpalpable breast lesions in a multicenter clinical trial: results from the radiologic diagnostic oncology group V. Radiology 2001;219(3):785–792

Schackmuth EM, Harlow CL, Norton LW. Milk fistula: a complication after core breast biopsy. AJR Am J Roentgenol 1993;161(5): 961–962

Shin HJ, Kim HH, Kim SM, et al. Papillary lesions of the breast diagnosed at percutaneous sonographically guided biopsy: comparison of sonographic features and biopsy methods. AJR Am J Roentgenol 2008;190(3):630–636

Simon JR, Kalbhen CL, Cooper RA, Flisak ME. Accuracy and complication rates of US-guided vacuum-assisted core breast biopsy: initial results. Radiology 2000;215(3):694–697

Soo MS, Baker JA, Rosen EL. Sonographic detection and sonographically guided biopsy of breast microcalcifications. AJR Am J Roentgenol 2003;180(4):941–948

Youk JH, Kim EK, Kim MJ, Oh KK. Sonographically guided 14-gauge core needle biopsy of breast masses: a review of 2,420 cases with long-term follow-up. AJR Am J Roentgenol 2008;190(1):202–207

6 Fine-Needle Aspiration Biopsy of Thyroid Nodules

Monzer M. Abu-Yousef

Classification

- Palpation-guided fine-needle aspiration biopsy (FNAB) – blind, less accurate; cannot see vessels or cystic versus solid
- Free-hand ultrasound-guided FNAB, without guiding system – cumbersome and less accurate
- Ultrasound-guided core needle biopsy (CNB) using 20-gauge cutting needle
- Ultrasound-guided FNAB with onsite cytopathology – do four aspirations, submit immediately to confirm adequacy
- Ultrasound-guided FNA with syringe using suction – not proven better than capillary aspiration

The purpose of this procedure is to differentiate benign from malignant nodules and to make a specific diagnosis.

Indications

- Solid nodules ≥1 cm with questionable ultrasound features
  - Nodules with microcalcifications
  - Nodules with irregular borders
  - Nodules with ill-defined margins
  - Solid nodule that is cold on scintigraphy
  - Recurrent thyroid mass
  - Nodules with cervical lymph nodes suspicious for or harboring thyroid cancer
- Solid nodules ≥1 cm in high-risk patients
  - History of neck radiation
  - Family history of thyroid neoplasia
  - History of multiple endocrine neoplasia (MEN II) syndromes
  - Single solid nodule in elderly patient
  - Single solid nodule in male patient ≤20 years of age
  - Past thyroid lobectomy for contralateral thyroid cancer
- Solid nodule ≥1.5 cm
- Complex solid and cystic nodule ≥2 cm
- Nodules showing interval increase in size
- Unsuccessful biopsy of palpable nodule

- Confirm a previously negative thyroid biopsy
- Solid nodule that is cold on scintigraphy
- Multinodular goiter – biopsy up to four nodules with the most suspicious features

Contraindications

Absolute Contraindications

- None

Relative Contraindications

- Completely cystic nodules
- Complex nodule with minimal solid component
- Nodules <0.5 cm in diameter
- Single solid nodules, hot on scintigraphy
- Nodules with colloid features (comet-tail artifacts)
- Microcystic nodules
- Nodules showing interval decrease in size

Preprocedural Evaluation

- Review patient's medical records and discuss case with referring physician if necessary
- Review previous imaging studies including ultrasound, positron emission tomography (PET), computed tomography (CT), or magnetic resonance imaging (MRI)
- If thyroid ultrasound exam was not obtained within last 3 months, perform a new one
- No need to check international normalized ratio (INR), prothrombin time (PT), partial thromboplastin time (PTT), or platelet count
- Check if patient is on Coumadin (Bristol-Myers Squibb, New York, NY); if so, check INR

Explain to the patient what procedure will be done, who will be doing it, why it will be done, how it will be done, potential complications, and alternative methods of diagnosis. Answer the patient's questions and have the patient sign the consent form before signing it yourself.

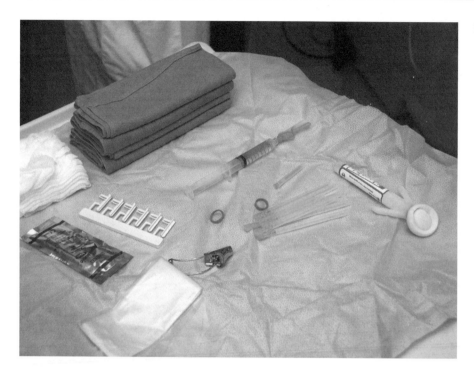

Fig. 6.1 Biopsy tray setup.

Equipment

Current ultrasound machines that are equipped with 6–8 MHz, phased, linear-array transducers are adequate for biopsy purposes.

Tray Setup (Fig. 6.1)

- 10-cc syringes
- Four 25-gauge needles and one 18-gauge needle
- Probe cover
- Pack of 4 × 4 sterile gauze
- Sterile probe cover
- Antiseptic soap/solution
- Ultrasound-guiding device
- Ultrasound-guiding adapters
- Sterile gel

Technique

- Place the patient supine with head extended and shoulders supported by a pillow (**Fig. 6.2**)
- Use 4–8 MHz frequency, transducer to select nodules that meet biopsy criteria
- Line-up nodule with needle tracks (**Fig. 6.3A**); mark needle entrance on skin (**Fig. 6.3B**)
- Biopsy can be done in either the axial or the sagittal plane (**Fig. 6.4**).
- Clean the patient's skin with antiseptic soap and drape the patient in a standard sterile fashion

- Draw 10 mL of 1% lidocaine and make a skin wheal using 1 mL
- Cover the probe with sterile plastic tubing; fit the guiding device and a 23-gauge adapter (**Fig. 6.5**)
- Using a 25-gauge spinal needle, inject 3 mL of 1% lidocaine in soft tissues along the needle path, including the thyroid capsule (**Fig. 6.6**)
- Have the patient hold breathing and swallowing; advance the 25-gauge spinal needle to the lesion surface, withdraw the stylet; then advance and withdraw the needle several times (**Fig. 6.7**).

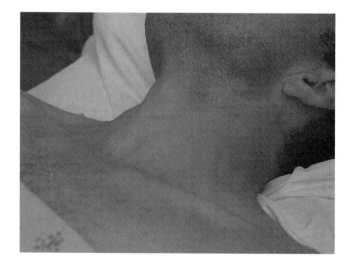

Fig. 6.2 Patient positioning.

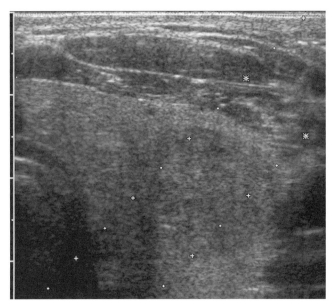 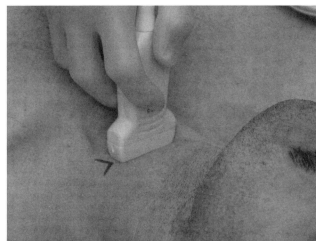

Fig. 6.3 (A) Nodule localization. **(B)** Needle entrance marking.

- Cover the needle hub as you take the needle out
- Make five consecutive passes, spread on slides, and prepare
- Submit to cytopathology
- Scan lateral neck and do ultrasound-guided biopsy of any suspicious cervical lymph nodes

Endpoints

- Do not exceed 10 aspirations.

Postprocedural Evaluation

- A postprocedure neck ultrasound exam is performed to check for hematoma.

- The patient is given an ice pack to apply to his or her neck for 5 minutes.
- Patient is then discharged with an instruction sheet to report any swelling, pain, redness, or discharge to the clinic.

Complications and Their Management

- Bleeding – uncommon and limited to subcutaneous tissues and muscles – compress biopsy site
- Infection – rare – follow standard sterile techniques; antibiotics as indicated
- Cord paralysis – rare and universally temporary – ensure needle tip visualization at all times

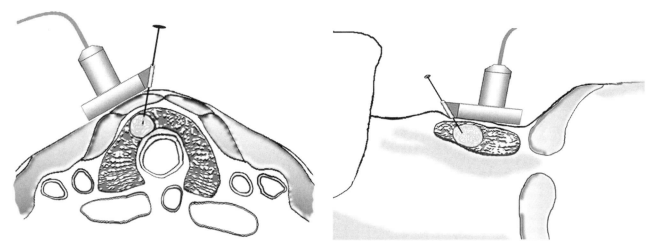

Fig. 6.4 (A) Scanning diagram demonstrating nodule localization in axial and **(B)** sagittal planes.

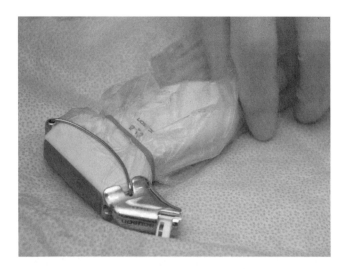

Fig. 6.5 Fitting the guide system on the ultrasound probe.

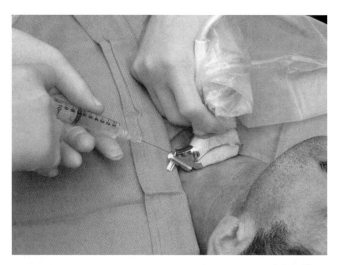

Fig. 6.6 Deep infiltration with lidocaine to include the thyroid capsule.

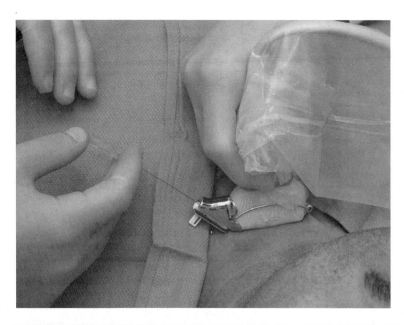

A

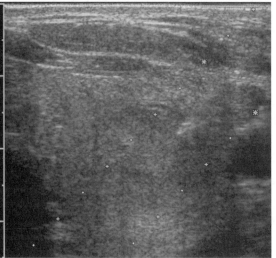

B

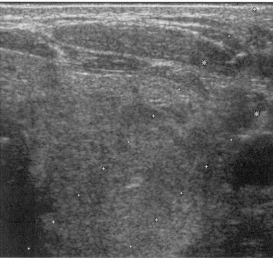

Fig. 6.7 Performing the biopsy. **(A)** Advancing the needle in the guiding system; **(B)** the needle tip stopped at the nodule surface, stylet withdrawn; **(C)** advancing the needle tip to and from back of nodule in rapid succession.

C

- Vasovagal reaction – uncommon – 0.5 mg atropine intramuscularly
- Allergic reaction to lidocaine – rare – antihistamines, prednisone ± epinephrine

Causes of Inadequate Biopsies

- Specimens contaminated by gel or diluted by blood or fluid
- Uncooperative patient as a result of pain or anxiety
- Excessive negative pressure with needle aspiration
- Vascular nodules
- Placing the needle tip in the back of the nodule prior to sampling
- Poor needle positioning in the cystic or vascular part of a nodule
- Size of nodule or solid part of cystic nodule too small to target

Techniques to Enhance Success Rate

- To minimize blood in aspirate
  - Use color Doppler or power Doppler to avoid large vessels in a nodule
  - Do 1–2 quick needle motions encompassing whole nodule width
  - Use minimal, ≤1 mL suction when syringe is used

- To avoid sample contamination with gel
  - Minimize ultrasound gel use
  - Alternatively, use saline as a coupling agent
- To improve sample cellularity
  - Avoid suction when in cystic part of nodule
  - Alternatively, use a 22-gauge needle
  - Be selective when sampling subcentimeter nodules
- To improve patient cooperation during biopsy
  - Reassure patient
  - Perform ultrasound-guided deep anesthesia along needle track including thyroid capsule
  - Administer conscious sedation if patient is still anxious
  - Ask patient to hold breath and swallowing during sampling

Diagnostic Efficacy

- Success rate: 97%
- Benign: 84%
- Malignant: 6%
- Possibly Malignant: 7.3%
- Inadequate: 2.7%

Further Reading

Accurso A, Rocco N, Palumbo A, Leone F. Usefulness of ultrasound-guided fine-needle aspiration cytology in the diagnosis of non-palpable small thyroid nodules. Tumori 2005;91(4):355–357

Bellantone R, Lombardi CP, Raffaelli M, et al. Management of cystic or predominantly cystic thyroid nodules: the role of ultrasound-guided fine-needle aspiration biopsy. Thyroid 2004;14(1):43–47

Cai XJ, Valiyaparambath N, Nixon P, Waghorn A, Giles T, Helliwell T. Ultrasound-guided fine needle aspiration cytology in the diagnosis and management of thyroid nodules. Cytopathology 2006;17(5):251–256

Ceresini G, Corcione L, Morganti S, et al. Ultrasound-guided fine-needle capillary biopsy of thyroid nodules, coupled with on-site cytologic review, improves results. Thyroid 2004;14(5):385–389

Frates MC, Benson CB, Charboneau JW, et al; Society of Radiologists in Ultrasound. Management of thyroid nodules detected at US: Society of Radiologists in Ultrasound consensus conference statement. Radiology 2005;237(3):794–800

Frates MC, Benson CB, Doubilet PM, et al. Prevalence and distribution of carcinoma in patients with solitary and multiple thyroid nodules on sonography. J Clin Endocrinol Metab 2006;91(9):3411–3417

Kim SJ, Kim EK, Park CS, Chung WY, Oh KK, Yoo HS. Ultrasound-guided fine-needle aspiration biopsy in nonpalpable thyroid nodules: is it useful in infracentimetric nodules? Yonsei Med J 2003;44(4):635–640

Mehrotra P, Hubbard JG, Johnson SJ, Richardson DL, Bliss R, Lennard TW. Ultrasound scan-guided core sampling for diagnosis versus freehand FNAC of the thyroid gland. Surgeon 2005;3(1):1–5

Orija IB, Piñeyro M, Biscotti C, Reddy SS, Hamrahian AH. Value of repeating a nondiagnostic thyroid fine-needle aspiration biopsy. Endocr Pract 2007;13(7):735–742

Rausch P, Nowels K, Jeffrey RB Jr. Ultrasonographically guided thyroid biopsy: a review with emphasis on technique. J Ultrasound Med 2001;20(1):79–85

Shin JH, Han BK, Ko K, Choe YH, Oh YL. Value of repeat ultrasound-guided fine-needle aspiration in nodules with benign cytological diagnosis. Acta Radiol 2006;47(5):469–473

Stacul F, Bertolotto M, Zappetti R, Zanconati F, Cova MA. The radiologist and the cytologist in diagnosing thyroid nodules: results of cooperation. Radiol Med (Torino) 2007;112(4):597–602

Tublin ME, Martin JA, Rollin LJ, Pealer K, Kurs-Lasky M, Ohori NP. Ultrasound-guided fine-needle aspiration versus fine-needle capillary sampling biopsy of thyroid nodules: does technique matter? J Ultrasound Med 2007;26(12):1697–1701

7 Superficial Lymph Node Biopsy

Beth S. Edeiken-Monroe, Brett J. Monroe, Bruno D. Fornage, and Suhas G. Parulekar

Classification

- Ultrasound and ultrasound-guided needle biopsy of the regional nodal basins are important components of the initial staging of cancer patients. They
  - Provide prognostic information
  - Help in the formulation of the treatment plan
  - Have proved accurate in diagnosing regional nodal involvement particularly in the groin, axilla, and neck
- Their major contribution and impact on management is the detection and diagnosis of early clinically occult ipsilateral or contralateral regional nodal metastasis that otherwise would not be included in the surgical dissection or radiation treatment field.

Indications

Indications for ultrasound guided biopsy of a lymph node include:

- Absence or displacement of the hilum
- Focal or diffuse thickening of the cortex
- Relative decreased echogenicity of the cortex
- Full or rounded shape of the lymph node
- Calcification within the lymph node
- Abnormal extrahilar vascular flow
- A cystic component
- Size is not a valid indication of an abnormal lymph node with the exception of asymmetric enlarged nodes in patients with lymphoma.

Technique

Ultrasound-guided fine-needle aspiration biopsy (FNAB) and core needle biopsy (CNB) are performed in the same room as ultrasound examinations in the outpatient facility. Ultrasound-guided FNAB is quick, relatively inexpensive, minimally invasive, and accurate when performed in the presence of an experienced cytopathologist.

Fine-Needle Aspiration Biopsy

- Focal metastatic deposits, as small as a few millimeters, can be targeted.

- In mixed solid/cystic lymph nodes, solid areas should be targeted.
- In patients with primary papillary thyroid cancer, fluid aspirate from a cystic lymph node may require determination of the thyroglobulin content of the fluid aspirate to diagnose metastatic disease.

Core Needle Biopsy

- May be technically difficult to perform on small lymph nodes that are close to vessels or locations difficult to reach
- More traumatic than FNAB and is associated with an increased risk of hematoma formation
- Rarely used to diagnose metastatic adenopathy
- May be needed to provide pretreatment information in patients with breast cancer such as histologic grade, expressions of estrogen and progesterone receptors and c-erbB2
- In patients with suspected lymphoma, CNB may be necessary to diagnose small cell lymphoma.

Contraindications

Absolute Contraindications

- There are no absolute contraindications to the performance of an ultrasound-guided needle biopsy of a superficial lymph node.

Relative Contraindications

- Anticoagulation – Risk of hemorrhage is reduced by halting anticoagulation therapy prior to biopsy for the recommended amount of time for each specific anticoagulant.

Preprocedural Evaluation

At our institution, the preprocedure evaluation includes:

- Allergy history
- Reconciliation of medications *and* vital signs with particular focus on blood pressure and anticoagulant medication
  - If the patient is allergic to the local anesthetic, the FNAB is performed without prebiopsy injection of Xylocaine (Abraxis Bioscience, Los Angeles, CA) 1%.

○ In a patient on anticoagulant therapy, a coagulation screen is performed in the morning on the day of the procedure.

○ In patients with hypertension, the procedure is delayed until the hypertension is addressed.

Equipment

Ultrasound-guided needle biopsy is performed with:

- Standard ultrasound equipment
- Standard hypodermic needles
- Syringe for FNA
- An automated or semiautomated CNB device for CNB
- Ultrasound examination is performed using a high resolution ultrasound scanner with color and power Doppler capability equipped with commercially available high-frequency (from 7 MHz) linear-array transducers.
- FNAB is performed with standard hypodermic needles varying from 20–25 gauge attached to a 10 or 20 mL syringe depending on the preference of the operator.
- We routinely perform FNAB with a 20-gauge needle attached to a 20 mL syringe. This allows sufficient aspiration on a minimum of passes, usually only one.
- Alternatively, an 18-gauge needle is employed in the case of fibrotic node or node with a thick necrotic content.

Various sizes of core biopsy needles can be used ranging from 14-gauge to 20-gauge with the length of the throw ranging from 1.1–2.3 cm and the core sample length from 0.7–1.7 cm; the selection of the needle often depends on the location and size of the targeted node.

Patient Positioning

- The preferred position of the patient for an ultrasound guided needle biopsy of a lymph node in the axilla or the soft tissues of the neck is the supine anterolateral position.
- Once the target area is determined, the patient can be obliqued on a wedge so that the target area is maximally exposed and the needle can be tracked from a superior angle.
- The preferred position of the patient for an ultrasound guided needle biopsy of a lymph node in the groin is the supine position.
- The comfort of the patient is important for compliance and of the operator for accuracy.

Technique

All ultrasound-guided biopsies at our institution are performed with free-hand technique and real-time ultrasound guidance. Needle guides may be used but in our experience, they are usually cumbersome.

Fine-Needle Aspiration Biopsy

- A preliminary ultrasound evaluation, including color Doppler imaging, should be performed to identify the suspicious lymph node targeted for biopsy.
- The patient is positioned by the operator for optimal exposure of the targeted node.
- The skin is cleansed with a local antiseptic.
- Local anesthesia (1% Xylocaine, 1–4 cc) is injected under ultrasound guidance along the planned tract of the needle course to the periphery of the targeted lesion.
- Under ultrasound guidance, the biopsy needle is inserted along the direction in which the local anesthetic was injected. The needle tip is placed in the abnormal area within the lymph node (usually in the cortex) (**Fig. 7.1**) and aspiration is performed, under constant ultrasound guidance, with several back and forth movements of the needle within the abnormal area as suction (~1.0–3 cc of negative pressure, but greater if necessary to obtain aspirate) is applied. During an ultrasound-guided FNAB, the needle should be redirected at different angles within the node for comprehensive sampling and to maximize the amount of cellular material sampled.
- In most cases, one or two passes are sufficient to obtain an adequate sample from the targeted lymph node.
- An image is obtained with the needle tip in the lesion to document accurate sampling.
- The FNAB aspirate is smeared on three to five slides, which are fixed in ethanol and then stained by the cytologist using the classic Papanicolaou technique. Some smears are also air-dried and stained with the Diff-quick method for immediate evaluation. When onsite evaluation is not possible, alcohol-fixed smears are preferable. Dependant on the cytopathologist's preferences and available resources, the aspirate can be divided between smears and other preparations, such as rinse for cytospin and cell block.
- The cytolopathologist reads the smears as malignant, suspicious, indeterminate, benign, or normal.
- In the case of inadequate sampling, the biopsy is repeated.

Core Needle Biopsy

The CNB technique is similar to the FNAB technique with the following differences:

- Prior to insertion of the core biopsy needle, a small incision is made in the skin when using a 14-gauge needle. This is not necessary with 18-gauge needles.

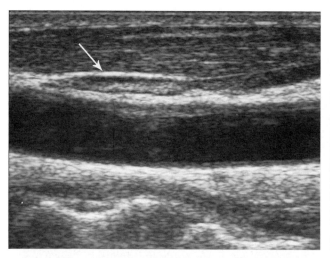

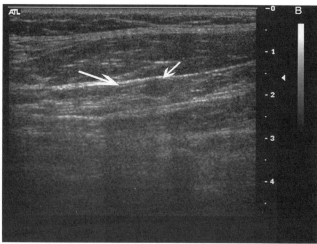

A

B

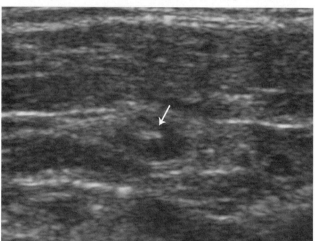

C

Fig. 7.1 (A) Comparison sonogram shows a 0.9-cm cervical lymph node (*long arrow*) in the longitudinal plane with a normal central echogenic hilum and hypoechoic cortex. **(B)** Sonogram of a cervical lymph node in the longitudinal plane shows a 0.7-cm lymph node with an abnormal bulge of the cortex (*short arrow*) with absence of the normal echogenic hilum of the medial portion that suggests metastatic infiltration of this region of the lymph node. The lateral portion of the lymph node is normal in appearance with a normal central echogenic hilum and thin echogenic cortex (*long arrow*). **(C)** Sonogram of the abnormal 0.7-cm cervical lymph node in the longitudinal plane with the biopsy needle tip (*short arrow*) placed in the abnormal portion of the lymph node.

- The biopsy needle tip is advanced under ultrasound guidance along the plane in which the local anesthetic was injected to a position just outside the margin of the target node and the position is documented with a static image.
- The automated biopsy device is activated so that the needle traverses the node to acquire the core sample. The location of the needle within the node is documented in both the longitudinal and transverse views after each pass to document accurate sampling.
- An average of two to four cores are obtained to allow for sufficient biopsy specimens.

Endpoints

The ultrasound-guided FNAB is concluded when specimen adequacy is confirmed by cytologic evaluation. The cytologic diagnosis is classified as malignant, suspicious, indeterminate, benign, or normal.

A CNB is completed once there has been acquisition of two to four cores of satisfactory quality.

Postprocedural Evaluation

Postprocedural evaluation includes vital signs, with a particular focus on blood pressure and evaluation for hemorrhage.

Limitations of Fine-Needle Aspiration Biopsy

The limitations of an ultrasound-guided FNAB include

- Nondiagnostic specimens
- Inconclusive results
- Incomplete classification of lymphoma

The leading causes of a nondiagnostic FNAB specimen are:

- A specimen of limited cellularity
- Poor preservation and fixation of the specimen

An inadequate/nondiagnostic FNAB requires a rebiopsy. Constant real-time monitoring of the needle tip within the target during vigorous aspiration guarantees that the sample is representative. The authors have found that the combination of a 20-gauge needle, visualization of the needle within the target throughout the aspiration, and vigorous aspiration can keep the rate of nondiagnostic specimens very low. The presence of an onsite cytopathologist who renders an immediate evaluation of the adequacy of the smears further reduces the rate of nondiagnostic specimens.

Complications

Ultrasound-guided needle biopsies of lymph nodes have a low rate of complications, the majority of which are related to bleeding.

- Pneumothorax is a very remote possibility in ultrasound-guided biopsy of axillary, and infraclavicular or supraclavicular lymph nodes, whereas it is more likely to occur with internal mammary lymph nodes.
- Injury to the trachea and the recurrent laryngeal nerve may occur during biopsies of the lymph nodes of the neck.
- The complication rate increases with the larger needle gauge and number of passes.

Complications associated with ultrasound-guided biopsy can be minimized by preprocedure precautions and cautious manipulation of the needles during and after the procedure.

- Hemorrhage of a major vessel or perforation of an organ may be avoided by keeping the biopsy needle under constant visualization during the entirety of the procedure.
- The needle should not be advanced until the tip is visible by ultrasound; simultaneously, there should be a conscious awareness of the outer length of the needle.
- Risk to the healthcare providers can be minimized by cautious manipulation of specimens from patients with infectious diseases such as hepatitis or acquired immunodeficiency syndrome (AIDS).

Conclusion

The increased use and improved technology of sonographic screening and FNA of the soft tissues has facilitated the diagnosis of lymph node metastases in the early stages. It has allowed an improved selection of patients for surgical treatment and helped in presurgical planning. In experienced hands, the reliability of ultrasound and ultrasound-guided FNA is now such that the surgical decision may be based solely on sonographic findings.

Further Reading

Abe H, Schmidt RA, Sennett CA, Shimauchi A, Newstead GM. US-guided core needle biopsy of axillary lymph nodes in patients with breast cancer: why and how to do it. Radiographics 2007;27(Suppl 1):S91–S99

Baloch ZW, Tam D, Langer J, Mandel S, LiVolsi VA, Gupta PK. Ultrasound-guided fine-needle aspiration biopsy of the thyroid: role of on-site assessment and multiple cytologic preparations. Diagn Cytopathol 2000;23(6):425–429

Buchbinder SS, Gurell DS, Tarlow MM, Salvatore M, Suhrland MJ, Kader K. Role of US-guided fine-needle aspiration with on-site cytopathologic evaluation in management of nonpalpable breast lesions. Acad Radiol 2001;8(4):322–327

Cheung YC, Wan YL, Lui KW, Lee KF. Sonographically guided core-needle biopsy in the diagnosis of superficial lymphadenopathy. J Clin Ultrasound 2000;28(6):283–289

Damera A, Evans AJ, Cornford EJ, et al. Diagnosis of axillary nodal metastases by ultrasound-guided core biopsy in primary operable breast cancer. Br J Cancer 2003;89(7):1310–1313

Gazelle GS, Haaga JR, Rowland DY. Effect of needle gauge, level of anticoagulation, and target organ on bleeding associated with aspiration biopsy. Work in progress. Radiology 1992;183(2):509–513

Kim KH, Son EJ, Kim EK, Ko KH, Kang H, Oh KK. The safety and efficiency of the ultrasound-guided large needle core biopsy of axilla lymph nodes. Yonsei Med J 2008;49(2):249–254

Kline TS, Kannan V, Kline IK. Lymphadenopathy and aspiration biopsy cytology. Review of 376 superficial nodes. Cancer 1984;54(6):1076–1081

Kouvaraki MA, Shapiro SE, Fornage BD, et al. Role of preoperative ultrasonography in the surgical management of patients with thyroid cancer. Surgery 2003;134(6):946–954, discussion 954–955

Krishnamurthy S, Sneige N, Bedi DG, et al. Role of ultrasound-guided fine-needle aspiration of indeterminate and suspicious axillary lymph nodes in the initial staging of breast carcinoma. Cancer 2002;95(5):982–988

Lemos S, Dias M, Gonçalo M, Pinto E, Fernandes G, Oliveira C. Detection of axillary metastases in breast cancer patients using ultrasound and colour Doppler combined with fine needle aspiration cytology. Eur J Gynaecol Oncol 2005;26(2):165–166

Oruwari JUN, Chung MA, Koelliker S, Steinhoff MM, Cady B. Axillary staging using ultrasound-guided fine needle aspiration biopsy in locally advanced breast cancer. Am J Surg 2002;184(4):307–309

Podkrajsek M, Music MM, Kadivec M, et al. Role of ultrasound in the preoperative staging of patients with breast cancer. Eur Radiol 2005;15(5):1044–1050

Screaton NJ, Berman LH, Grant JW. Head and neck lymphadenopathy: evaluation with US-guided cutting-needle biopsy. Radiology 2002;224(1):75–81

8 Endovaginal Procedures
Dean A. Nakamoto

Classification

Endovaginal ultrasound-guided interventional procedures are an important tool for the interventionist. These procedures are typically well tolerated by women and can be performed with local anesthesia or no anesthesia at all. Lesions located within the central pelvis, which can be difficult to access by the usual percutaneous transabdominal or transsciatic methods, can often be easily and safely accessed with the endovaginal technique. Real-time needle visualization and no ionizing radiation are additional benefits of endovaginal ultrasound guidance.

Endovaginal Ultrasound-Guided Interventional Procedures

Indications

- Biopsies of adnexal masses, iliac nodes, and vaginal cuff
- Aspirations and drainages of endometrial fluid collections
- Pelvic fluid collections and abscesses

Contraindications
Absolute Contraindication

- Prepubescent girls and women with vaginal stenosis

Relative Contraindication

- Women who are not sexually active

Patient Preparation

- For most fine-needle aspirations and biopsies, antibiotic prophylaxis is usually not necessary. Antibiotic prophylaxis may be prudent in certain patients, such as patients with prosthetic heart valves and artificial joint replacements because it can be difficult to sterilize the vaginal vault.
- In patients undergoing a pelvic abscess drainage procedure, appropriate antibiotic coverage is usually recommended prior to starting the procedure.

Patient Positioning

- Place the patient on a cart in lithotomy position, lying supine with feet placed in stirrups or other foot supports.
- If a cart with foot supports is not available, the patient should flex hips and bend knees so that feet are close to hips.
- The patient should spread her legs and relax her hips.
- Place several folded towels or sheets under the patient's hips to raise the hips ~10 cm above the bed, allowing more freedom of motion of the ultrasound probe within the vagina.

Positioning is particularly important if the target is located in the anterior aspect of the pelvis. To direct the probe tip toward the anterior pelvis, the probe handle must be moved posteriorly. Raising the patient's hips with the folded sheets makes it easier to move the probe handle posteriorly. Otherwise, the cart or table that the patient is lying on will prohibit the interventionist from moving the probe handle posteriorly.

Endovaginal Ultrasound-Guided Biopsy

Preprocedural Evaluation and Preparation of the Patient

- Perform initial endovaginal ultrasound exam to
  - Verify location and accessibility of the target
  - Identify loops of bowel, urinary bladder, and major blood vessels to avoid
- Ensure proper alignment of the needle guide with the lesion
- Place the endovaginal probe as close as possible to the lesion
- Use a hysterosalpingogram tray setup (**Fig. 8.1**)
- Prep the perineum with povidone–iodine-soaked sponge swabs
- Insert the speculum and prep the vagina with the povidone–iodine solution, by gently instilling 15–20 cc of povidone–iodine solution into the vagina using a syringe with connecting tubing

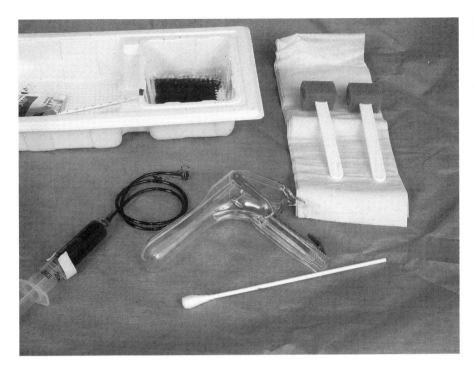

Fig. 8.1 Hysterosalpingogram tray. The contents include a syringe and connecting tubing (which should be filled with ~15 cc of povidone–iodine solution), a plastic speculum, a long cotton swab, and sponge swabs to clean the perineum. The sponge swabs should be soaked in the povidone–iodine solution and then used to clean the perineum.

- After flooding the vaginal canal with the povidone–iodine, remove the tubing and then insert a long cotton swab into the vagina and carefully remove the speculum, leaving the long cotton swab in the vagina
- Gently swirl the cotton swab around the vagina while pulling the cotton swab out of the vagina. This coats the entire vaginal wall with the povidone–iodine solution, including the portions of the vaginal wall that were initially covered by the speculum.

Equipment

Fine-Needle Aspiration or Cutting Needle Biopsy

- Use one of the commercially available guides. Most will accept up to 18-gauge needles.
- The redundant vaginal wall can be difficult to penetrate. Exert enough pressure on the endovaginal probe to "tent" the vaginal wall (easier for the needle to penetrate the vaginal wall).
- With the commercially available guide, use 20-cm or longer needles. Be sure needle length extending beyond the needle guide is sufficient to reach the target by measuring the distance to the lesion before placing the needle.
- For lesions that are beyond the reach of the 20-cm needle, get a 30-cm (or longer) single-step trocar-based catheter, discard the outer catheter, and use only the metal stiffener with the trocar needle in the needle guide of the endovaginal probe.

Endovaginal Ultrasound-Guided Biopsy for Adnexal/Pelvic Masses and Endometrium

- Use a 20-gauge Chiba needle
- Instill 1–2 cc 1% lidocaine as a local anesthetic in the appropriate site in the vaginal wall

It can be difficult to have subsequent needle passes enter the vaginal wall at the same site; therefore, it is important to use other landmarks in the pelvis (i.e., vessels, the bladder wall) to help ensure needle penetration at or near the lidocaine wheal. A fine-needle aspiration (FNA) also allows one to assess the vascularity of a lesion directly. With most FNAs, only a few drops of blood or no blood at all may come out while the needle is within the lesion. If several milliliters or more of blood are aspirated during the performance of the FNA, then this suggests that the lesion is quite vascular. For such vascular lesions, it may be prudent to defer performing a cutting needle biopsy to avoid a potential bleeding complication. Alternatively, if a cutting needle is needed, one could perform a core needle biopsy, but with a small needle, such as a 20-gauge cutting needle or smaller.

Endovaginal Ultrasound-Guided Biopsies of the Adnexa, Iliac Nodes, or Vaginal Cuff

- Localize the solid portions of the lesions
- Use 20-gauge cutting needles to verify metastases (if there is a known primary malignancy)

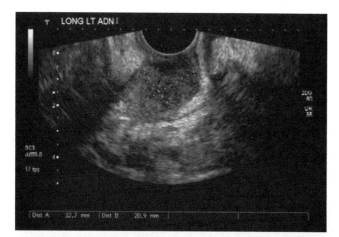

A

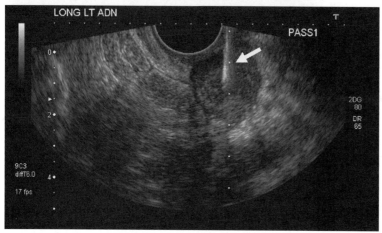

B

Fig. 8.2 Left adnexal mass in a patient with endometrial carcinoma status post total abdominal hysterectomy/bilateral salpingo-oophorectomy. **(A)** Image from the endovaginal ultrasound demonstrates the adnexal mass. **(B)** Endovaginal ultrasound-guided fine-needle aspiration with a 20-gauge Chiba needle (*arrow*). The biopsy proved an endometrial carcinoma recurrence.

- If there is no known primary malignancy, an 18-gauge cutting needle may be needed.
- If there is concern for lymphoma, then an 18-gauge or larger cutting needle may be necessary. The probe can be

oriented in either the sagittal or the transverse plane to obtain the best pathway to the lesion (**Figs. 8.2, 8.3, 8.4**).

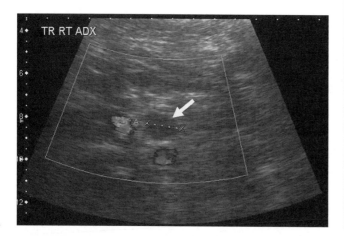

A

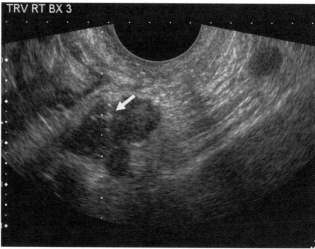

B

Fig. 8.3 Iliac node biopsy in a patient with a history of ovarian carcinoma and colon carcinoma. **(A)** Image from a transabdominal pelvic ultrasound demonstrates the left external iliac node (*arrow*). **(B)** Endovaginal ultrasound-guided cutting needle biopsy of the node with a 20-gauge Temno needle (Cardinal Health, Dublin, OH) (*arrow*). The biopsy result was an ovarian carcinoma metastasis.

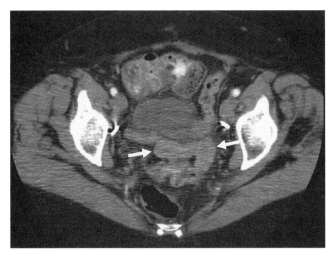

A

B

Fig. 8.4 A 66-year-old female with a history of ovarian carcinoma status post total abdominal hysterectomy/bilateral salpingo-oophorectomy, with recurrent tumor at the vaginal cuff. **(A)** CT scan showing soft tissue mass at vaginal cuff (*arrows*). **(B)** Endovaginal ultrasound-guided biopsy of the soft tissue mass with a 20-gauge Temno cutting needle (Cardinal Health, Dublin, OH) (*arrow*).

Aspiration of fluid from the endometrial canal can be performed in patients when the gynecologist is unable to access the stenosed uterine cervix.

Endovaginal Ultrasound-Guided Aspiration of the Endometrium or Endometrial Cavity

- Target the lower uterine body, near the cervix
- Using a 19-gauge catheter sheath needle, puncture the myometrium
- Aspirate fluid from the endometrial canal (**Fig. 8.5**)

Postprocedural Evaluation

- Observe the patient and monitor the vitals for
  - 2 hours after uncomplicated FNA
  - 4 hours after a cutting needle biopsy procedure

Endovaginal Ultrasound-Guided Pelvic Abscess Drainage

Causes of central or deep pelvic abscess:

- Tuboovarian abscess
- Sigmoid diverticular abscess

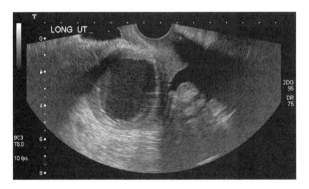

A

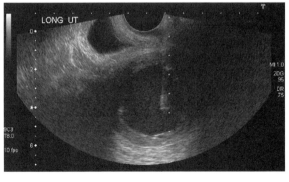

B

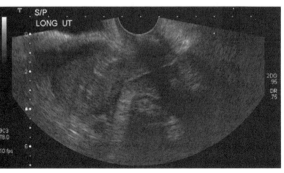

C

Fig. 8.5 A 53-year-old female with history of low-grade cervical carcinoma and hydrometrocolpos. Due to location of the cervix and cervical stenosis, the gynecologist was unable to access the cervix. **(A)** Endovaginal ultrasound image of the uterus with complex fluid within the endometrial canal. **(B)** Endovaginal ultrasound-guided aspiration of the fluid in the endometrial canal using a 19-gauge Yueh centesis needle (Cook Medical, Bloomington, IN). The approach is through the myometrium near the cervix. **(C)** Endovaginal ultrasound image after the aspiration shows nearly complete evacuation of the endometrial canal.

- Ruptured appendicitis
- Postsurgical abscess

General Principles and Approaches

Transabdominal Approach

Most preferred approach is the anterior transabdominal route. Catheter is placed through the anterior abdominal wall into the abscess. This can be performed with computed tomography (CT) or ultrasound guidance. Some central pelvic abscesses are not amenable to this approach due to intervening structures, such as loops of bowel, major vessels, the uterus, and bladder.

Transrectal Approach

The transrectal and/or transvaginal approaches are the next best option. A catheter is placed within the rectum or vagina and directed through the wall of the rectum or vagina into the abscess. The transrectal approach can be performed with either CT or ultrasound guidance.

Transvaginal Approach

The transvaginal approach is typically performed with ultrasound guidance.

Endovaginal Ultrasound-Guided Abscess Drainage

Equipment

The initial patient preparation is the same as for pelvic biopsies.

- Use either a single-step trocar catheter or the modified Seldinger technique
- A needle/catheter guide for the endovaginal probe must be used such that the needle/catheter guide can be easily removed from the catheter once the catheter is placed in the abscess. There are various methods to do this.
  ○ Method 1 for catheter preparation: use sheath that comes with the trocar-based catheters
  ○ Method 2 for catheter preparation: use a standard angiographic peel-away sheath

Techniques

- Method 1 for catheter preparation (**Fig. 8.6**)
  ○ Sheath is cut to a length of ~10 cm.
  ○ Using a pair of scissors or a scalpel, a longitudinal cut is made down the length of the sheath. This will allow for later removal of the sheath from the catheter.
  ○ Fix sheath to the ultrasound probe with rubber bands
  ○ Place the probe with the guide into the vagina
  ○ Place the catheter into the sheath guide

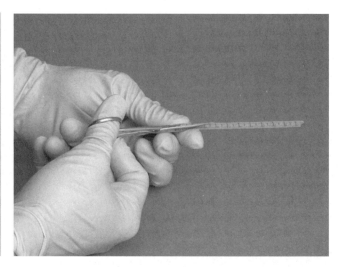

A   B

Fig. 8.6 Technique for abscess drainage using endovaginal ultrasound-guidance and a single-step trocar catheter. To perform this procedure, a catheter guide must be fashioned such that it can be easily removed from the catheter once the catheter is placed within the abscess. This method uses the plastic sheath that comes packaged with the trocar-based catheter. Alternatively, a plastic sheath from a Chiba needle can be used. **(A)** The sheath is cut to a length of ~10 cm. Note using the sterile scissors to make a beveled edge, which allows for easier insertion of the guide and catheter. **(B)** Using the pair of scissors, a single cut is then made along the length of the sheath. The guide will later be pulled off of the catheter along this longitudinal cut.

C

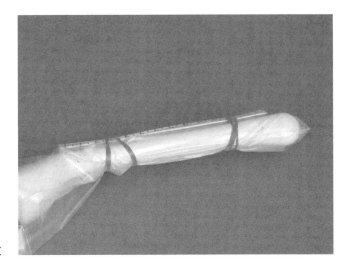

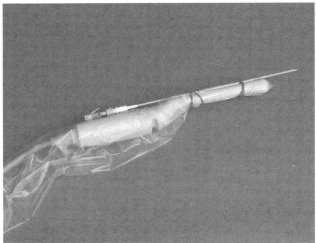

D

E

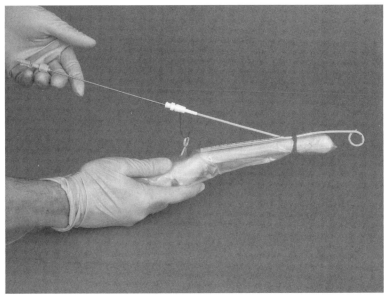

Fig. 8.6 *(Continued)* **(C)** The sheath is then fixed to the endovaginal probe with rubber bands. It is important that the distal beveled edge of the sheath does not extend beyond the distal tip of the endovaginal probe. The sheath and probe assembly is then advanced into the vagina. **(D)** A single-step trocar catheter is then inserted into the sheath, and the abscess can be punctured. Be sure that the catheter is long enough to go through the sheath and form the pigtail in the abscess. **(E)** Once the pigtail of the catheter is formed within the abscess, the endovaginal probe is removed. The catheter is pulled through the longitudinal cut made in the sheath in **Fig. 8.6B**. Leaving the metal stiffener partially within the catheter makes it easier to pull the catheter through the longitudinal cut in the sheath. As the probe and sheath are withdrawn from the vagina, carefully cut the rubber bands that secure the sheath to the probe.

- Exerting enough pressure to tent the vaginal wall, puncture vaginal wall and abscess
- Once catheter is inserted and fixed into the abscess, pull sheath off catheter along the longitudinal cut in the sheath
- Method 2 for catheter preparation
  - Use a peel-away sheath that is large enough to fit over the intended catheter
  - A peel-away sheath is fixed to the ultrasound probe with rubber bands.
  - Once the catheter is in the abscess, the peel-away sheath is removed from the catheter (**Fig. 8.7**).

Depending on operator preference and catheter selection, either a one-step-trocar catheter technique or the modified Seldinger technique can be used. It is typically easier to use the trocar-based catheters with ultrasound.

- Single-step technique for catheter placement
  - For 6–10-French trocar-based catheters, place through the vaginal wall with endovaginal ultrasound guidance (**Figs. 8.8, 8.9**).

12-French or larger trocar-based catheters are difficult to place through the vaginal wall with the single-step technique due to patient discomfort. If a 12-French or larger catheter is desired, then the modified Seldinger technique may be necessary:

- Modified Seldinger technique
  - Use a catheter sheath needle (such as a 19-gauge Yueh centesis needle [Cook Medical, Bloomington, IN]) to access the abscess using the appropriate needle guide
  - Once the abscess is punctured, withdraw the needle from the catheter sheath

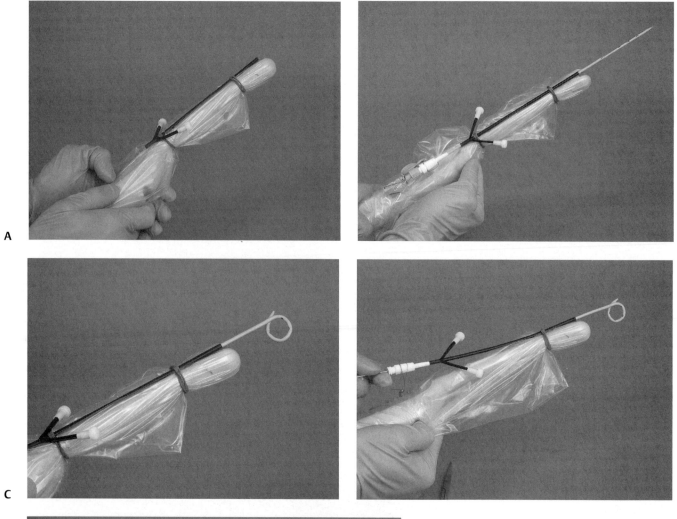

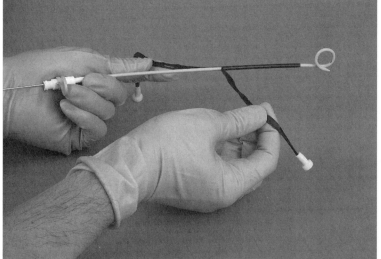

Fig. 8.7 Endovaginal drainage using a peel-away sheath. **(A)** The peel-away sheath is attached to the probe by rubber bands. Be sure the tip of the sheath does not protrude beyond the tip of the probe. **(B)** The single-step trocar-based catheter is inserted into the sheath and then into the abscess. Be sure that the catheter is long enough to puncture the abscess. If necessary, the peel-away sheath can be shortened by pulling on the tabs. **(C)** Form the pigtail within the abscess. **(D)** Slowly remove the probe from the vagina without pulling on the catheter. Carefully cut the rubber bands supporting the peel-away sheath. **(E)** Remove the peel away sheath from the catheter by gently pulling on the tabs.

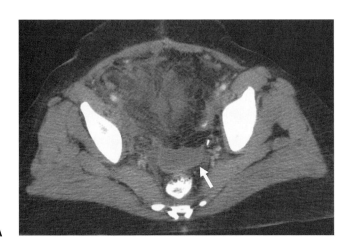
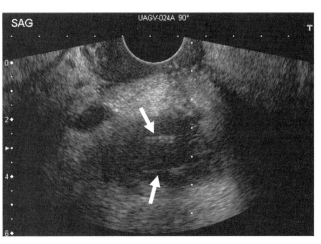

Fig. 8.8 A 45-year-old patient status post total abdominal hysterectomy, now with a central pelvic abscess. The procedure was performed in the intensive care unit. **(A)** An initial computed tomography scan demonstrates a central pelvic abscess (arrow). **(B)** Endovaginal ultrasound demonstrates a 8-French single-step trocar pigtail catheter in the abscess (*arrows*).

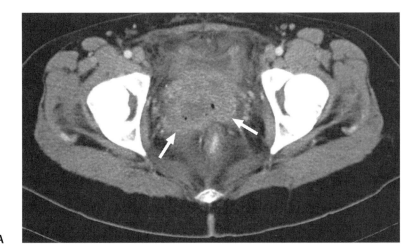

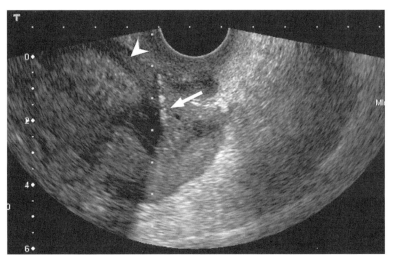

Fig. 8.9 A 43-year-old patient status post total abdominal hysterectomy with fever and pelvic pain. **(A)** A computed tomography scan demonstrates the small fluid collection just superior to the vaginal cuff (*arrows*). Because of the small size of the fluid collection, only an endovaginal ultrasound-guided aspiration was performed using a 19-gauge catheter sheath needle. **(B)** Endovaginal ultrasound demonstrates 19-gauge Yueh centesis needle (Cook Medical, Bloomington, IN) (*arrow*) in the small fluid collection. Note the proximity of bowel (*arrowhead*).

○ A standard 0.035-inch (0.889-mm) angiographic guidewire is advanced through the catheter sheath into the abscess.

○ Use a relatively stiff guidewire, such as a Rosen wire, to avoid losing access to the abscess

○ Soft guide wires may be inadvertently kinked while attempting dilation.

○ A super-stiff Amplatz guidewire could also be used; however, one must be careful not to perforate the abscess wall with the super-stiff wire.

- Modified Seldinger technique used under ultrasound guidance

○ Important to visualize the wire and catheter as manipulations are performed

○ A two-person procedure, with one person performing the wire and catheter manipulations and the other person scanning with the endovaginal probe

○ Care must be taken while scanning to keep the probe and needle guide as close to the puncture site in the vaginal wall as possible.

○ Excess motion of the endovaginal probe may inadvertently dislodge the guidewire from the abscess.

○ Having fluoroscopy available once the guidewire is in the abscess may make the subsequent dilations and catheter placement easier.

- Fluoroscopy entails either performing the ultrasound-guided puncture of the abscess on a fluoroscopy table, or moving the patient to the fluoroscopy table from the ultrasound cart after the abscess is accessed with a guidewire.

- Can be uncomfortable for the patient to perform the entire procedure on the fluoroscopy table due to lack of stirrups and hardness of the table

- Avoid inadvertently dislodging the guidewire while moving the patient to the fluoroscopy table after the abscess is accessed with a guidewire

- Once the patient is on the fluoroscopy table, the tract can be dilated over the guidewire to the desired size and the catheter can be placed under direct fluoroscopic visualization.

- Once the catheter is placed, the pigtail is formed in the abscess and the remaining catheter is taped to the patient's inner thigh.

Transperineal Approach

A catheter is directed superiorly through the perineum into the abscess. CT is typically used here.

Transsciatic Approach

This is the least preferred approach. A catheter traverses the gluteus muscles and sciatic notch. If this route is utilized, it is important to have the catheter traverse the inferior medial portion of the sciatic notch, that is, close to the inferior aspect of the sacrum. Typically, CT guidance is used. Possible complications include fasciitis and sciatic nerve injury, as well as patient discomfort from the catheter's location.

Postprocedural Care

- Daily flushing the catheter with a small amount of saline is recommended; however, one must be careful to avoid dislodging the catheter.
- Monitor output from the drain
- Output from the tube should gradually decrease over time.
- The character of the fluid should become more serous, and the patient's white blood cell count should normalize.
- Once the output is 10–15 cc per 24 hours, the tube may be pulled.
- Most abscesses resolve in 3–5 days.

We recommend imaging prior to removing the tube to verify the abscess has resolved. If the output from the drain changes to feculent material or bowel succus, then one should consider a communication with the colon or small bowel. At this point, a sinogram could be performed to evaluate for a fistulous tract to colon or bowel.

Conclusion

Endovaginal ultrasound-guidance can be used to perform a variety of procedures easily. These procedures can be performed quickly and are relatively inexpensive – with very few contraindications. Most of these procedures can be performed with little or no sedation, and the majority of women tolerate the procedures well.

Further Reading

Harisinghani MG, Gervais DA, Maher MM, et al. Transgluteal approach for percutaneous drainage of deep pelvic abscesses: 154 cases. Radiology 2003;228(3):701–705

Nakamoto DA, Haaga JR. Emergent ultrasound interventions. Radiol Clin North Am 2004;42(2):457–478

O'Neill MJ, Rafferty EA, Lee SI, et al. Transvaginal interventional procedures: aspiration, biopsy, and catheter drainage. Radiographics 2001;21(3):657–672

Scanlan KA, Propeck PA, Lee FT Jr. Invasive procedures in the female pelvis: value of transabdominal, endovaginal, and endorectal US guidance. Radiographics 2001;21(2):491–506

Zanetta G, Lissoni A, Franchi D, et al. Safety of transvaginal fine needle puncture of gynecologic masses: a report after 500 consecutive procedures. J Ultrasound Med 1996;15:401–404

9 Transrectal Prostate Biopsy

Ahmet Tuncay Turgut and Vikram S. Dogra

Classification

Transrectal ultrasound- (TRUS-) guided prostate biopsy is a common outpatient procedure with an annual performance of ~500,000 in the United States, and is the gold standard for the diagnosis of prostate cancer. Combined use of prostate biopsy and digital rectal examination yields the best diagnostic outcome for prostate cancer. Controversies still exist regarding the optimal number biopsy samples to be taken and their localization. In general, 12 core biopsy of the prostate has replaced the old sextant biopsy.

Indications

Absolute Indications

- Abnormal digital rectal examination (DRE), elevated serum total prostate-specific antigen (PSA) levels >4 ng/mL
- A serum PSA velocity higher than 0.75 mg/mL per year and suspicious finding(s) on TRUS examination (**Table 9.1**)

Relative Indications

- Free PSA level less than 20% with serum total PSA level being in the gray zone

Table 9.1 Indications for Transrectal Ultrasound-Guided Prostate Biopsy

Absolute
Abnormal digital rectal examination
Elevated serum total PSA level
PSA velocity >0.75 ng/mL/year
Suspicious TRUS finding(s)
Relative
Free PSA <20% when total PSA is in gray zone
Ratio of pro-PSA to free PSA >1.8%
Prior to surgery for BPH
Prior to the use of salvage local therapy to diagnose and stage recurrence of prostate cancer after failed radiation therapy

Abbreviations: PSA, prostate-specific antigen; TRUS, transrectal ultrasound; BPH, benign prostatic hyperplasia

- A ratio of pro-PSA to free PSA higher than 1.8%
  - Performing the biopsy before surgical treatment of benign prostatic hyperplasia (BPH) and before the use of salvage local therapy to diagnose and stage the recurrence of prostate cancer in patients suspected of failing radiation therapy are further relative indications for prostate biopsy.

Digital Rectal Examination

DRE can

- Identify localized cancer in a prostate with an irregular and hard consistency and asymmetric shape (inherently subjective)
- Has high false-negative and false-positive rates

Classically, a total PSA level exceeding 4 ng/mL is accepted as an indication for prostate biopsy, though controversy still exists regarding the upper limit for a normal PSA.

Prostate-Specific Antigen

- PSA has similar problems as DRE such as low specificity. Because of its low specificity, the following additional parameters are used to identify high-risk individuals who are to be referred to biopsy:
  - Total PSA value of >2–6 ng/mL for patients younger than 50 years of age
  - PSA velocity exceeding 0.75 ng/mL
  - Free PSA/total PSA ratio less than 0.20 ultrasound features
  - Suspicious gray-scale TRUS findings such as hypoechoic nodule, heterogenous echotexture of the peripheral zone (PZ), and hypervascularity detected by color Doppler TRUS are also indications for TRUS-guided prostate biopsy.

Indications for Repeat Biopsy (Table 9.2)

Postinitial Negative Biopsy

- A persistently elevated or rising PSA level (>4 ng/mL)
- A histopathologic outcome involving high-grade prostatic intraepithelial neoplasia (HGPIN)

85

Table 9.2 Indications for Repeat Prostate Biopsy

Persistently elevated or rising PSA level (>4 ng/mL)

Suspicious histopathology (HGPIN, ASAP, or suspicious but nondiagnostic cellular changes)

Increased prostate volume (>60 mL)

Family history of prostate cancer

PSA velocity > 0.75 ng/mL per year

Free PSA/total PSA ratio <0.20

Abbreviations: PSA, prostate-specific antigen; HGPIN, high-grade prostatic intraepithelial neoplasia; ASAP, atypical small acinar proliferation

- Atypical small acinar proliferation (ASAP)
- Suspicious but nondiagnostic cellular changes necessitate a repeat biopsy.

Additional Factors

- Increased prostate volume higher than 60 mL
- Family history of prostate cancer
- PSA velocity >0.75 ng/mL per year
- Free PSA/total PSA ratio <0.20

Contraindications (Table 9.3)

Absolute Contraindications

- Bleeding diathesis
- Acute prostatitis
- Urinary tract infections

Relative Contraindications

- Failure to take antibiotic prophylaxis
- Intractable patient anxiety
- Acute painful perianal disorders are considered as relative contraindications.

Table 9.3 Contraindications for Prostate Biopsy

Absolute
Bleeding diathesis
Acute prostatitis
Urinary tract infections
Relative
Failure to take antibiotic prophylaxis
Intractable patient anxiety
Acute painful perianal disorders

Table 9.4 Protocol for Preprocedural Evaluation for Prostate Biopsy

Informed consent

Questioning of medical history (bleeding diathesis, blood clotting medication)

Periprocedural antibiotic prophylaxis

Rectal administration of bowel cleansing enema

Achievement of an empty urinary bladder

Preprocedural Evaluation and Patient Preparation (Table 9.4)

- A written informed consent must be obtained from the patient.
- Medical history of the patient must be questioned for bleeding diathesis and intake of any medication altering blood clotting.
- Discontinuation of anticoagulants, nonsteroidal antiinflammatory drugs 7–10 days prior to procedure
- Stopping of low-dose aspirin (<300 mg per day) is not needed.
- Periprocedural antibiotic prophylaxis of Cipro (ciprofloxacin), 500 mg twice daily beginning before the day of the procedure and continuing for 3 consecutive days

Day of the Biopsy (Early)

- Request the patient to self-administer a bowel-cleansing enema (precaution against infectious complications)
- Instruct the patient not to empty his urinary bladder completely. It helps define a clear interface with the prostate's superior margin.

Equipment

- A color Doppler ultrasound scanner equipped with a transrectal probe is essential for
  - TRUS-guided prostate biopsy
  - Biplane probes for transrectal prostate scanning with a combination of end-viewing or side-viewing transducers in the 5–8 MHz range
- Use ultrasound gel inside and over a latex condom covering the probe to eliminate the air.

Room Setup

- Anticipate a high level of anxiety in a patient scheduled for TRUS-guided prostate biopsy (worry over pain, discomfort)
- Ensure procedure is performed in an uncrowded, warm, and quiet room

Technique

Patient Positioning and Probe Insertion

- Place the patient in a left lateral decubitus position with the knees and hips fully flexed
- A DRE performed before the insertion of the probe may reveal any physical examination abnormality correlating with ultrasound findings.
- Instruct the patient to take a deep breath, relax for maximum comfort
- Insert probe through rectum

Anesthesia Considerations

- The preferred method is TRUS-guided periprostatic injection of a local anesthetic.
  - Proven to be efficient for increasing patient tolerance during the subsequent prostate biopsy

Injection of the anesthetic agent preferably is performed in the prebiopsy period (allowing time for effect) with a 22-gauge needle. Infiltration of the anesthetic agent (lidocaine without epinephrine) is done at the white pyramidal site between the prostate and the seminal vesicle laterally. This site is called the "Mount Everest sign" because of its white, peaked appearance created by the fat in this location on a sagittal plane – 5 mL of lidocaine is injected on each side. An ultrasound wheal is seen as hypoechoic filling the Mount Everest area.

- Conscious sedation with intravenous midazolam – recommended as an alternative and efficient means of anesthesia to counteract the aforementioned limitations for periprostatic anesthetic injection

This method involves the intravenous injection of midazolam 5–10 minutes before the biopsy procedure is performed by an anesthetist and should be accompanied by routine noninvasive monitoring.

- Intrarectal administration of lidocaine gel – another suitable form of anesthesia before prostate biopsy

Transrectal Ultrasound Evaluation

- Main role of TRUS for a suspected prostate cancer involves guiding prostate biopsies.
- The entire prostate gland can be evaluated systematically in transverse and semicoronal planes beginning from the level of seminal vesicles adjacent to the prostate base and continuing with the demonstration of the zonal prostate anatomy down to the level of the apex (**Fig. 9.1**).

- The prostate with its neighboring structures should also be scanned from right to left in the sagittal plane.
- The prostate volume can be calculated from the measurements of the three longest orthogonal diameters of the prostate by means of the ellipsoid formula (Volume of prostate $= 0.52 \times td \times apd \times ccd$, where td is the transverse diameter of the prostate, apd is the anteroposterior diameter of the prostate, and ccd is the craniocaudal diameter of the prostate).

Biopsy

- A stabilizing needle guide is attached to the transrectal probe through which an 18-gauge 20-cm-long biopsy needle located within and extending from the tip of a spring-loaded biopsy gun is passed before "firing" for sampling the prostate (**Fig. 9.2**).
- Not infrequently, 22- to 25-cm-long needles may be necessary for an adequate sampling of a gland with prostatic hyperplasia.
- Additionally, a 22-gauge Chiba needle is needed in case the injection of a local anesthetic agent to the periprostatic region is to be performed for lessening the anticipated pain with subsequent prostate biopsy.

Owing to the multicentric character of prostate cancer, TRUS-guided prostate biopsy involves zone-based systematic sampling of the prostate rather than being lesion-directed alone, contrary to the other image-guided biopsies. Biopsies are taken

- In a spatially oriented fashion from the regions of the prostate where the tumors are most likely to be located
  - Sampling of the regions with focal gray-scale or color Doppler abnormalities is performed (**Figs. 9.3, 9.4**).
    - Sampling strategy is directed to PZ as most (80%) of the prostate cancers are located in PZ and have a higher Gleason grade and risk for metastasis compared with the inner gland cancers.
- Biopsies are performed either in sagittal or axial scanning mode depending on the transducer design.
- Firing of the biopsy gun should be performed after indenting the prostate capsule with the biopsy needle so that contamination with the periprostatic tissue can be avoided and a longer tissue can be extracted during sampling.
- Length of the needle trajectory within the gland should be predicted with the help of the trajectory line on the ultrasound screen to avoid inadvertent penetration of structures such as urethra and periprostatic tissue, which would otherwise increase the morbidity of the procedure.

Lobes of Prostate

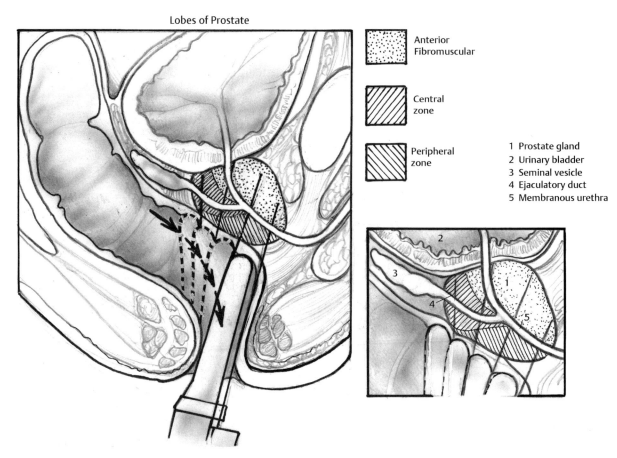

Anterior
Fibromuscular

Central
zone

Peripheral
zone

1 Prostate gland
2 Urinary bladder
3 Seminal vesicle
4 Ejaculatory duct
5 Membranous urethra

Fig. 9.1 Schematic drawing in sagittal plane depicting the movement of transrectal probe for TRUS examination beginning from the level of seminal vesicles adjacent to the prostate base and continuing with the demonstration of the zonal prostate anatomy down to the level of the apex. Note that the stabilizing needle attached to the probe enables the sampling of the gland at the aforementioned levels consecutively.

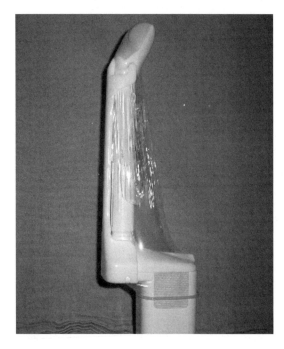

Fig. 9.2 Biplane transrectal probe with an attached stabilizing needle guide through which a biopsy needle or Chiba needle is passed for sampling of the prostate or injection of local anesthetic agent.

A systematic sampling approach first was introduced with a sextant sampling protocol.

- Involves obtaining core biopsies at the midway between the lateral border and the median plane at the levels of base, midgland, and apex of the prostate, respectively.
- Several modifications of sextant sampling aimed to increase the diagnostic yield by increasing the number of cores and directing the cores more laterally have been developed (**Fig. 9.5**).
- Currently, extended sampling protocols with 10–12 cores are preferred in most centers (**Fig. 9.6**).
- No consensus has been provided yet for optimal sites and number of biopsies.

Inner gland (IG) sampling is

- Not routinely performed during primary prostate biopsies as its cancer detection rate is usually lower and involves less aggressive cancers

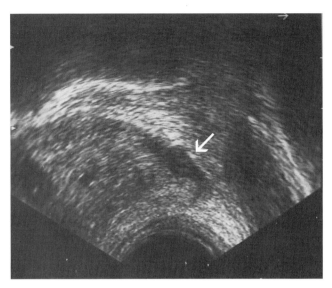
A

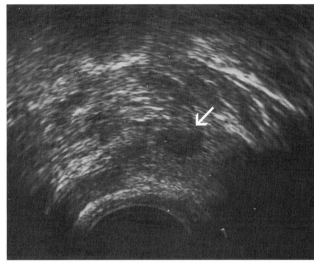
B

Fig. 9.3 A 60-year-old man, total prostate-specific antigen (PSA): 3.25 ng/mL, free PSA/total PSA: 0.17. **(A)** Transrectal ultrasound examination in axial and **(B)** sagittal planes revealed a well-defined, hypoechoic nodule showing slight capsular bulging located at the lateral part of the basal region of left lobe (*arrows*). The nodule was biopsied in addition to 12-core systematic sampling. Histopathologic analysis of the sample from the nodule revealed adenocarcinoma (Gleason grade 2 + 2 = 4), whereas cancer was not detected in any of the cores from either lobe included in the systematic sampling protocol.

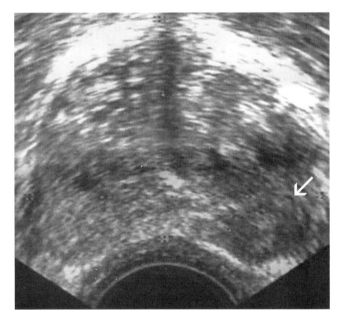
A

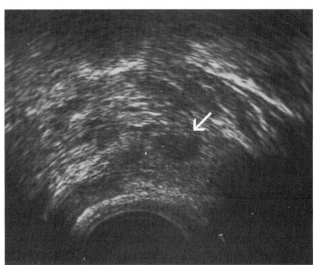
B

Fig. 9.4 A 65-year-old man, total prostate-specific antigen (PSA): 5.33 ng/mL, free PSA/total PSA: 0.08. **(A)** Transrectal ultrasound examination in axial and **(B)** sagittal planes revealed an ill-defined lesion with heterogenous echotexture and slight capsular bulging located at the mid- to lateral part of the basal region of the left lobe. The nodule was biopsied in addition to having 12-core systematic sampling. Histopathologic analysis of the samples from the lesion and from the left-lateral basal region, respectively, revealed adenocarcinoma (Gleason grade 3 + 2 = 5); however, cancer was not detected in any of the samples from the right lobe.

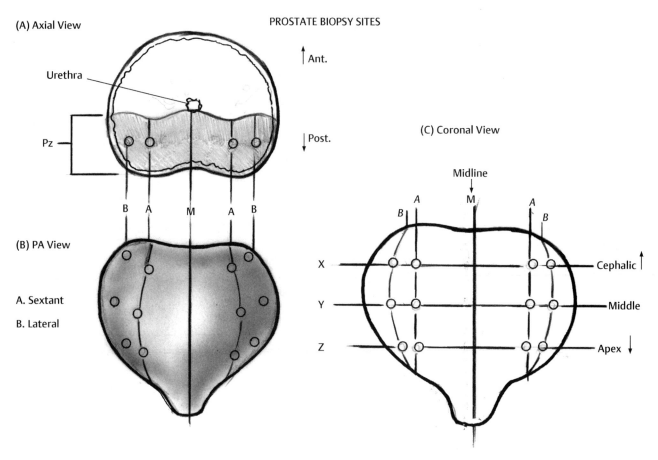

Fig. 9.5 (A) Axial, **(B)** posteroanterior, and **(C)** coronal views of the prostate demonstrating the anatomic localizations of the biopsy cores in sextant (A) and lateral (B) sampling protocols. In the extended sampling protocol, additional cores lateral to the sites for the classic sextant biopsy at the base (X), middle part (Y), and apex (Z) of the prostate are targeted.

- Regions in the prostate not routinely sampled in the initial biopsy such as the anterior horn of the PZ, lateral areas, and the IG should be sampled during a repeat biopsy.
- Diagnosis of HGPIN in the initial biopsy, which is regarded to be either precancerous or concurrent with cancer having a remote location, necessitates the sampling of both the PZ and IG.
- A previous diagnosis of nondiagnostic cellular changes necessitates a site-specific approach in repeat biopsy as the diagnosis might be associated with small cancer volume or inappropriate sampling.
- A minimum interval of 6 weeks should be considered between the initial and repeat biopsies. In cases with repeated negative biopsies and persistence of the suspicion for malignancy, saturation biopsies involving sampling of more than 20 cores in the prostate gland without considering any zonal pattern are recommended.

Endpoints

- Obtaining successful 12 core samples

Postprocedural Evaluation

- The extracted samples should be sent to the laboratory for histopathologic analysis in separate containers filled with formalin solution.
- The patient should be observed for complications during the procedure and immediate postprocedural period.

- For patients having sedation with intravenous midazolam, blood pressure and pulse monitoring must be performed for half an hour after the biopsy procedure and the patients must be observed for 2 hours.
- For those patients who discontinued oral anticoagulants before the biopsy, the medication can be restarted 24 hours after the procedure.

Complications

Major complications are very rare; however, at least one minor complication can be detected in 70% of the patients.

- Mild, self-limiting bleeding is the most common complication and may be in the form of hematuria, hemospermia, or rectal bleeding. All patients should be asked to void before leaving the department.

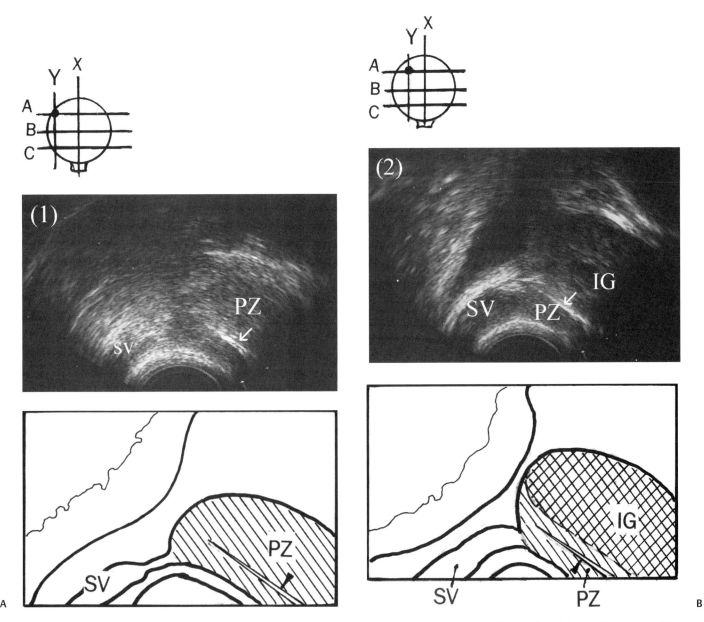

A   B

Fig. 9.6 Serial sagittal ultrasound scans and the relevant schematic drawings demonstrating the systematic sampling of the peripheral zone of the prostate with the biopsy needle (*arrows*) at **(A)** lateral-basal, **(B)** medial-basal, (*Continued on page 92*)

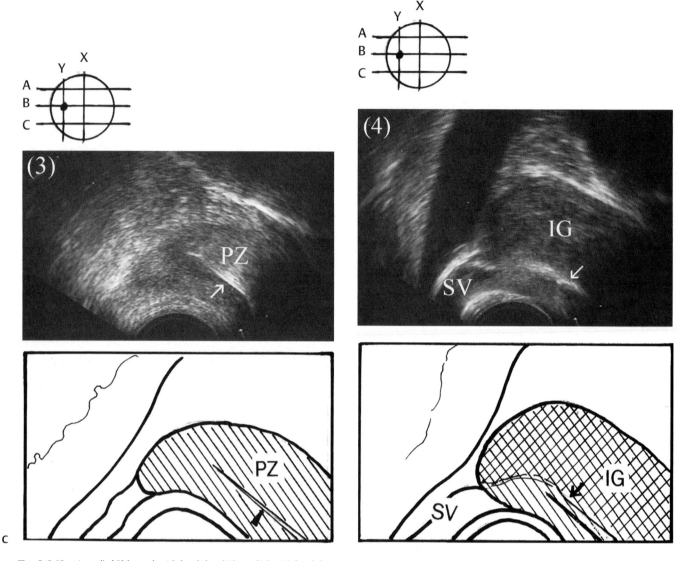

Fig. 9.6 *(Continued)* **(C)** lateral-midglandular, **(D)** medial-midglandular,

- Infectious complications with their associated findings such as fever, bacteremia, and bacteriuria may occur.
- Postprocedural pain or discomfort may be encountered. Vasovagal symptoms, urinary retention, urinary incontinence, epididymitis, periprostatic hematoma, and disseminated intravascular coagulopathy may be rarely detected in the immediate and late postbiopsy period.

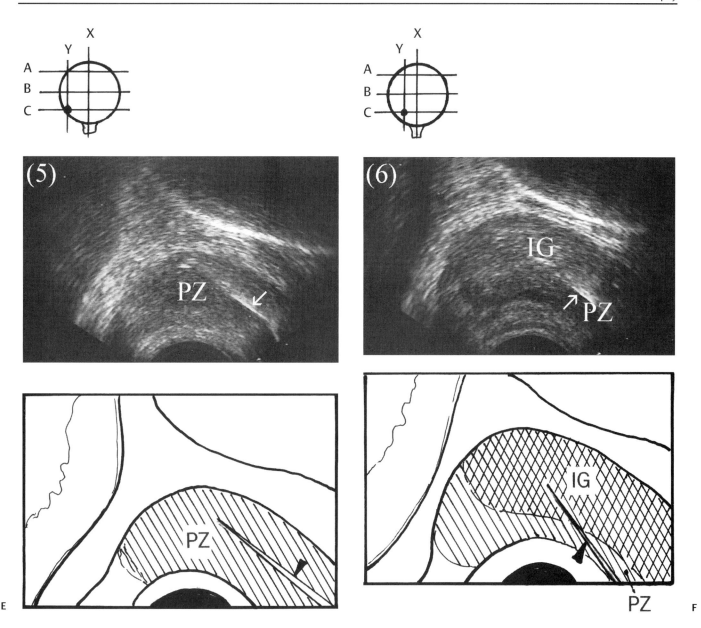

Fig. 9.6 *(Continued)* **(E)** lateral-apical, and **(F)** medial-apical regions (IG, inner gland; PZ, peripheral zone; SV; seminal vesicle).

Further Reading

Boczko J, Messing E, Dogra V. Transrectal sonography in prostate evaluation. Radiol Clin North Am 2006;44(5):679–687, viii

Djavan B, Margreiter M. Biopsy standards for detection of prostate cancer. World J Urol 2007;25(1):11–17

Papatheodorou A, Ellinas P, Tandeles S, et al. Transrectal ultrasonography and ultrasound-guided biopsies of the prostate gland: how, when, and where. Curr Probl Diagn Radiol 2005;34(2):76–83

Raja J, Ramachandran N, Munneke G, Patel U. Current status of transrectal ultrasound-guided prostate biopsy in the diagnosis of prostate cancer. Clin Radiol 2006;61(2):142–153

Sadeghi-Nejad H, Simmons M, Dakwar G, Dogra V. Controversies in transrectal ultrasonography and prostate biopsy. Ultrasound Q 2006;22(3):169–175

Turgut AT, Olçücüoğlu E, Koşar P, Geyik PO, Koşar U. Complications and limitations related to periprostatic local anesthesia before TRUS-guided prostate biopsy. J Clin Ultrasound 2008;36(2):67–71

II Ultrasound-Guided Access and Drainage

10 Vascular Access
Wael E.A. Saad

Classification

Vascular access is usually the "opening" step to myriad vascular procedures managing enumerable vascular and nonvascular diseases. Broadening this matter for discussion is the number of vessels, both arterial and venous, that can be used for access. Unfortunately, the scope of this book does not allow us to cover all of these procedures in detail. Indications, contraindications, and endpoints in this chapter are focused on vascular entry (access) only.

Indications

Vascular access is usually the "opening" step to myriad vascular procedures managing enumerable vascular and nonvascular diseases. As a result, indications are broad. They depend on intent and vessel type. The following is a briefing.

Indications Based on Intent

The intent of vascular access, in its simplest definition, is entry to the target vessel at a trajectory and in a particular vascular segment to be able to fulfill the greater aim of the procedure embarked on. Vascular access procedures can be classified into

- Vascular entry for diagnostic purposes
- Vascular entry with the intent of placing an indwelling tube/catheter
- Vascular entry with the intent of implanting a long-term prosthesis or implantable device
- Vascular entry with a remote therapeutic intent

Indications Based on Vessels: Venous

- Small upper extremity veins – radial and ulnar forearm veins
  - Peripheral intravenous (IV) access for medication – popular/common
  - Upper extremity venography/mapping (e.g., preop planning for fistula)
- Larger upper extremity veins – brachial and axillary veins
  - Peripheral IV access for blood transfusions and rapid medication delivery – popular/common

- Upper arm, subclavian, and central venous venography
  - Long-term central venous access (peripherally inserted central catheter [PICC – popular/common] and arm port-a-catheters/reservoir catheters)
  - Access for central venous therapeutic purposes
    - Vena caval filter placement
    - Upper extremity and central venous thrombolysis ± stent placement
- Subclavian vein
  - Long-term central venous access for implants (tunneled, nontunneled, and port-a-catheters/reservoir catheters, cardiac pacers)
  - Access for central venous therapeutic purposes
    - Vena caval filter placement
    - Central venous venoplasty/stent placement
  - Central venous venography
- Jugular vein
  - Long-term central venous access (tunneled, nontunneled, and port-a-catheters/reservoir catheters – popular/common)
  - Access for central venous therapeutic purposes
    - Vena caval filter placement – popular/common
    - Central venous venoplasty/stent placement
    - Transjugular hepatic procedures (transjugular intrahepatic portosystemic shunt [TIPS], liver biopsy, hepatic venography–portography) – popular/common
    - Transjugular renal procedures (renal biopsy)
    - Transjugular cardiac procedures (endocardial biopsy, Swan-Ganz catheter placement, pacers)
    - Gonadal vein embolization/sclerosis
  - Central venous venography
- Femoral vein
  - Access for central venous therapeutic purposes
    - Vena caval filter placement – popular/common
    - Central venous venoplasty/stent placement – popular/common
    - Transfemoral hepatic procedures – not common, only when above-diaphragm veins are exhausted
    - Gonadal vein embolization/sclerosis
  - Central venous venography
  - Long-term central venous access (tunneled, nontunneled, and port-a-catheters/reservoir catheters) when above-diaphragm veins are exhausted/occluded
  - Endocrine venous sampling

- Popliteal and below-knee (tibial) veins
  - Access for central venous therapeutic purposes
    - Lower extremity venous thrombolysis ± veno-plasty/stent placement ± vena cava filter placement – popular/common

Indications Based on Vessels: Arterial

- Radial artery
  - Arterial line for real-time pressure transduction – popular/common
  - Quick access ABG (arterial, blood, gas)
- Brachial or axillary artery – popular/common with cardiologists, considered a second-line arterial access for radiologists and vascular surgeons
  - Diagnostic arteriography
    - Cardiac arteriography – popular/common
    - Aortography ± lower extremity runoff when femoral arteries occluded
    - Visceral/mesenteric arteriography when femoral arteries occluded
  - Access for arterial therapeutic purposes
    - Cardiac catheterization (angioplasty/stent placement) – popular/common
    - Visceral/mesenteric angioplasty/stent placement when femoral arteries occluded or when femoro-visceral angles are not favorable for available wires/platforms/operator talent
    - One access as part of complicated thoracoabdominal endograft repairs
  - Arterial line for real-time pressure transduction
- Carotid artery
  - Access for arterial therapeutic purposes
    - One access as part of complicated thoracic arch endograft repairs
- Femoral artery – popular/common with radiologists and vascular surgeons
  - Diagnostic arteriography – popular/common

- Aortography ± lower extremity runoff
- Visceral/mesenteric arteriography
- Upper extremity and cerebral arteriography
- Cardiac arteriography
  - Access for arterial therapeutic purposes – popular/common
    - Visceral/mesenteric angioplasty/stent placement
    - Main access of thoracoabdominal endograft repairs
    - Upper extremity and cerebral angioplasty/stent placement
    - Arterial thrombolysis procedures
    - Cardiac catheterization (angioplasty/stent placement)
  - Arterial line for real-time pressure transduction – popular/common
  - Long-term implantable arterial access (arterial Port-a-catheters/reservoir catheters or pumps for chemo-infusion) – popular/common in Japan and South Korea

Contraindications

There are no true absolute contraindications. All contraindications are relative to the type and urgency of the procedure. In addition, the location and longevity of the access affect the coagulopathy threshold. **Table 10.1** gives some idea about suggested coagulation parameters. There are no clear values set based on evidence-based research. These are suggested thresholds and personal opinion of the author.

Preprocedural Evaluation

Evaluate prior cross-sectional imaging and laboratory values. Obtain informed consent and document a baseline vascular exam.

Table 10.1 Suggested Coagulation Parameters

	Vascular Entry without Implant/ Dwell Catheters and Emergent	Vascular Entry without Implant/ Dwell Catheters and Elective	Vascular Entry with Implant and Elective
Arterial	INR: ≤2.2* PLT: ≥50,000 aPTT: ≤90 s	INR: ≤1.4 PLT: ≥50,000 aPTT: ≤65 s	INR: ≤1.2 PLT: ≥70,000 aPTT: ≤35 s
Venous	INR: ≤4.2* PLT: ≥30,000 aPTT: ≤90 s	INR: ≤2.2 PLT: ≥50,000 aPTT: ≤65 s	INR: ≤2.0 PLT: ≥50,000 aPTT: ≤65 s

*In emergent arterial (and even venous) vascular access, operators can tolerate greater coagulation parameters than those in the table. This can be achieved by keeping the vascular access sheath in and not pulling it out. However, this requires greater postprocedural patient care than that available on a general medical/surgical hospital floor. Patients should be in an intensive care unit (ICU) or a step-down unit depending on institutional policy.

Abbreviations: INR, international normalized ratio; PLT, platelets; aPTT, activated partial thromboplastin time; s, seconds

- Look for vascular anomalies and anatomic variations
  - Some anomalies/variations may preclude accessing a particular vessel. For example, a sciatic artery should be identified as an anatomic anomaly.
  - Other anomalies may make the subsequent vascular procedure more difficult/impossible despite an initially successful access. For example, when planning a transjugular liver biopsy or TIPS procedure, a patent jugular vein may allow initial access, but an occluded superior vena cava would make it impossible to approach the liver from that successful jugular access.
- Look for adjacent structures that can be inadvertently traversed
  - This helps to plan the needle trajectory and evaluate other access vessels altogether.
    - For example, an enlarged inguinal hernia when planning a femoral vessel access
- Look for preexisting vascular injuries
  - Avoid accessing where there is a vascular injury from a prior access
  - These vascular injuries include pseudoaneurysms, arteriovenous fistulas, and large hematomas.

All coagulation parameter thresholds are relative to the type and urgency of the procedure. In addition, the location and longevity of the access affect the coagulopathy threshold. **Table 10.1** lists suggested coagulation parameters. There are no clear values based on evidence-based research. These are suggested thresholds based on my experience; they should aid in the decision-making process regarding implants versus no implants (dwell catheters) and the urgency of the procedure.

Indications

- Consent, not only to access (unless it is the only procedure), but to the entire procedure; part of it is its access.
- See above for indications

Alternatives

- To refuse the access or the procedure
- The alternative to vascular access for diagnostic purposes is noninvasive cross-sectional imaging such as computed tomography angiography (CTA), computed tomography venography (CTV), magnetic resonance angiography (MRA), and magnetic resonance venography (MRV).

Procedural Risks

- Major complications (**Tables 10.2, 10.3, and 10.4**)
  - Bleeding with large expansile hematomas
    - Pain, drop in hematocrit, need for blood transfusion (an issue with arterial access, especially

Table 10.2 Complications of Diagnostic Arteriography without Contrast Complications (Closest to Arterial Vascular Access)

Complication	Incidence
All hematomas*	Up to 10%
Major hematomas†	0.0–0.7%
Vessel thrombosis	0.0–0.8%
Distal emboli	0.0–0.1%
Pseudoaneurysm/AVF	0.04–0.2%
Dissection	0.0–0.4%

*Frequency after arterial access is subject to definitions. Asymptomatic hematomas depend on size of hematoma and the site of access. Small axillary artery hematomas can be symptomatic due to nerve injury/compression.

†Major hematomas are defined as hematomas dropping hematocrit and requiring blood transfusion and/or hematomas requiring surgical evacuation.

Abbreviations: AVF, arteriovenous fistula

femoral artery access if high above the inguinal ligament)
- Patient instability (an issue with arterial access, especially femoral artery access if high above the inguinal ligament)
- Hematomas may grow and compress adjacent nerves and cause neuropathy (an issue with arterial access, especially axillary artery access if high above the inguinal ligament).
  - Arterial injuries
    - Pseudoaneurysms
    - Dissection
    - Arteriovenous fistula
  - Infections
    - Especially concerning implants such as tunneled central catheters and port-a-catheters
- Minor complications
  - Inadvertent transgression of adjacent vessel(s)
  - Minor infections not involving implants and not creating discharge or collections
  - Hematomas not requiring blood transfusion, surgical evacuation, or leading to patient instability

Table 10.3 Complications of Jugular or Subclavian Access

Complication	Incidence
Pneumothorax	0.0–1.0%
Hemothorax	0.0–1.0%
Site hematoma	0.0–1.0%
Air emboli	0.0–1.0%
Wound infection and dehiscence	0.0–1.0%
Sepsis	0.0–1.0%
Venous thrombosis	4.0%

Table 10.4   Complications of PICC-Line/Upper Extremity Vein Access

Complication	Incidence
Pneumothorax/hemothorax	0.0%
Arterial injury	0.0–0.5%
Site hematoma	0.0–1.0%
Wound infection and dehiscence	0.0–1.0%
Sepsis	0.0–1.0%*
Venous thrombosis	3.0%*
Phlebitis	4.0%*

*These complications are due to indwelling catheters (PICC line) and are far lower in incidence in venous access without indwelling catheters/implants.

Abbreviations: PICC, peripherally inserted central catheter

- This is for arterial access exams and not for venous access.
- A neurologic exam is required for carotid access or whenever the catheter reaches the aortic arch.
- This is to compare with the postaccess or postangiogram vascular exam.
- The mainstay of the distal vascular exam is examination of the distal artery pulses (palpation, auscultation, Doppler ultrasound), skin color, temperature, and capillary refill.

Equipment

Ultrasound Guidance

- Ultrasound machine
- Doppler capability is not necessary, but is good to have in case vascular injuries are encountered.
- A linear higher frequency transducer (7.5–9 MHz) is usually good for all vascular accesses.
- A multiarray 4–5 MHz ultrasound transducer is usually not required unless in the case of femoral vessel access in morbidly obese patients.
- A transducer guide bracket is usually not required. Access/target vessels are usually superficial enough; they do not need needle guide brackets.
- Sterile transducer cover

Standard Surgical Preparation and Draping

- Chlorhexidine skin preparation/cleansing fluid
- Fenestrated drape

Local Infiltrative Analgesia Administration

- 21-gauge infiltration needle
- 10–20 mL 1% lidocaine syringe

Sharp Access

- 11-blade incision scalpel
- Access needle (21- to 18-gauge, usually 21- or 18-gauge)
- A 21-gauge needle accepts a 0.018-inch coaxial wire
- A 18-gauge needle accepts a 0.035- to 0.038-inch coaxial wire

Coaxial Wires and Tubular Access

- A coaxial access wire is required to convert.
- Access needle (21- to 18-gauge, usually 21- or 18-gauge)

Tubular Access Devices

- Telescoped graduate dilation system to upsize 0.018-inch wire to 0.035-inch wire. This comes with micropuncture kit sets. It usually has a 2.5- to 3-French inner dilator and a 4- to 5-French outer dilator.
- A fascial dilator that can be passed over a 0.035-inch guidewire may be used to dilate the soft tissue and fascia. The sizes of the dilators used go up as much as the subsequent catheter being placed.
- A peel-away sheath is required for tunneled central venous catheters or implantable port-a-catheters.
- A side-port vascular sheath (usually 4- to 5-French) is required for a stable arterial or venous access when contemplating diagnostic venography or angiography with or without interventions.

Technique

Intravenous Access and Medication

- Required for moderate sedation and fluid replenishment/resuscitation
- The vascular access that is being placed may be for this purpose. The patient may have a difficult venous access and only lidocaine can be given locally until the vascular access is established.

Preaccessment Ultrasound Exam

- Determine easiest visibility of the target vessel
- Identify the target segment of the vessel
- Rule out any superficial structures in the way, especially arterial branches that can be injured by the needle on its way to the target vessel
- The traditional/common transducer orientation is transverse to the vessel.
- Differentiate between veins and adjacent arteries
  - This can be performed by pressing down on the vessels transversely using the transducer (compression) (**Figs. 10.1, 10.2, 10.3, 10.4, and 10.5**).

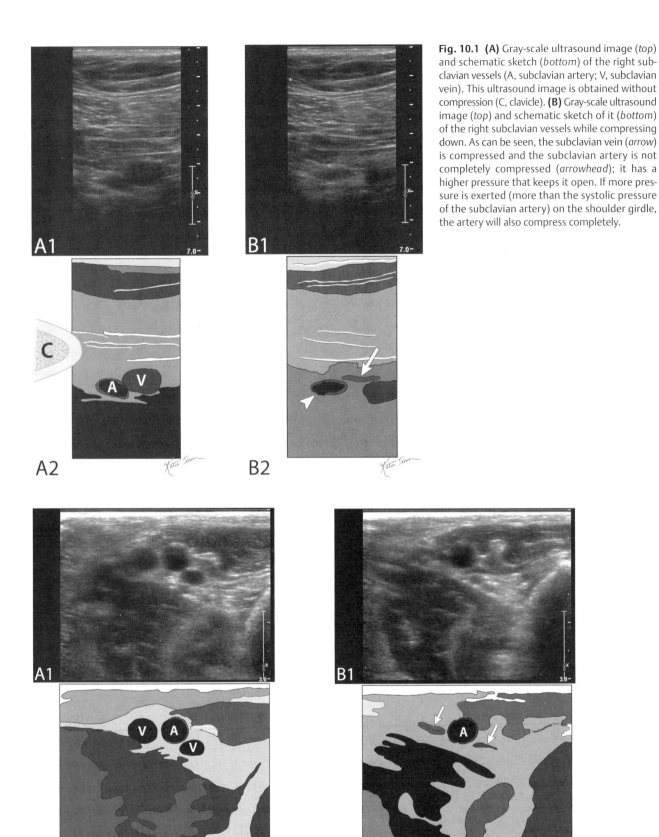

Fig. 10.1 **(A)** Gray-scale ultrasound image (*top*) and schematic sketch (*bottom*) of the right subclavian vessels (A, subclavian artery; V, subclavian vein). This ultrasound image is obtained without compression (C, clavicle). **(B)** Gray-scale ultrasound image (*top*) and schematic sketch of it (*bottom*) of the right subclavian vessels while compressing down. As can be seen, the subclavian vein (*arrow*) is compressed and the subclavian artery is not completely compressed (*arrowhead*); it has a higher pressure that keeps it open. If more pressure is exerted (more than the systolic pressure of the subclavian artery) on the shoulder girdle, the artery will also compress completely.

Fig. 10.2 **(A)** Gray-scale ultrasound image (*top*) and schematic sketch (*bottom*) of the brachial vessels (A, brachial artery; V, brachial veins). This ultrasound image is obtained without compression. **(B)** Gray-scale ultrasound image (*top*) and schematic sketch of it (*bottom*) of the brachial vessels while compressing down. As can be seen, the brachial veins (*arrows*) are compressed and the brachial artery (A) is not completely compressed; it has a higher pressure that keeps it open. If more pressure is exerted (more than the systolic pressure of the brachial artery) on the arm, the artery will also compress completely.

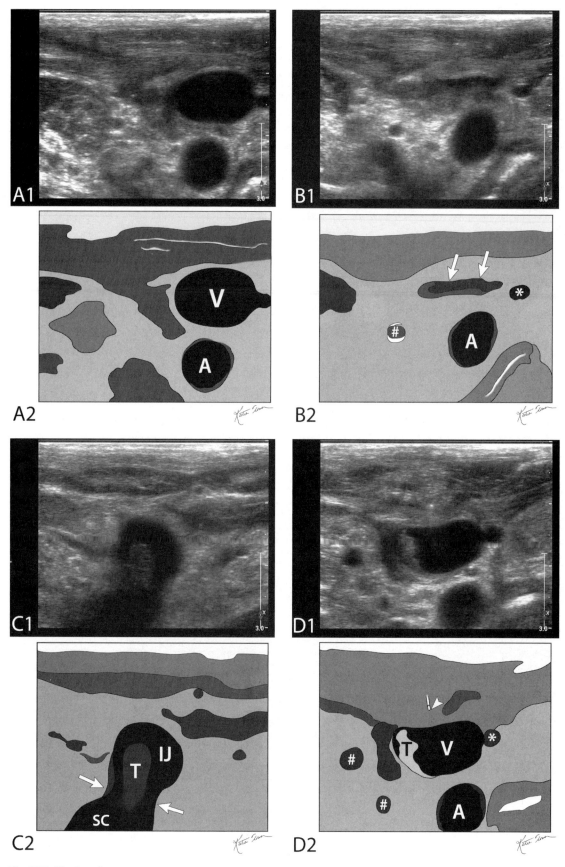

Fig. 10.3 (Continued)

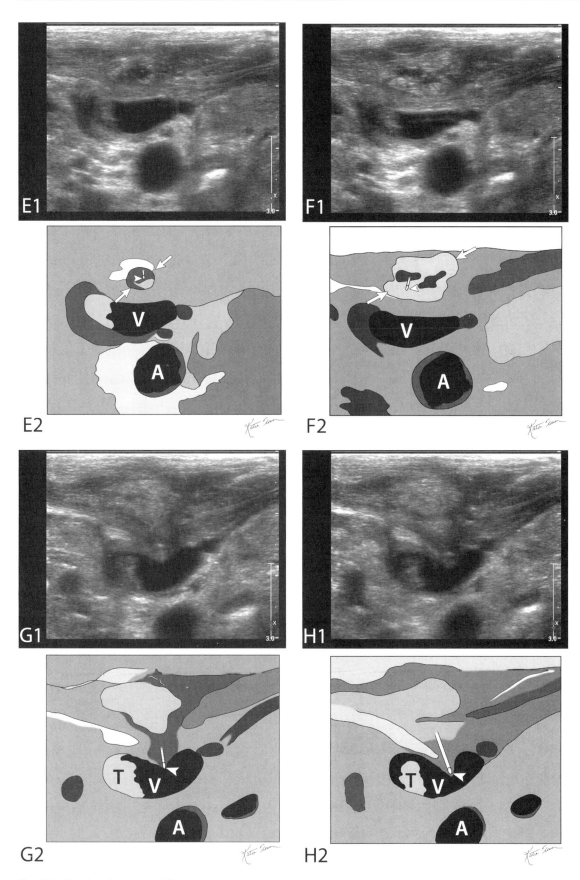

Fig. 10.3 (Continued on page 104)

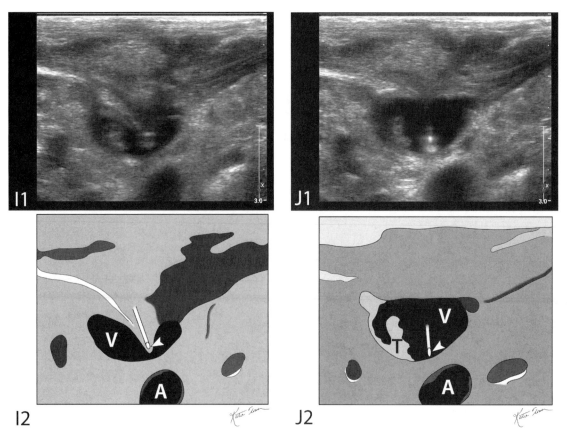

Fig. 10.3 *(Continued)* Ultrasound-guided jugular vein access. **(A)** Gray-scale ultrasound image *(top)* and schematic sketch *(bottom)* of a right jugular vein (V) and its adjacent carotid artery (A). This ultrasound image is obtained without compression. **(B)** Gray-scale ultrasound image *(top)* and schematic sketch *(bottom)* of a right jugular vein and its adjacent carotid artery (A) with compression using the linear ultrasound transducer. As can be seen, the jugular vein collapses *(arrows)* and the carotid artery is open. This helps the operator differentiate between vein and artery. Incidentally noted is a venous collateral *(asterisk)* and an external carotid artery branch (#). **(C)** Gray-scale ultrasound image *(top)* and schematic sketch *(bottom)* of a right internal jugular vein (IJ) to right subclavian vein junction (SC). The operator has paned down behind the clavicle to evaluate the distal internal jugular vein. This is where most internal jugular vein occlusions or stenoses occur. A nonocclusive thrombus (T) is seen in the jugulo-subclavian vein junction *(between arrows)*. **(D)** Gray-scale ultrasound image *(top)* and schematic sketch *(bottom)* of a right jugular vein and its adjacent carotid artery (A). A lidocaine needle is seen approaching the jugular vein *(arrowhead)*. Lidocaine has not yet been injected. Incidentally noted is a nonocclusive thrombus (T) in the jugular vein (V). Nonocclusive thrombus should not preclude jugular venous access. Also incidentally noted are venous collateral *(asterisk)* and external carotid artery arterial branches (#). **(E)** Gray-scale ultrasound image *(top)* and schematic sketch *(bottom)* of a right jugular vein (V) and its adjacent carotid artery (A). A lidocaine needle is seen near the jugular vein *(arrowhead)*. Lidocaine is being injected and forming a wheal *(between arrows)*. **(F)** Gray-scale ultrasound image *(top)* and schematic sketch *(bottom)* of a right jugular vein (V) and its adjacent carotid artery (A). The lidocaine needle tip is again seen near the jugular vein *(arrowhead)*. Lidocaine continues to be injected and creates a larger wheal *(between arrows)*. **(G)** Gray-scale ultrasound image *(top)* and schematic sketch *(bottom)* of the right jugular vein (V). A 21-gauge needle has been advanced by the operator and the needle tip is pushing down and indenting the superficial wall of the jugular vein *(arrowhead at needle tip)*. Again noted is a nonocclusive thrombus in the jugular vein. The carotid artery (A) is deeper than the jugular vein. **(H)** Gray-scale ultrasound image *(top)* and schematic sketch *(bottom)* of the right jugular vein (V). The 21-gauge needle has been advanced further by the operator and the needle tip is still pushing down and indenting the superficial wall of the jugular vein *(arrowhead at needle tip)* and has not yet impaled the superficial wall. Again noted is a nonocclusive thrombus in the jugular vein (T). The carotid artery (A) is deeper than the jugular vein. **(I)** Gray-scale ultrasound image *(top)* and schematic sketch *(bottom)* of the right jugular vein (V). The 21-gauge needle has been advanced even further by the operator and the needle tip is still pushing down and indenting the superficial wall of the jugular vein *(arrowhead at needle tip)* and has not yet impaled the superficial wall. The needle tip *(arrowhead)* has been pushed almost down to the deep wall of the jugular vein. Again noted is a nonocclusive thrombus in the jugular vein. The carotid artery (A) is deeper than the jugular vein. **(J)** Gray-scale ultrasound image *(top)* and schematic sketch *(bottom)* of the right jugular vein (V). The 21-gauge needle has been advanced deeper by the operator into the lumen of the jugular vein. The superficial wall of the jugular vein (V) has rebounded to its normal/original position once it has been impaled by the 21-gauge needle *(arrowhead at needle tip)*. The needle tip is inside the lumen adjacent to the deep wall of the jugular vein. At this time, the procedure is converted to a fluoroscopy. Again incidentally noted is the nonocclusive thrombus (T) in the jugular vein.

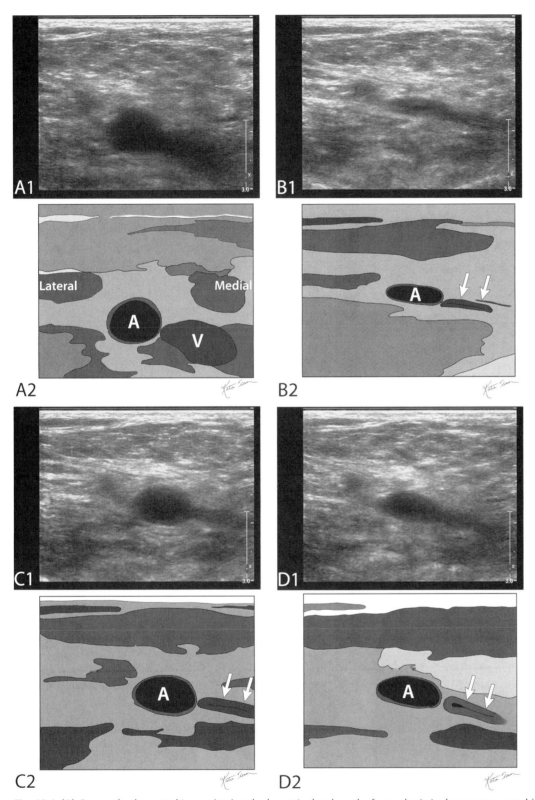

Fig. 10.4 **(A)** Gray-scale ultrasound image (*top*) and schematic sketch (*bottom*) of the right femoral vessels (A, femoral artery – seen lateral; V, femoral vein – seen medial). This ultrasound image is obtained without compression. **(B,C,D)** Gray-scale ultrasound images (*top*) and schematic sketches (*bottom*) of the right femoral vessels while compressing down. The pressure exerted is higher than the diastolic pressure and lower than the systolic pressure. **Figures 10.4B–10.4D** are in series. As can be seen, the femoral vein is always compressed (*arrows*) and the femoral artery partly compresses depending on what stage in the cardiac cycle the image was obtained. **Figure 10.4B** was obtained during diastole, **Fig. 10.4C** was in systole, and **Fig. 10.4D** was in the end of systole (starting to collapse). The pressure exerted by the ultrasound probe is high to compress the vein at all times, and is high enough to compress the artery during diastole but not in systole.

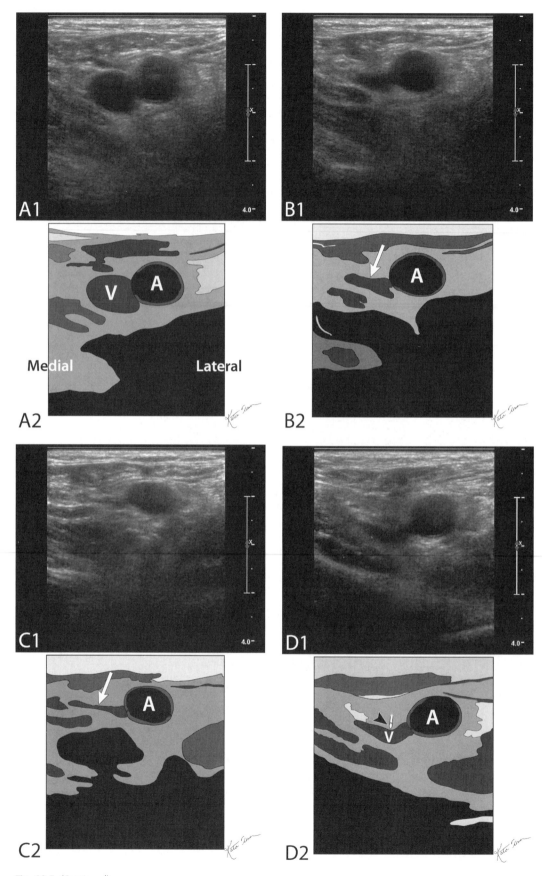

Fig. 10.5 (Continued)

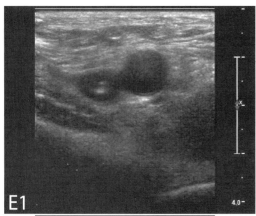

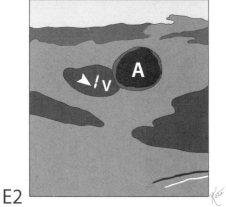

Fig. 10.5 *(Continued)* **(A)** Gray-scale ultrasound image *(top)* and schematic sketch *(bottom)* of the left femoral vessels (A, femoral artery – seen lateral; V, femoral vein – seen medial). This ultrasound image is obtained without compression. **(B,C)** Gray-scale ultrasound images *(top)* and schematic sketches *(bottom)* of the femoral vessels while compressing down. As can be seen, the femoral vein *(arrow)* is compressed and the adjacent femoral artery (A) is not completely compressed; it has a higher pressure that keeps it open. The operator has now identified/confirmed which vessel is a vein and which is an artery, and that the femoral vein is not thrombosed. Thrombosed veins do not compress. **(C)** The operator has exerted more pressure compared with **(B)**. **(D)** Gray-scale ultrasound image *(top)* and schematic sketch *(bottom)* of the left femoral vessels (A, femoral artery; V, femoral vein). A 21-gauge needle has been advanced by the operator and is now tenting the superficial wall of the femoral vein *(arrowhead at needle tip)*. **(E)** Gray-scale ultrasound image *(top)* and schematic sketch *(bottom)* of the left femoral vessels (A, femoral artery; V, femoral vein). A 21-gauge needle has been advanced by the operator into the femoral vein. The superficial wall of the femoral vein has rebounded to its normal/original position once it has been impaled by the 21-gauge needle *(arrowhead at needle tip)*. At this time, the procedure is converted to a fluoroscopy. **(F)** Fluoroscopic image of the left hip and pelvis after the 21-gauge needle has been placed into the left femoral vein *(arrowhead at needle tip)*. A radiopaque ruler is placed to aid in femoral access for an inferior vena cava filter placement. **(G)** Fluoroscopic image of the left hip and pelvis after the 21-gauge needle has been placed into the left femoral vein *(arrowhead at needle tip)*. A 0.018-inch wire has been passed coaxially through the needle. The leading tip of the wire *(arrow)* is seen projecting in the vicinity of the left iliac vein. *(Continued on page 108)*

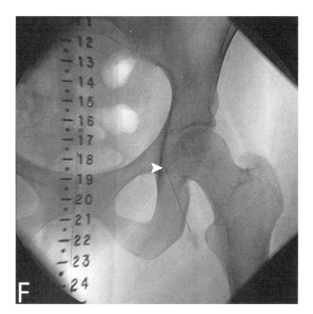

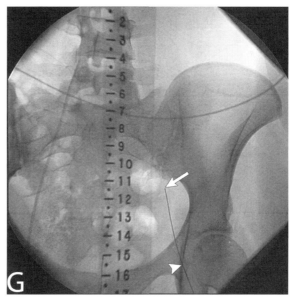

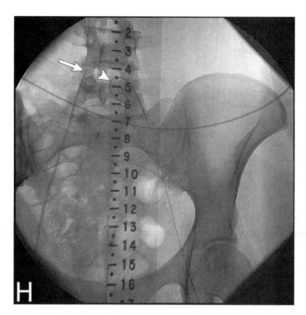

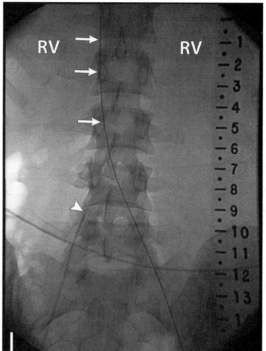

Fig. 10.5 *(Continued)* **(H)** Fluoroscopic image of the left hip and pelvis. The 0.018-inch wire has been advanced further and has curled in the specious left iliac vein (*arrowhead*). Incidentally noted is a right femoral vein central line (*arrow at central catheter tip*), which delineates the anatomy of the confluence of the common iliac veins. **(I)** Fluoroscopic image of the upper pelvis and lumbar spine. The 0.018-inch wire has been advanced further and is now in the inferior vena cava (IVC; *arrows*). Wires that go smoothly to the right side of the vertebral column are most likely venous (IVC is to the right of midline) and less likely arterial (aorta is to the left of midline). Again, incidentally noted is the right femoral vein central line (*arrow at central catheter tip*), which delineates the anatomy of the confluence of the common iliac veins. RV refers to the level of the renal veins.

- Veins compress first.
- Arteries are seen pulsating under compression exerting pressure greater than the diastolic pressure and less than the systolic pressure (**Fig. 10.4**).
- It is difficult to compress veins due to thrombosed veins, tense extremity edema, and extremity tenderness (or simply because the patient does not allow you to).
- By anatomy, for example, the femoral vein is medial to the femoral artery and the carotid is medial to the internal jugular vein (**Figs. 10.4, 10.5, 10.6, 10.7, 10.8, and 10.9**).
- Arteries usually have a discernible wall and veins have an imperceptible wall by high-frequency ultrasound.
- The operator should follow the target vessel distally as much as he or she can to assess patency. For example, it is typical to assess the patency of the internal jugular vein all the way down to the jugulo-subclavian junction. The internal jugular vein may be patent throughout its course and be occluded distally at its junction with the subclavian vein. This is typical of patients who have a history of indwelling jugular catheters.

- Manipulating the transducer is used to choose and triangulate the skin entry site, the target vessel segment, and the trajectory to achieve access of the target vessel.
- The operator must not only think of successfully "hitting" the target blood vessel, but also of hitting it at an ideal angle so that a wire can be passed through the vessel, allowing passage of the vascular sheath.

Standard Surgical Preparation and Draping

- Skin preparation/cleansing in the region that was chosen as an ultrasound imaging portal and a needle access needle portal
- Place a fenestrated drape at the chosen and prepared skin region

Local Infiltrative Analgesia Administration

- Utilizing a 21- to 23-gauge (by at least a 3.7-cm-long) infiltration needle, 1% lidocaine infiltration is performed.
- The operator uses the 21- to 23-gauge needle as a rehearsal and uses it to determine the angle of needle entry.

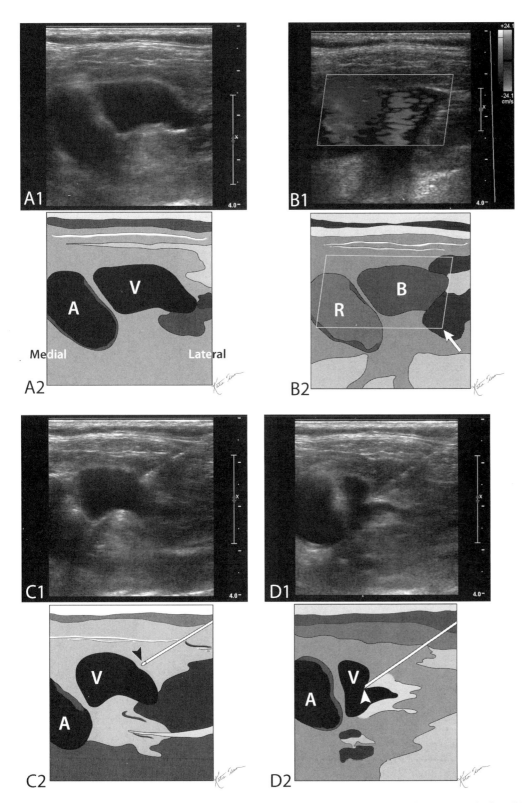

Fig. 10.6 **(A)** Gray-scale ultrasound image (*top*) and schematic sketch (*bottom*) of a right jugular vein (V) and its adjacent carotid artery (A). The carotid artery usually runs posteromedial to the jugular vein. This ultrasound image is obtained without compression. **(B)** Doppler ultrasound image (*top*) and schematic sketch (*bottom*) of the same right jugular vein (B, blue) and its adjacent carotid artery (R, red). Note is the Doppler box (*arrow*) is placed over the jugular and carotid. **(C)** Gray-scale ultrasound image (*top*) and schematic sketch (*bottom*) of the right jugular vein (V). A 21-gauge needle has been advanced by the operator so as to impale the

jugular vein from its lateral side wall (*arrowhead at needle tip*). The needle tip is seen approaching the wall. The needle is perpendicular to the long axis of the jugular vein and is along the long axis of the ultrasound transducer, which is transverse to the jugular vein (A, carotid artery). **(D)** Gray-scale ultrasound image (*top*) and schematic sketch (*bottom*) of the right jugular vein (V). The 21-gauge needle has been advanced by the operator further. The lateral wall of the jugular vein is indenting inwards as the jugular vein compresses (*arrowhead at needle tip*), which is pushing up against the jugular vein wall (A, carotid artery). *(Continued on page 110)*

109

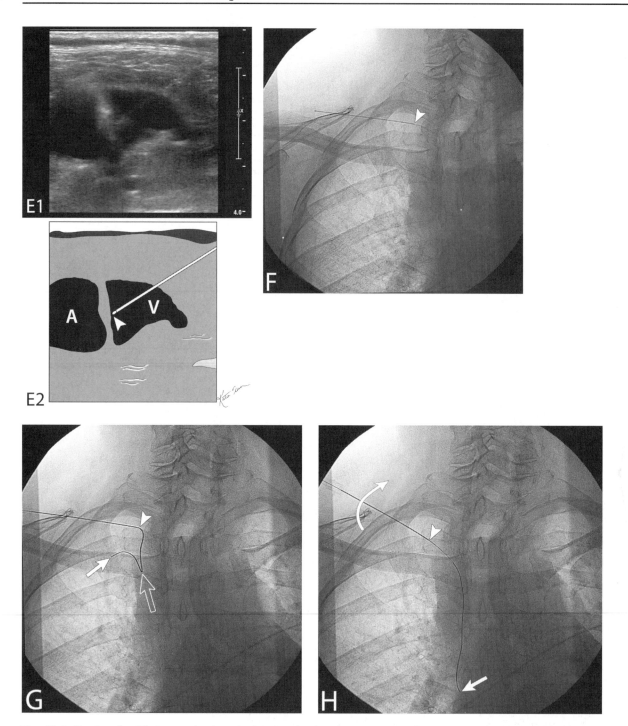

Fig. 10.6 *(Continued)* **(E)** Gray-scale ultrasound image *(top)* and schematic sketch *(bottom)* of the right jugular vein (V). The 21-gauge needle has been advanced by the operator into the lumen of the jugular vein. The lateral wall of the jugular vein has rebounded to its normal/original position once it has been impaled by the 21-gauge needle *(arrowhead at needle tip)*. The needle tip is inside the lumen adjacent to the medial wall of the jugular vein. At this time, the procedure is converted to a fluoroscopy. **(F)** Fluoroscopic image of the 21-gauge needle that has been placed into the right jugular vein **(Figs.10.6C–10.6E)** *(arrowhead at needle tip)*. As can be seen the 21-gauge needle is oriented parallel to the clavicle and both are perpendicular to the normal course of the right jugular vein. This approach has a higher likelihood of the wire pointing upwards toward the sigmoid sinus. It usually requires needle and wire manipulation. **(G)** Fluoroscopic image of the right supraclavicular fossa. A 0.018-inch wire has been passed coaxially through the 21-gauge needle *(arrowhead at needle tip)*. The tip of the wire *(solid arrow)* has caught on the subclavian vein as it joins with the jugular vein. Further wire advancement has caused the wire to buckle into the right brachiocephalic vein *(hollow arrow)*. **(H)** Fluoroscopic image of the right supraclavicular fossa. The 0.018-inch wire has been passed further through the 21-gauge needle *(arrowhead at needle tip)*. The tip of the wire *(solid arrow)* has passed through the brachiocephalic vein and is entering the superior vena cava (SVC). The *curved directional arrow* shows the operator's needle motion that aligns the needle with the wire and helps advance the wire in the desired direction, which is straight down into the SVC and right atrium.

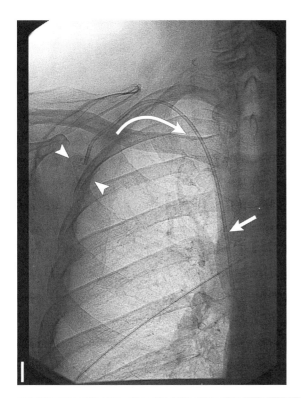

Fig. 10.6 *(Continued)* **(I)** Fluoroscopic image of the upper right chest after a port-a-catheter has been placed. The *arrowheads* point to the reservoir of the port-a-catheter and the *arrow* points to the intravenous catheter itself. The *curved arrow* signifies the smooth curvature of the port-a-catheter as it traverses from lateral to medial entering the jugular vein through it lateral wall. What helps with achieving this smooth curve is the low puncture (closest to the clavicle) and the lateral jugular wall puncture.

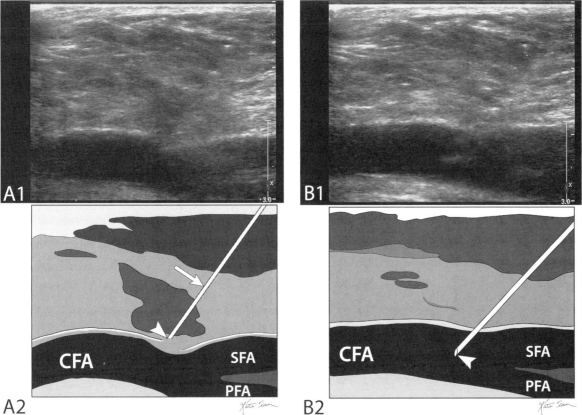

Fig. 10.7 (A) Gray-scale ultrasound image (*top*) and schematic sketch (*bottom*) of a right femoral artery. The transducer is long on the longitudinal axis of the femoral artery. This is why the entire shaft (*arrow*) of the needle is seen. Access of the femoral vessels is usually with the transducer being transverse to the artery and not long on it as in this case (this is not typical). The 18-gauge needle tip (*arrowhead*) is pushing against the common femoral artery. At this time, the operator should feel the pulsations of the common femoral artery through the needle (CFA, common femoral artery; SFA, superficial femoral artery; PFA, profunda femoral artery). **(B,C)** Gray-scale ultrasound image (*top*) and schematic sketch (*bottom*) of a right femoral artery. The transducer is still long on the longitudinal axis of the femoral artery (not typical) in **(B)** and transverse (typical) to the femoral artery in **(C)**. *(Continued on page 112)*

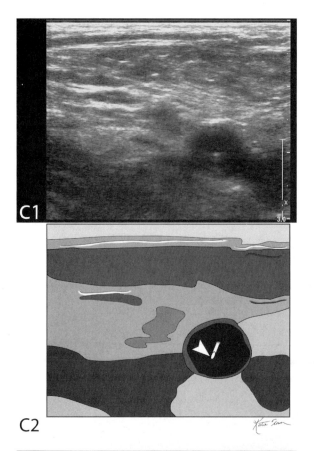

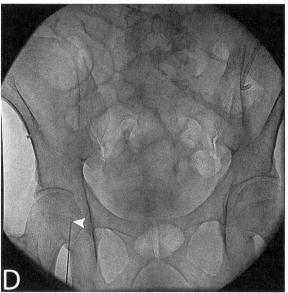

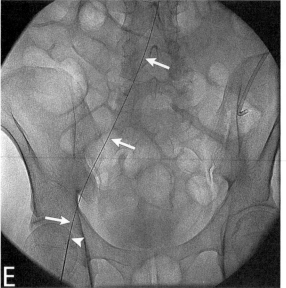

Fig. 10.7 *(Continued)* Access of the femoral vessels is usually with the transducer being transverse to the artery and not long on it as in this case (this is not typical). The 18-gauge needle tip *(arrowhead)* has impaled the femoral artery and is now in the common femoral artery lumen *(arrowhead)*. At this time, the procedure is converted to fluoroscopic guidance (CFA, common femoral artery; SFA, superficial femoral artery; PFA, profunda femoral artery). **(D)** Fluoroscopic image of the 18-gauge needle that has been placed into the right femoral artery *(arrowhead at needle tip)*. As can be seen, the 18-gauge needle shaft is oriented parallel to the femoral shaft and along the long axis of the femoral artery. The tip of the needle projects over the medial aspect of the femoral head, which is the typical fluoroscopic/radiographic landmark signifying the location of the right common femoral artery. **(E)** Fluoroscopic image of the right hip over the 18-gauge needle. A 0.035-inch wire *(arrows)* has been passed coaxially through the 18-gauge needle *(arrowhead at needle tip)*.

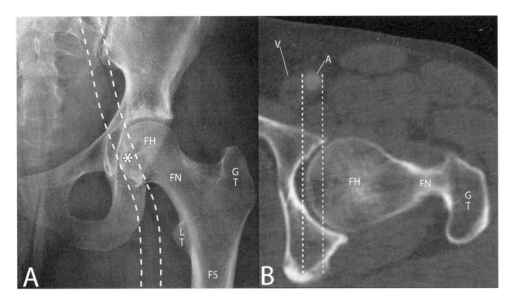

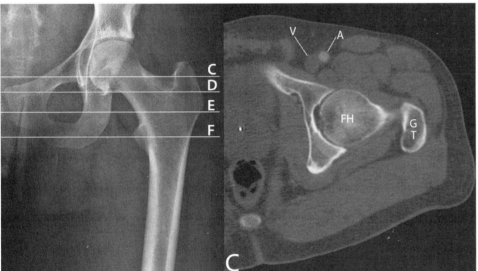

Fig. 10.8 **(A)** Radiograph of the left hip. The dotted lines represent the course of the main arterial flow (from proximal to distal: external iliac artery, common femoral artery, and superficial femoral artery) of the left lower extremity. The asterisk marks the level of the common femoral artery (FH, femoral head; FN, femoral neck; GT, greater trochanter; LT, lesser trochanter; FS, femoral shaft). **(B)** Computed tomography (CT) of the left hip. The dotted lines help show how the projection of the common femoral artery (A) at the level of the femoral head (*asterisk in* **Fig. 10.8A**) projects over the medial aspect of the femoral artery on radiographs. The femoral vein (V) is medial to the femoral artery (A) (FH, femoral head; FN, femoral neck; GT, greater trochanter). **(C)** CT of the left hip. It should be compared with the key radiograph; the horizontal line (C) represents the axial level. Again noted is the femoral artery (A) projecting over the medial aspect of the femoral artery on radiographs. The femoral vein (V) is medial to the femoral artery (A) (FH, femoral head; GT, greater trochanter).   *(Continued on page 114)*

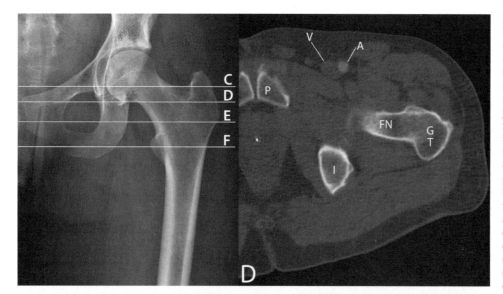

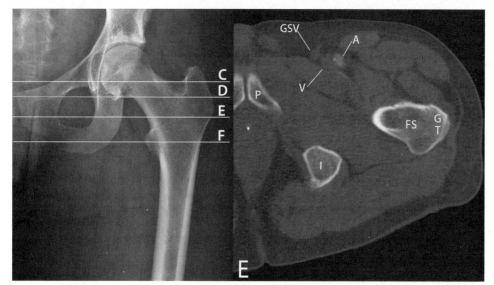

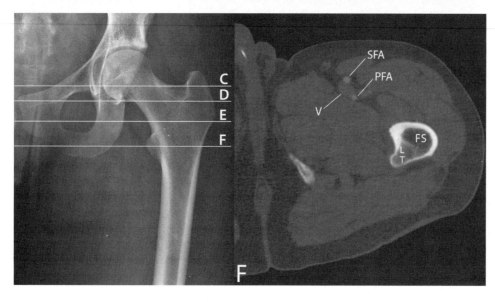

Fig. 10.8 *(Continued)* **(D)** CT of the left hip. It should be compared with the key radiograph; the horizontal line (D) represents the axial level. The axial level is at the level of the lowermost aspect of the femoral artery. Again noted is the femoral artery (A) projecting over the medial aspect of the femoral artery on radiographs. The femoral vein (V) is medial to the femoral artery (A) (FN, femoral neck; GT, greater trochanter; I, ischium; P, pubis). **(E)** CT of the left hip. It should be compared with the key radiograph; the horizontal line (E) represents the axial level. The axial level is at the level of the base of the femoral neck and greater trochanter. The femoral artery (A) is still lateral to the femoral vein (V), but it is starting to "slip" to become superficial to the femoral vein and becoming the superficial femoral artery. The greater saphenous vein (GSV) is approaching the femoral vein anteromedially in this axial image (FS, femoral shaft; GT, greater trochanter; I, ischium; P, pubis). **(F)** CT of the left hip. It should be compared with the key radiograph; the horizontal line (F) represents the axial level. The axial level is at the level of the lesser trochanter (LT). The femoral vein (V) sits between the superficial femoral artery (SFA) and the deeper profunda femoris artery (PFA). The vein is now deeper to the main lower extremity flow (SFA, superficial femoral artery; FS, femoral shaft).

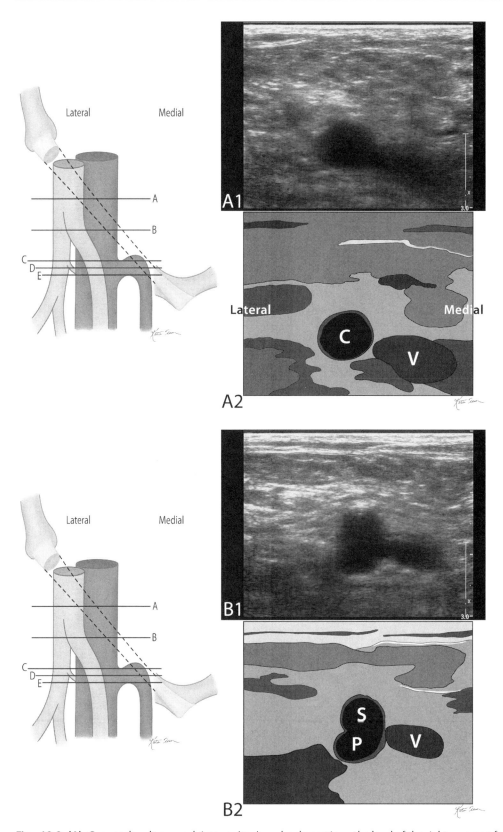

Fig. 10.9 (A) Gray-scale ultrasound image (*top*) and schematic sketch (*bottom*) of the right femoral vessels at the level of the right common femoral artery (C). Medial to the common femoral artery is the femoral vein (V). **Fig. 10.9 (B)** Gray-scale ultrasound image (*top*) and schematic sketch (*bottom*) of the right femoral vessels just below the level of the right common femoral artery in **Fig. 10.9A**. This is just at the level of the bifurcation of the common femoral artery into the superficial femoral artery (S) and the profunda femoris artery (P). Medial to the common femoral artery is the femoral vein (V).   *(Continued on page 116)*

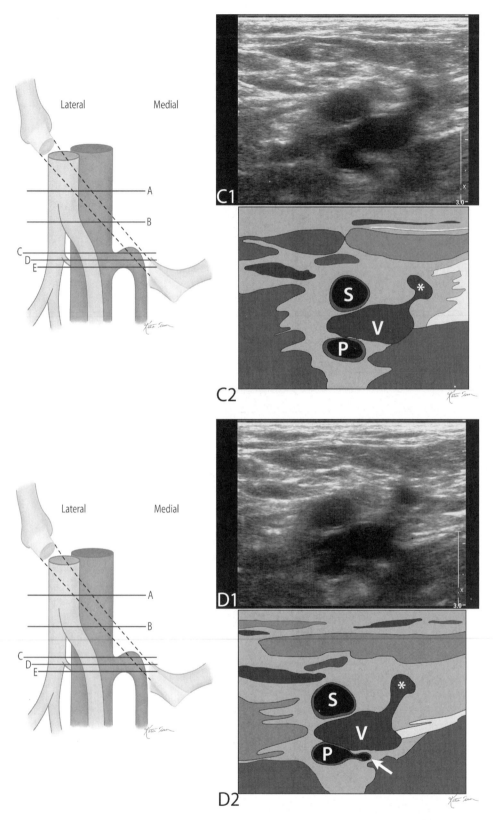

Fig. 10.9 *(Continued)* **(C)** Gray-scale ultrasound image *(top)* and schematic sketch *(bottom)* of the right femoral vessels just below the level of **Fig. 10.9B**. The common femoral artery has split completely into the superficial femoral artery (S) and the profunda femoris artery (P). The femoral vein (V) is now positioned in between the superficial femoral artery and the profunda femoris. The greater saphenous vein *(asterisk)* is entering the femoral vein at this level. **(D)** Gray-scale ultrasound image *(top)* and schematic sketch *(bottom)* of the right femoral vessels just below the level of **Fig. 10.9C**. The common femoral artery has split completely into the superficial femoral artery (S) and the profunda femoris artery (P). The femoral vein (V) is still positioned in-between the superficial femoral artery and the profunda femoris. The greater saphenous vein *(asterisk)* is entering the femoral vein at this level. In **Fig. 10.9D**, a small arterial branch *(arrow)* is seen coming off the profunda femoris artery.

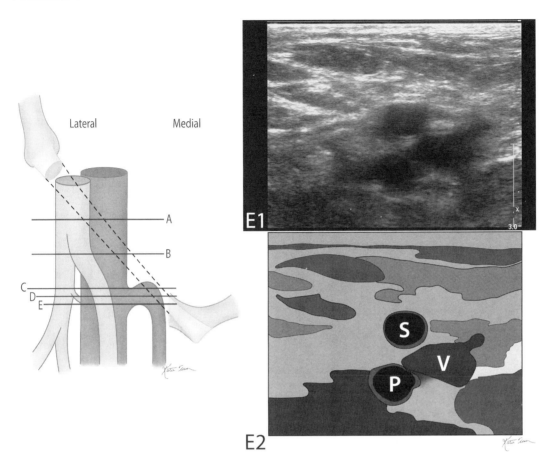

Fig. 10.9 *(Continued)* **(E)** Gray-scale ultrasound image *(top)* and schematic sketch *(bottom)* of the right femoral vessels just below the level of **Fig. 10.9D**. The common femoral artery has split completely into the superficial femoral artery (S) and the profunda femoris artery (P).

Technical aspects regarding entry to the vessel depends on the type and location of the vessel. Hence, each vessel will be discussed separately. All the technical descriptions described below are modifications to a technique termed the modified Seldinger technique.

Ultrasound-Guided Sharp Access and Fluoroscopic-Guided Wire and Tube/Catheter Access: Upper Extremity Veins

- It is important to identify veins for adjacent arteries when attempting to access upper extremity veins by ultrasound guidance. Upper extremity arteries are probably the most difficult to differentiate for adjacent veins especially in
  - Infants and small children
  - Patients with ventricular-assisted devices (VAD) where there is little pulse pressure
- A 21-gauge beveled tip access needle is passed free hand under real-time ultrasound guidance.

- The transducer is usually placed transverse to target vein segment (transverse to the long axis of the target vein segment).
- Panning the transducer down as the needle is advanced allows the operator to watch the needle tip as it is advanced. Experienced operators can triangulate the transducer probe angle, the needle trajectory, and the target vascular segment, and then await the needle tip at the vascular wall as the needle is advanced.
- The needle may often be seen tenting (indenting) the superficial wall of the arm veins inwards toward the lumen. The needle is not in until it is seen in the jugular lumen and the impaled superficial wall has rebounded to its normal position.
- Once the needle tip is seen in the jugular vein lumen, the 0.018 wire is placed into the needle.
  - Some operators aspirate from the needle to confirm that the needle is in the vein. This is not unreasonable when dealing with small veins and especially if the operator is not sure whether he/she has successfully accessed the vein by imaging.

- Once the needle tip is in the vein lumen, and the wire has been placed through its hub, the procedure is converted to real-time fluoroscopy.
- The wire is advanced gently without resistance under fluoroscopy into the subclavian vein.
- Once the wire is in the subclavian vein, an incision is made utilizing an 11-blade scalpel usually by a 1- to 2-mm-depth stab of the 11-blade. The blade incision is made over the needle so not to damage the wire.
- A 4- to 5-French transitional sheath (micropuncture dilator) is passed over the wire while holding counter-tension on the wire so not to kink the wire.
- Contrast does not need to be injected to perform a venogram unless there is trouble passing the wire centrally in the vena cava.
  - Venography is not usually performed by using the access needle. This way carries a high risk of losing access and creating a dissecting contrast stain/infiltrate, which may complicate subsequent access attempts.
  - Venography is better performed using a 2.5- to 3-French "inner" micropuncture sheath, which is placed over the same 0.018-inch wire that cannot be advanced centrally.
- Details of PICC and regular transducer sheath placement and management will not be included in this chapter.

Ultrasound-Guided Sharp Access and Fluoroscopic-Guided Wire and Tube/Catheter Access: Subclavian Vein

- A 21-gauge beveled tip access needle is passed free hand under real-time ultrasound guidance.
  - Some operators like using an ultrasound guide when accessing this vein.
  - This vein may be the more difficult of veins to access under imaging.
  - The target segment may not be too lateral or too medial. The ideal subclavian vein segment lies just over the outer/lateral edge (one third) of the first rib.
    - Too medial: The catheter would pass through the scalene muscles/ligaments and cause pain and pinching of the catheter with the motion of the patient's shoulder girdle ("pinch-off syndrome"). Pinch-off syndrome causes kinking compression of the catheter lumen and poor catheter flow. With time, pinch-off syndrome may cause a break of the catheter due to material fatigue (catheter material wear-and-tear).
    - Too lateral: The catheter would come out of the skin closer to the armpit/axilla leading to (1) a higher risk of infection, (2) patient discomfort, and (3) difficulty (little room) for catheter tunneling if a tunneled catheter is the intention.

- The transducer is usually placed transverse to the subclavian vein (transverse to the long axis of the subclavian vein).
- Panning the transducer down as the needle is advanced allows the operator to watch the needle tip as it is advanced. Experienced operators can triangulate the transducer probe angle, the needle trajectory, and the target vascular segment, and then await the needle tip at the vascular wall as the needle is advanced.
- The needle may hit the top surface of the first rib. The operator should make sure that the needle tip has adequately impaled the subclavian vein.
- Aspirating from the needle to confirm that the needle is in the vein is advised.
  - This is a vein that is not easily seen, not as superficial and not as collapsible as other veins.
  - Connecting the beveled 21-gauge micropuncture kit to a syringe for aspiration through a connector tube allows aspiration to be performed by an assistant while giving a free range of motion to the needle in the primary operator's hand.
- Once the needle tip is in the vein lumen, and the wire has been placed through its hub, the procedure is converted to real-time fluoroscopy.
- The wire is advanced gently under fluoroscopy into the superior vena cava (SVC) and without resistance.
- If the wire points upwards toward the head:
  - The wire should be pulled back and the needle manipulated so that it points downward and the bevel points downward as well, and then the wire is advanced.
  - Sometimes the exact opposite works. The bevel and needle tip are pointed upward and the 0.018-inch wire is advanced so that it hits the cephalad wall of the subclavian vein near its junction with the jugular vein and "bounces off" that wall to enter the vena cava.
- Once the wire is in the SVC, an incision is made utilizing an 11-blade scalpel usually by a 3-mm-depth stab of the 11-blade. The blade incision is made over the needle so not to damage the wire.
- A 4- to 5-French transitional sheath (micropuncture dilator) is passed over the wire while holding counter-tension on the wire so not to kink the wire. This allows the operator to pass a more robust wire.
  - The wire required is usually 0.035 inch for port-a-catheter and tunneled central catheter peel-away sheaths.
  - Low flow/small-bore catheters (5- to 8-French) may need 0.021- to 0.025-inch wires.
- Contrast does not need to be injected to perform a venogram unless there is trouble passing the wire centrally in the vena cava.

- Venography is not usually performed by using the access needle. This way caries a high risk of losing access and creating a dissecting contrast stain/infiltrate that may complicate subsequent access attempts.
- Venography is better performed using a 2.5- to 3-French "inner" micropuncture sheath that is placed over the same 0.018-inch wire that cannot be advanced centrally.
- Details of port-a-catheter and tunneled central catheters or transjugular procedures will not be discussed further in this chapter.

Ultrasound-Guided Sharp Access and Fluoroscopic-Guided Wire and Tube/Catheter Access: Jugular Vein

- A 21-gauge beveled tip access needle is passed free hand under real-time ultrasound guidance (**Figs. 10.3, 10.6, and 10.10**).
- The transducer is usually placed transverse to the jugular vein (transverse to the long axis of the jugular vein).
- The needle can be passed along (parallel) the long axis of the jugular vein (transverse to the transducer) (**Figs. 10.3 and 10.10**) or the needle can be passed perpendicular to the long axis of the jugular vein (**Fig. 10.6**).

- The former is most common (**Figs. 10.3 and 10.10**).
- The latter is resorted to by some authors when placing tunneled central catheters/port-a-catheters in morbidly obese patients (**Fig. 10.6**).
- The latter allows the needle access to the vein to be as close to the clavicle as possible. In addition, it helps form a smooth transition curve of the catheter over the clavicle between the tunneled part of the catheter and the venous part of the catheter.
- The problem with the latter is that the lateral wall approach has a higher risk of having the subsequent wire advancement going up toward the head instead of the wire going down centrally into the superior vena cava (see below) (**Figs. 10.11 and 10.12**).
- Panning the transducer down as the needle is advanced allows the operator to watch the needle tip as it is advanced. Experienced operators can triangulate the transducer probe angle, the needle trajectory, and the target vascular segment, and then await the needle tip at the vascular wall as the needle is advanced.
- The needle may be seen tenting (indenting) the superficial wall of the jugular vein inwards toward the lumen (**Figs. 10.3, 10.6, and 10.10**). The needle is not in until it is seen in the jugular lumen and the impaled superficial

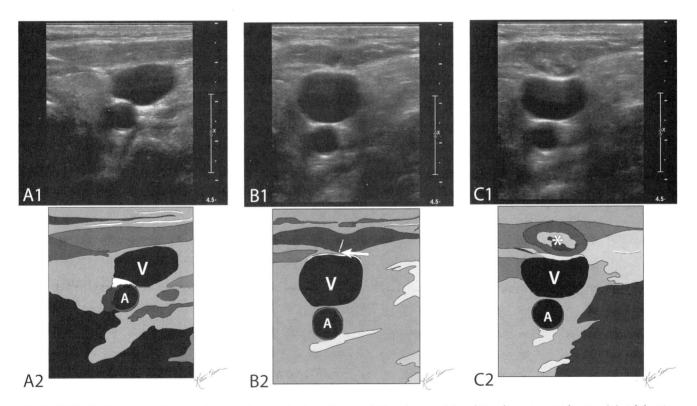

Fig. 10.10 (A,B) Gray-scale ultrasound image (*top*) and schematic sketch (*bottom*) of a right jugular vein (V) and its adjacent carotid artery (A). This ultrasound image is obtained without compression. **(C)** Gray-scale ultrasound image (*top*) and schematic sketch (*bottom*) of a right jugular vein (V) and its adjacent carotid artery (A). A lidocaine needle has been advanced and lidocaine is being injected and forming a wheal (*asterisk*). (Continued on page 120)

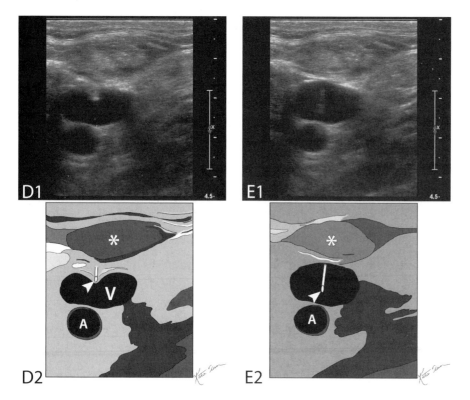

Fig. 10.10 *(Continued)* **(D)** Gray-scale ultrasound image *(top)* and schematic sketch *(bottom)* of the right jugular vein (V). A 21-gauge needle has been advanced by the operator and the needle tip is pushing down and indenting the superficial wall of the jugular vein *(arrowhead at needle tip)*. The carotid artery (A) is deeper than the jugular vein. The asterisk signifies the overlying lidocaine wheal. **(E)** Gray-scale ultrasound image *(top)* and schematic sketch *(bottom)* of the right jugular vein (V). The 21-gauge needle has been advanced deeper by the operator into the lumen of the jugular vein. The superficial wall of the jugular vein (V) has rebounded to its normal/original position once it has been impaled by the 21-gauge needle *(arrowhead at needle tip)*. At this time, the procedure is converted to a fluoroscopy. The asterisk signifies the overlying lidocaine wheal.

wall has rebounded to its normal position (**Figs. 10.3, 10.6, and 10.10**).

- Once the needle tip is seen in the jugular vein lumen, the 0.018 wire is placed into the needle.
- Some operators aspirate from the needle to confirm that the needle is in the vein. This is unnecessary because the operator has seen the needle tip in the lumen.
    ○ Aspiration is done when the operator is unsure of needle entry or his or her imaging of the needle tip entry is unclear.
    ○ Aspiration adds manipulation to the needle and the operator may inadvertently lose access.
- Once the needle tip is in the vein lumen, and the wire has been placed through its hub, the procedure is converted to real-time fluoroscopy.
- The wire is advanced gently under fluoroscopy into the SVC and without resistance.
- If the wire points upward toward the head:
    ○ This is typical of a side wall access (see above) (**Figs. 10.6, 10.11, and 10.12**)
    ○ The wire should be pulled back and the needle manipulated so that its hub is more vertical (closer to patient's ear) (**Figs. 10.11 and 10.12**), then the wire is advanced.
- Once the wire is in the SVC, an incision is made utilizing an 11-blade scalpel usually by a 3-mm-depth stab of the 11-blade. The blade incision is made over the needle so not to damage the wire.
- A 4- to 5-French transitional sheath (micropuncture dilator) is passed over the wire while holding countertension on the wire so not to kink the wire. This allows the operator to pass a more robust wire.
    ○ The wire required is usually 0.035 inch for port-a-catheter and tunneled central catheter peel-away sheaths.
    ○ Low flow/small-bore catheters (5- to 8-French) may need 0.021- to 0.025-inch wires.
- Contrast does not need to be injected to perform a venogram unless there is trouble passing the wire centrally in the vena cava.
    ○ Venography is not usually performed by using the access needle. This way carries a high risk of losing access and creating a dissecting contrast stain/infiltrate, which may complicate subsequent access attempts.

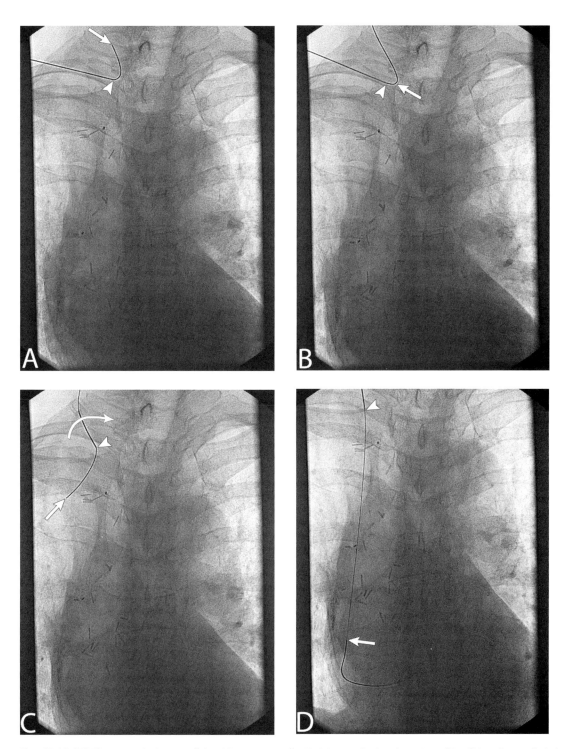

Fig. 10.11 (A) Fluoroscopic image of the 21-gauge needle that has been placed into the right jugular vein via its lateral wall (*arrowhead at needle tip*). As can be seen, the 21-gauge needle is oriented parallel to the clavicle and both are perpendicular to the normal course of the right jugular vein. This approach has a higher likelihood of the wire pointing upwards toward the sigmoid sinus. The 0.018-inch wire (*arrow*) has been passed and is actually heading cephalad toward the sigmoid sinus. It usually requires needle and wire manipulation. **(B)** Fluoroscopic image of the 21-gauge needle that has been placed into the right jugular vein via its lateral wall (*arrowhead at needle tip*). As can be seen, the 21-gauge needle is still oriented parallel to the clavicle and perpendicular to the normal course of the right jugular vein. The 0.018-inch wire has been passed further and has curved off (*arrow*) the medial wall of the jugular vein and is still heading cephalad toward the sigmoid sinus. It usually requires needle and wire manipulation. **(C)** Fluoroscopic image of the 21-gauge needle that has been maneuvered as depicted by the *curved directional arrow* so that the needle is parallel to the jugular vein and is in line with the desired direction of the 0.018-inch wire (which is straight down) (*arrowhead at needle tip*). The wire has been pulled back and redirected downward into the right brachiocephalic vein (*straight arrow*). **(D)** Fluoroscopic image of the 21-gauge needle that has been maneuvered so that the needle is parallel to the jugular vein and is in line with the desired direction of the 0.018-inch wire (which is straight down) (*arrowhead at needle tip*). The wire has been pushed downward into the right atrium (*arrow at superior vena cava junction with the right atrium*).

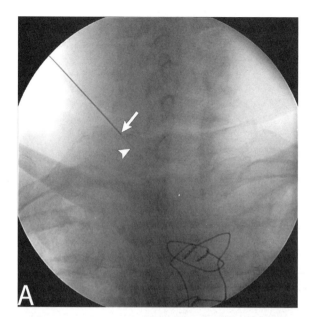

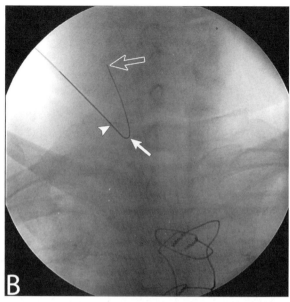

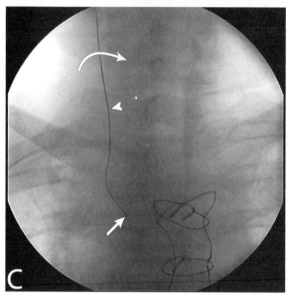

Fig. 10.12 (A) Fluoroscopic image of the 21-gauge needle that has been placed into the right jugular vein (*arrowhead at needle tip*). The 0.018-inch wire (*arrow at leading tip*) is still in the needle. **(B)** Fluoroscopic image of the 21-gauge needle. The 0.018-inch wire curves inside the jugular lumen, probably off the medial wall of the jugular vein (*solid arrow and arrowhead at needle tip*). The wire is heading cephalad (*hollow arrow*). **(C)** Fluoroscopic image of the 21-gauge needle that has been maneuvered as depicted by the *curved directional arrow* so that the needle is parallel to the jugular vein and is in line with the desired direction of the 0.018-inch wire (which is straight down) (*arrowhead at needle tip*). The wire has been pulled back and redirected downward into the right brachiocephalic vein (*straight arrow*).

- ○ Venography is better performed using a 2.5- to 3-French "inner" micropuncture sheath, which is placed over the same 0.018-inch wire that cannot be advanced centrally.
- • Details of port-a-catheter and tunneled central catheters or transjugular procedures will not be discussed further in this chapter.

Ultrasound-Guided Sharp Access and Fluoroscopic-Guided Wire and Tube/Catheter Access: Femoral Vein

- • Utilizing fluoroscopy the level of the femoral vein access is chosen to be at the level of the femoral head (**Figs. 10.8 and 10.9**).

- ○ This allows the operator
  - • To achieve hemostasis by compressing the femoral vein against a noncompliant/hard structure (femoral head)
  - • To avoid the femoral artery – at the femoral head the artery and vein are next to one another. The femoral artery runs deep to the femoral vein higher up (see the section below on femoral artery access for anatomy details) (**Figs. 10.8 and 10.9**).
- ○ If fluoroscopy is not available, puncture the femoral vein where it runs adjacent to the common femoral before it bifurcates into the profunda femoris and the superficial femoral artery.
- • A 21- to 18-gauge single-wall puncture beveled tip access needle is passed free hand under real-time ultrasound guidance.

- The transducer is usually placed transverse to the femoral vein (transverse to the long axis of the femoral vein) (**Fig. 10.5**).
- Having the patient bear down (Valsalva maneuver) engorges the femoral vein and increases its blood pressure.
  - This enlarges the target segment of the femoral vein. A bigger target is easier to hit, which is more important with nonimage-guided femoral vein access.
  - It adds structure (increase engorged pressure) to the vein and makes it easier to impale with the needle – not just tenting/indenting its more superficial wall.
- If intending advanced transfemoral interventions with large sheaths (filters, large vein stents, etc.), the operator should be cognizant to come in at an obtuse angle (cephalad) so that subsequent introductory sheaths do not kink at the vein entry site and prostheses (filters or stents) do not jam inside their introductory sheaths.
- Panning the transducer down as the needle is advanced allows the operator to watch the needle tip as it is advanced. Experienced operators can triangulate the transducer probe angle, the needle trajectory, and the target vascular segment, and then await the needle tip at the vascular wall as the needle is advanced.
- The needle may be seen tenting (indenting) the superficial wall of the femoral vein inwards toward the lumen. The needle is not in until it is seen in the femoral vein lumen and the impaled superficial wall has rebounded to its normal position (**Fig. 10.5**).
- Once the needle tip is seen in the femoral vein lumen, the 0.018-inch wire is placed into the 21-gauge needle or a 0.035-inch wire is advanced through the 18-gauge needle.
- Some operators aspirate from the needle to confirm that the needle is in the vein. This is unnecessary because the operator has seen the needle tip in the lumen.
  - Aspiration is done when the operator is unsure of needle entry or his or her imaging of the needle tip entry is unclear.
  - Aspiration adds manipulation to the needle and the operator may inadvertently lose access.
- Once the needle tip is in the vein lumen, and the wire has been placed through its hub, the procedure is converted to real-time fluoroscopy (**Fig. 10.5**).
- The wire is advanced gently under fluoroscopy into the inferior vena cava (IVC) and without resistance. The wire should project over the right of the vertebral column (**Fig. 10.5**).
- Once the wire is in the IVC, an incision is made utilizing an 11-blade scalpel usually by a 3-mm-depth stab of the 11-blade. The blade incision is made over the needle so not to damage the wire.

- In cases of using a 0.018-inch access needle, a 4- to 5-French transitional sheath (micropuncture dilator) is passed over the wire while holding counter-tension on the wire so not to kink the wire. This allows the operator to pass a more robust wire.
- Contrast does not need to be injected to perform a venogram unless there is trouble passing the wire centrally in the vena cava.
  - Venography is not usually performed by using the access needle. This way carries a high risk of losing access and creating a dissecting contrast stain/infiltrate, which may complicate subsequent access attempts.
  - Venography is better performed using a 4- to 5-French micropuncture sheath, which is placed over the same 0.018-inch wire that cannot be advanced centrally.
- Details of tunneled central catheters or transfemoral procedures will not be discussed further in this chapter.

Ultrasound-Guided Sharp Access and Fluoroscopic-Guided Wire and Tube/Catheter Access: Popliteal or Tibial Veins

- The indication for accessing the popliteal vein is for the treatment of acute or chronic deep venous thrombosis. The intent is venous thrombolysis/clot removal. This requires certain objectives for success.
  - Establish/clear up inflow. This requires the operator to access proximal to the clot in nonthrombosed veins. As a result, if the popliteal vein is thrombosed, the operator may want to access more proximally (proximal to flow) into the hopefully nonthrombosed tibial veins.
  - Mechanical and pharmaceutical thrombolysis
  - Resolving outflow stenosis or chronic thrombus using balloon venoplasty ± stent placement
- A 21-gauge single-wall puncture beveled tip access needle is passed free hand under real-time ultrasound guidance.
- The transducer is usually placed transverse to the popliteal vein (transverse to the long axis of the vein).
- Large vascular sheaths (for filters, large vein stents, mechanical thrombectomy devices, etc.) are required. In addition, these sheaths will be dwelling for 24–72 hours and a sharp angle may be uncomfortable for the patient. Hence, the operator should come in at an obtuse angle (cephalad) so that subsequent introductory sheaths do not kink at the vein entry site and prostheses (filters or stents) do not jam inside their introductory sheaths.
- The needle may be seen tenting (indenting) the superficial wall of the popliteal vein inwards toward the lumen. The needle is not in until it is seen in the

femoral vein lumen and the impaled superficial wall has rebounded to its normal position.

- Once the needle tip is seen in the femoral vein lumen, the 0.018-inch wire is placed into the 21-gauge needle.
- Once the needle tip is in the vein lumen, and the wire has been placed through its hub, the procedure is converted to real-time fluoroscopy.
- The wire is advanced gently under fluoroscopy into the femoral vein without resistance.
- Once the wire is in the femoral vein, an incision is made utilizing an11-blade scalpel usually by a 3-mm-depth stab of the 11-blade. The blade incision is made over the needle so not to damage the wire.
- A 4- to 5-French transitional sheath (micropuncture dilator) is passed over the wire while holding counter-tension on the wire so not to kink the wire. This allows the operator to pass a more robust wire.
- Contrast is then injected to perform a venogram for the following purposes:
  ○ Confirm adequate placement of the access in the popliteal or tibial vein(s)
  ○ Assess the age and extent of the clot
  ○ Obtain a baseline venogram to compare after thrombolysis
- Details of venous thrombolysis from this point in the procedure onward will not be included in this chapter.

Ultrasound-Guided Sharp Access and Fluoroscopic-Guided Wire and Tube/Catheter Access: Upper Extremity (Radial, Brachial, and Axillary) Arteries

- It is important to identify veins for adjacent arteries when attempting to access upper extremity veins by ultrasound guidance. Upper extremity arteries are probably the most difficult to differentiate for adjacent veins especially in
  ○ Infants and small children
  ○ Patients with VADs where there is little pulse pressure.
- A 21-gauge beveled tip access needle is passed free hand under real-time ultrasound guidance.
- The transducer is usually placed transverse to a small artery (transverse to the long axis of the artery).
- Panning the transducer down as the needle is advanced allows the operator to watch the needle tip as it is advanced. Experienced operators can triangulate the transducer probe angle, the needle trajectory, and the target vascular segment, and then await the needle tip at the vascular wall as the needle is advanced.
- Tenting of the wall is usually not encountered in arteries.
- Once the needle tip is seen in the artery lumen, an immediate arterial blood return is seen. It should not

be seen pulsating out of the needle hub in small arteries and a 21-gauge needle.

- On blood return, the 0.018-inch wire is placed into the needle.
- At this time, the procedure is converted to real-time fluoroscopy.
- The wire is advanced gently under fluoroscopy without resistance.
- Once the wire is secure in the artery, an incision is made utilizing an11-blade scalpel, usually by a 3-mm-depth stab of the 11-blade.
  ○ The blade incision is made over the needle so not to damage the wire.
  ○ It should not be deep enough to injure the underlying artery.
  ○ If the artery is superficial, the needle can be pulled and torqued to raise (tent) the skin away from the underlying artery.
  ○ A 4- to 5-French transitional sheath (micropuncture dilator) is passed over the wire while holding counter-tension on the wire so not to kink the wire.

Ultrasound-Guided Sharp Access and Fluoroscopic-Guided Wire and Tube/Catheter Access: Femoral Artery

- The following is referred to as the modified Seldinger technique (**Fig. 10.7**).
- Utilizing fluoroscopy, the level of the femoral artery access is chosen to be at the level of the femoral head (**Figs. 10.8 and 10.9**).
  ○ This allows the operator
    - To achieve hemostasis by compressing the femoral artery against a noncompliant/hard structure (femoral head) (**Figs. 10.8 and 10.9**).
    - To avoid the femoral vein – at the level of femoral head the artery and vein are next to one another. The femoral artery runs deep to the femoral vein higher up (**Figs. 10.8 and 10.9**).
  ○ If fluoroscopy is not available, puncture the femoral artery where it runs adjacent to the femoral vein before the common femoral artery bifurcates into the profunda femoris and the superficial femoral artery (**Figs. 10.8 and 10.9**).
- A 21- to 18-gauge single-wall puncture beveled tip access needle is passed free hand under real-time ultrasound guidance. I prefer using an 18-gauge needle and a 0.035-inch wire.
- The transducer is usually placed transverse to the femoral artery (transverse to the long axis of the femoral artery) (**Fig. 10.7**).
- Panning the transducer down as the needle is advanced allows the operator to watch the needle tip as it is advanced. Experienced operators can triangulate

the transducer probe angle, the needle trajectory, and the target vascular segment, and then await the needle tip at the vascular wall as the needle is advanced (**Fig. 10.7**).

- Tenting of the wall is usually not encountered in arteries.
- Once the needle tip is seen in the artery lumen, an immediate arterial blood return is seen. Blood may be seen pulsating at but not out of the needle hub when using a 21-gauge needle. However, it should pulsate out of an 18-gauge needle.
- However, I prefer to "double wall" the common femoral artery from the beginning.
  - Going through-and-through the femoral artery prevents arterial bleeding from the needle. It buys time for the operator to let down the transducer and hold the 0.035-inch wire.
  - When ready with the wire in one hand, the needle is pulled out slowly as it is torqued down. Once the needle tip is pulled into the lumen and pops off the posterior wall, a flash of pulsating blood should be seen. The wire is then advanced into the needle under fluoroscopy.
- The wire is advanced gently under fluoroscopy without resistance.
- Once the wire is secure in the artery, an incision is made utilizing an 11-blade scalpel usually by a 3-mm-depth stab of the 11-blade.
  - The blade incision is made over the needle so not to damage the wire.
  - It should not be deep enough to injure the underlying artery.
  - If the artery is superficial, the needle can be pulled and torqued to raise (tent) the skin away from the underlying artery.
  - A 4- to 5-French transitional sheath (micropuncture dilator) is passed over the wire while holding counter-tension on the wire so not to kink the wire.
- A vascular side-port sheath is advanced over the 0.035-inch wire.

Hemostasis

- Venous access sites
  - Upper extremity and jugular vein access usually require 5 minutes of compression unless there is distal venous obstruction.
  - Coughing may increase bleeding for a jugular venous access.
  - Purse-string sutures may help control venous access sites.
- Axillary artery access site
  - Pressure can be exerted on the axillary artery access site to obtain hemostasis. Pressure is enough to stop bleeding, but not too much to occlude the axillary artery.
  - Pressure is held while the arm is in midabduction. Pressure is exerted against the humeral head for ~10–15 minutes in the noncoagulopathic patient.
  - The patient's arm is then placed overnight in a sling to support it in a neutral position. Distal pulses should be compared with baseline pulses.
  - Percutaneous closure devices can reduce the time of compression to achieve hemostasis.
- Femoral artery access site
  - Pressure is exerted on the femoral artery access site to obtain hemostasis. Pressure is enough to stop bleeding, but not too much to occlude the femoral artery.
  - Pressure is held while the patient is flat on his or her back. Pressure is exerted against the femoral head for ~12–20 minutes in the noncoagulopathic patient.
  - The patient is to remain in bed for at least 4–6 hours. If a therapeutic procedural has been performed (access sheath ≥6-French), a patient can be left straight on his or her back in bed for up to 12 hours (4–12 hours) per protocol.
  - Distal pulses are compared with baseline pulses during and after compression for hemostasis.
  - Numerous percutaneous closure devices are available. These reduce the time of compression to achieve hemostasis and reduce the bed-rest time (time to ambulation). This allows earlier patient discharge.

Endpoints

As discussed before, the endpoint of vascular access (whether it is the end or the means of the procedure) is intraluminal entry of the needle and wire into the desired vascular segment in the appropriate direction.

Postprocedural Evaluation and Management

Initial Postprocedural Observation Period and Admission

- If vascular access is part of a larger procedure, the length of the hospital stay depends on the type of procedure.
- In general, the length of the postprocedural stay varies from one practice to the other.
- After a venous access only procedure (this includes tunneled and implantable venous catheters/reservoirs), patients can be discharged. They are usually observed for 1 hour from the venous access procedure/catheter placement. This is mostly due to sedation issues.

- The procedure can be performed on an outpatient basis.
- The patient can be discharged 1 hour after the procedure.
- A responsible adult should stay with the patient overnight.
- For patients who have undergone arterial access procedures for diagnostic purposes only (angiograms):
  - The procedure can be performed on outpatient basis.
  - Patients can be discharged 6–8 hours after the procedure.
  - In cases of a femoral access procedure, the above two points apply if the car ride home is less than 1 hour (no sitting in the car and flexing the hip). The patient's home should be less than 1 hour from the nearest emergency department and someone (a responsible adult) should stay with the patient overnight.
- For patients who have undergone an arterial access procedure for therapeutic purposes (angioplasty, stent placement, embolization, arterial port-a-catheter implant, chemoinfusion pump):
  - Almost all practices admit the patient for at least 24 hours/overnight stay.
  - The patient needs to lay flat for 4–12 hours after the procedure.
  - Closure devices may reduce time to ambulation down to 1–2 hours.

Intravenous Fluid, Diet, and Activity

- Intravenous access should be kept until just before the patient's discharge.
- Some institutions start clear liquid diet immediately and advance it as tolerated. Other institutions/operators commence a clear liquid diet after a period of abstinence of oral intake. This period could be 1 hour, for example.
- Give intravenous fluid until oral intake is adequate.
- For patients who have undergone venous access procedure for diagnostic or therapeutic purposes:
  - Bed rest for $1/_2$ to 1 hour after the procedure.
  - Activity is then as tolerated by the patient.
- For patients who have undergone arterial access procedures for diagnostic or therapeutic purposes:
  - The patient needs to lay flat for 4–12 hours after the procedure. Instructions during this period include
    - Keep accessed leg(s) straight for 4–8 hours
    - Do not actively raise head from pillow
    - If the patient coughs, sneezes, strains, or laughs, he or she must apply pressure to the groin.

- No bathroom privileges (the patient must use a urinal or bedpan)
- Activity is then as tolerated by the patient.

Pain Management and Medications

- The patient may have mild to moderate pain for 24 hours postprocedure.
- As far as vascular access is concerned only, narcotics are usually not required during the postaccess stay of the patient prior to discharge. Occasionally, some patients require oral narcotic analgesics such as acetaminophen and a hydrocodone combination medication. Rarely does a patient require intravenous narcotics such as fentanyl.
- Patients who have undergone embolization procedures, especially where a soft tissue mass (that includes viscera such as the liver, kidney, or uterus) may very well require a narcotic analgesic for 24–48 hours (usually 12–24 hours) including a morphine patient-controlled analgesia (PCA) pump.
- On discharge, patients usually tolerate the procedure well and do not require analgesics more potent than over-the-counter medications.
- Medication for pain management is described above.
- Antiemetics are given if patients are symptomatic and can be expected to be given for 24 hours (more common with embolization procedures).
- Antibiotics (metronidazole: Flagyl; Pfizer Pharmaceuticals, New York, NY) are given by some institutions for 5–7 days for embolization procedures.

Monitoring Vital Signs and Vascular Exam

- Vital sign monitoring includes blood pressure and heart rate. Occasionally, oxygen saturation monitoring is required in cases of shortness of breath and/or chest pain.
- Vitals are obtained every 15 minutes for 1 hour.
- Sedation/anesthesia may promote a softer blood pressure than a patient's baseline blood pressure. This is the most likely due to sedation with or without dehydration. Patients usually respond in time with hydration and as the sedatives wear off.
- Continued hypotension and more importantly, a rise in heart rate may indicate hypovolemia (bleeding). If signs of hypovolemia occur, an intravenous volume bolus is given and a noncontrast computed tomography (CT) exam is performed to confirm the clinical suspicion of bleeding. A retroperitoneal bleed may be physically unapparent.
- A vascular exam (distal pulses by palpation and/or Doppler ultrasound)

- ○ Should be made with the vital signs
- ○ Should be compared with baseline vascular exam (preprocedure) and immediate postprocedure vascular exams
- ○ A neurology exam should be scheduled for patients who have had aortic arch or branch vessels diagnostic or therapeutic exams.

Postprocedural Imaging

- Some institutions/operators routinely perform a chest x-ray (CXR) of patients who have undergone jugular or subclavian vein access.
  - ○ This is not necessary and probably dates back to when central lines were done blindly (without imaging). (However, my institution performs a CXR.)

Complications and Their Management

Management of Bleeding Complications

- Intravenous access should be kept until just after discharge in an outpatient setting in case fluid resuscitation is required.
- Bleeding can take several forms and have different sources.
  - ○ Skin bleeding (external)
  - ○ Site bleeding depending on procedure and site of procedure
    - Site hematomas (associated neuropathy in upper axillary artery punctures)
    - Retroperitoneal bleeding
    - Hemothorax
- Significant bleeding affecting vital signs and patient stability should be managed by
  - ○ Fluid resuscitation starting with crystalloid fluid bolus
  - ○ Type and cross
  - ○ Repeat hematocrit to compare with baseline
  - ○ Check international normalized ratio (INR), prothrombin time (PT), and partial thromboplastin time (PTT); correct if needed
  - ○ Stop heparin if it is being administered
  - ○ Blood transfusion to maintain hematocrit at or above 30%
  - ○ Surgical consult
- Imaging
  - ○ CXR to rule out hemothorax
  - ○ Noncontrast CT to rule out retroperitoneal bleeding

Management of Pleural/Thoracic Complications

- If chest pain with or without reduced oxygen saturation is encountered, a CXR should be obtained to rule out pneumothorax or hemothorax.
- Clinically significant hemo- and/or pneumothorax require chest tube placement, increased nasal cannula oxygenation, and fluid resuscitation/bleeding management in case of the former (see above).
- If an asymptomatic pneumothorax is encountered a chest tube is not required. A repeat CXR is obtained in an hour. A chest tube is placed if the patient is symptomatic at any time or there is an expanding pneumothorax. For details, see the postthoracentesis pneumothorax algorithm in Chapter 17.

Abscess Formation

- Abscess formation in the vascular access site should be evacuated surgically.
- Infections (from the simple skin infections to a flocculent abscess) related to implants, such as catheters and port-a-catheters, should prompt removal of the implants in addition to abscess drainage.
- Antibiotics should be given according to culture and sensitivity of the cultures obtained (blood and site cultures)

Vascular Injuries

- Vascular injuries – a collective term of the following vascular pathologies that can be due to prior (usually arterial) vascular access:
  - ○ Arterial dissection
  - ○ Arteriovenous fistulas
  - ○ Pseudoaneurysms
  - ○ Combinations of the above
- Arterial dissection should be noted intraprocedurally. If it is flow-limiting it should be stented. If not flow limiting, observation with imaging follow-up with or without anticoagulation should be performed.
- Arteriovenous fistulas can be seen intraprocedurally. However, if from a vascular access, it is probably seen later either as an imaging incidental during an angiogram/venogram or clinically. Clinically significant fistulas are either treated endoluminally (if feasible) or surgically (second-line treatment).
- The management of postcatheterization pseudoaneurysms is discussed in Chapter 22.

Further Reading

Lewis CA, Allen TE, Burke DR, et al; Society of Interventional Radiology Standards of Practice Committee. Quality improvement guidelines for central venous access. J Vasc Interv Radiol 2003;14(9 Pt 2): S231–S235

Singh H, Cardella JF, Cole PE, et al; Society of Interventional Radiology Standards of Practice Committee. Quality improvement guidelines for diagnostic arteriography. J Vasc Interv Radiol 2003;14(9 Pt 2): S283–S288

11 Percutaneous Nephrostomy
Wael E.A. Saad

Indications

The following is generally the order from the most common indication to the least common indication for a percutaneous nephrostomy.

- Drainage of an obstructed renal pelvicalyceal system (renal collecting system)
  - Pyonephrosis (infection/pus in the renal collecting system)
  - Worsening renal function due to obstructive uropathy
- Providing a portal (percutaneous access) for minimal invasive urologic interventions
  - For percutaneous nephrolithotripsy (PCNL)
  - For ureteric interventions
    - Balloon dilation of ureteric strictures
    - Coil embolization of debilitating ureteric fistulas
    - Traversal of transected (strictured/leaking) ureters
- Urine diversion
  - Ureteric leaks/fistulas
  - Hemorrhagic cystitis
- Relief of pain related to renal calculi and/or pregnancy

Notice that there is no mention of hydronephrosis. Hydronephrosis is not an indication to percutaneous nephrostomy. Hydronephrosis is not synonymous with urinary obstruction and urinary obstruction does not necessarily lead to hydronephrosis. Acute high-grade urinary obstruction shuts down the kidney's ability to form urine; thus, it does not lead to the backing-up of urine to cause enlargement/engorgement of the pelvicalyceal system by urine. Dilation of the pelvicalyceal system can be seen for months after an obstruction has been resolved. In addition, there are several causes of nonobstructive hydronephrosis:

- Lingering hydronephrosis for months after an obstruction has resolved
- Physiologic hydronephrosis
  - Polydipsia and polyuria and their causes
  - Pregnancy

Contraindications

Relative Contraindication

- Uncorrected coagulopathy. Relative versus absolute contraindication depends on the degree of coagulopathy, the clinical setting, and the degree of urgency of the percutaneous nephrostomy procedure.

Preprocedural Evaluation

Evaluate Prior Cross-Sectional Imaging

- Look for abnormalities and anatomic variations of the target kidney
  - Evaluate the orientation of the kidney that is going to be accessed including any rotational abnormality
  - Evaluate the site of the kidney. It might be a pelvic kidney, for example.
  - In severe cases the malrotation and/or the malposition of the target kidney may require a transabdominal access and not the traditional transretroperitoneal access.
    - The above helps in planning the positioning of the patient on the angiography suite.
    - The above reduces the intraprocedural ultrasound scan time in finding the target kidney.
  - Evaluate if there is duplication of the collecting system. If there is duplication, is it partial or complete? And which moiety is obstructed/affected? Accessing the wrong moiety is obviously not desired and would subject the patient to two procedures; the mistaken first moiety and the proper second moiety (**Figs. 11.1, 11.2, 11.3, and 11.4**).
  - Evaluate for renal cysts and less commonly calyceal diverticula. Under ultrasound, cysts may be mistaken for dilated calyces. Inadvertently targeting a cyst will obviously not lead to draining/accessing the collecting system.
  - Evaluate for renal tumors. Renal tumors may be hypervascular and may cause bleeding. Having a percutaneous nephrostomy drain indwelling through a tumor theoretically may cause tumor dissemination.

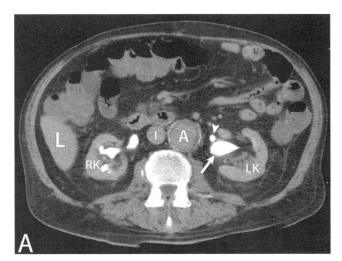

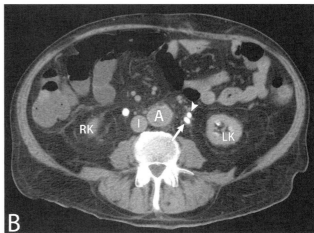

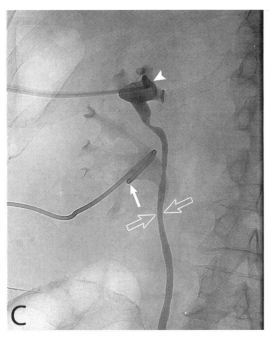

Fig. 11.1 Duplicated collecting system. **(A)** Delayed contrast enhance (pyelogram phase) axial computed tomography (CT) image of the midabdomen at the level of the renal pelvis. The left kidney (LK) exhibits a duplicated collecting system. The *arrowhead* points to the upper moiety (*upper pole*) ureter, which passes adjacent to the lower moiety renal pelvis (*arrow*) that is leading to a separate ureter (L, liver; RK, right kidney; LK, left kidney; I, inferior vena cava; A, abdominal aorta). **(B)** Delayed contrast-enhanced (pyelogram phase) axial CT image at a lower level than in **Fig. 11.1A**. The left kidney (LK) exhibits a duplicated collecting system. There are two separate ureters (*arrowhead: upper moiety; arrow: lower moiety*). If they both continue separately to the urinary bladder then it is a complete duplication. If they fuse, then this is a partial duplication. This is a complete duplicated collecting system (*not shown*) (RK, right kidney; LK, left kidney; I, inferior vena cava; A, abdominal aorta). **(C)** Fluoroscopic image of the same patient as **Figs. 11.1A and 11.1B** demonstrating a nephrostomy tube in each moiety (*arrowhead: upper; arrow: lower*) of the completely duplicated collecting system. The *hollow arrows* point to the upper moiety ureter. The lower moiety ureter is not seen. The ureters do not fuse. The purpose of this image is not to show complete ureteric separation, but to show the requirement of the two nephrostomy tube placements.

○ Evaluate for stones. Stones can be used as fluoroscopic landmarks if the operator has difficulty accessing the collecting system by ultrasound. In addition, calyces that are completely occupied by a single calculus that sits in it like a cast may provide technical difficulty to the operator where he or she finds it difficult to pass a wire from the needle into the infundibulum and onwards into the renal pelvis.
○ Evaluate for residual contrast, for example, a delayed or persistent nephrogram or pyelogram (**Figs. 11.3 and 11.5**). These can be used as fluoroscopic land-

marks if the operator has difficulty accessing the collecting system by ultrasound.
• Look for adjacent organs that can be inadvertently traversed
○ This helps plan the needle trajectory for the percutaneous nephrostomy.
○ This can help reduce transgression of adjacent organs with a subsequent potentially major complication.
○ Particular organs that may be traversed include the colon, spleen, and liver for native kidneys and small bowel for transplant kidneys.

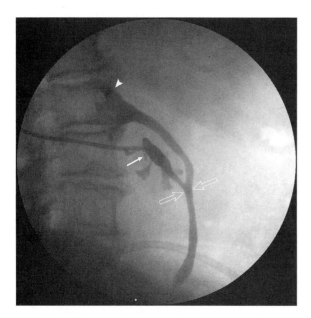

Fig. 11.2 Fluoroscopic image during a nephrostogram demonstrating a partially duplicated collecting system. The upper moiety (*arrowhead*) does not have a nephrostomy tube. The nephrostomy tube is in the lower moiety collecting system (*arrow*) and drains both moieties because their ureters fuse close by the renal pelvises (*hollow arrows*). The only stipulation for the system to be drained by one nephrostomy tube is that the proximal ureters be patent.

Evaluate Prior Nuclear Renal Scan

- In cases where there is hydronephrosis by cross-sectional imaging without evidence of worsening or poor renal function and in the absence of sepsis, it is not unreasonable to ask for a renal scan to evaluate for (or prove) renal obstruction.
- A renal scan evaluates function of the kidneys.
    - There is no need to drain an unobstructed poorly functioning kidney in cases of poor renal function. Only the obstructed functioning kidney should be drained (at least first).
    - Furthermore, in institutions that stage bilateral nephrostomies to reduce patient morbidity (see below), the renal scan helps the operator pursue the least functioning and/or the most obstructed kidney first.

Evaluate Preprocedure Laboratory Values

- Laboratory value evaluation mostly involves ruling out coagulopathy.
    - Suggested coagulopathy thresholds are
        - International normalized ratio (INR): ≤1.4–1.5
        - Platelets (PLT): ≥50,000–70,000

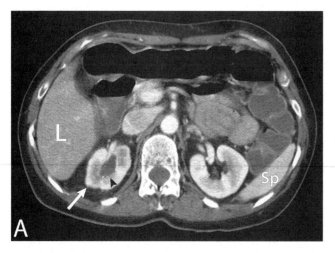

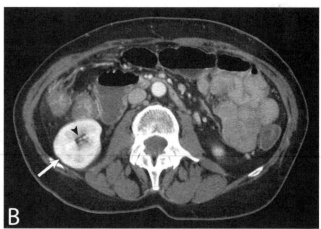

Fig. 11.3 (A,B,C) Duplicated collecting system with upper moiety obstruction. Contrast-enhanced (nephrogram phase) axial computed tomography (CT) images through the upper, mid-, and lower portions of the right kidney. These images are to be compared with the delayed images (pyelogram phase) in **Figs. 11.3D, 11.3E, and 11.3F.** There is slight hydronephrosis of the upper pole moiety (**Fig. 11.3A,** *arrowhead*) compared with the lower pole moiety (**Fig. 11.3B,** *arrowhead*). In addition, there is a slight delay in the nephrogram phase of the upper moiety (**Fig 11.3A,** *arrow*) compared with the lower moiety (**Figs. 11.3B and 11.3C,** *arrows*) (L, liver; Sp, spleen). **(D,E,F)** Delayed contrast-enhanced (pyelogram phase) axial CT images through the upper, mid-, and lower portions of the right kidney. These images are to be compared with the earlier images (nephrogram phase) in **Figs. 11.3A, 11.3B, and 11.3C.** There is a delay of the nephrogram of the upper pole moiety (**Fig. 11.3D,** *arrow*). The upper pole is still in the nephrogram phase (**Fig. 11.3D,** *arrow*) compared with the lower pole moiety (**Figs. 11.3E and 11.3F,** *arrow*). The lower moiety is well within the pyelogram phase with contrast in the lower moiety renal pelvis (asterisk, **Fig. 11.3E**). In **Fig. 11.3F,** the contrast is seen in the left singular ureter and the right lower moiety ureter (*arrows*) (L, liver; RK, right kidney; LK, left kidney). **(G,H)** Maximum intensity projection (MIP; **Fig. 11.3G**) and a three-dimensional reconstruction (**Fig. 11.3H**) of the same CT examination partly shown in **Figs. 11.3A–11.3F**); both demonstrating the singular renal collecting system on the left (*hollow arrow*) and the duplicated collection system on the right (*solid arrow in the upper moiety; arrowhead in the lower moiety*). The left collecting system (*hollow arrow*) and the lower moiety right collecting system (*arrowhead*) are synchronized (same contrast phase). However, the obstructed upper moiety on the right (*solid arrow*) is delayed and is still in the nephrogram phase. Notice the shadow of a ureterocele (U)

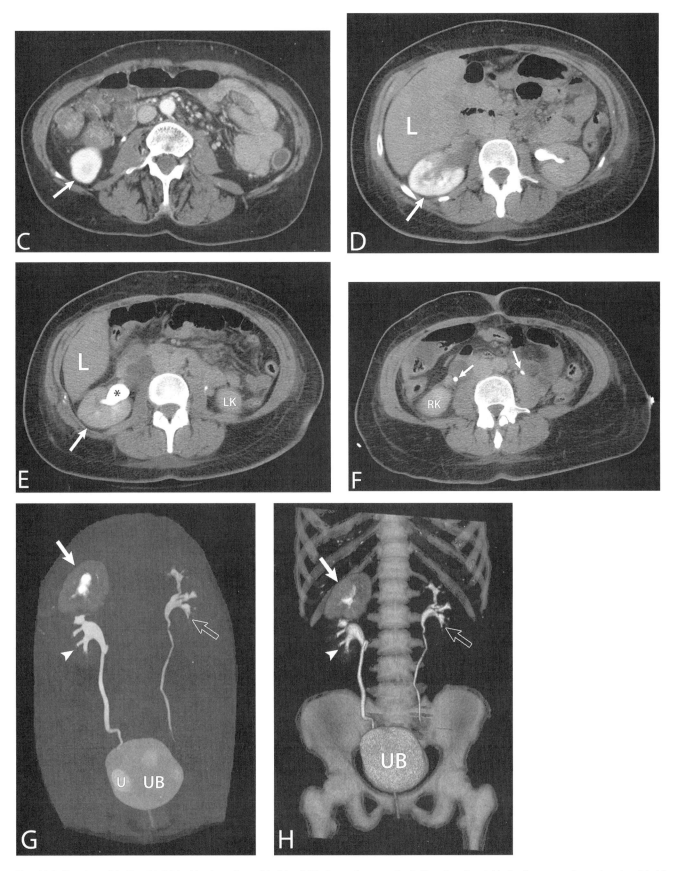

Fig. 11.3 *(Continued)* in **Fig. 11.3G** inside the urinary bladder (UB). Remember, "Vowels stay together and constants stay together" – Upper pole: Obstructed, Ectopic, Ureterocele, enters bladder Inframedial Lower pole: Reflux, Dominant (drains larger renal mass), enters bladder supralateral. *(Continued on page 132)*

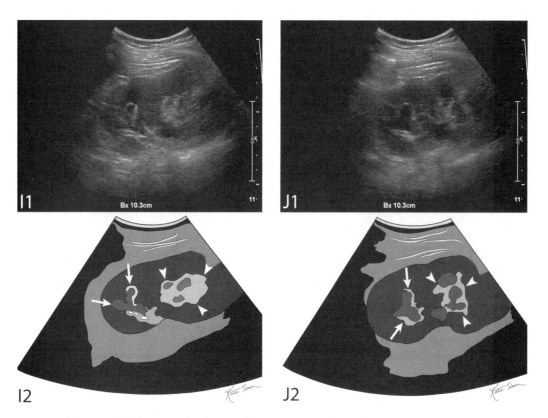

Fig. 11.3 *(Continued)* **(I,J)** Gray-scale ultrasound images *(top)* and schematic sketches *(bottom)* of the same duplicated system on the right side. Again noted is the mild hydronephrosis in the upper pole moiety *(arrows)* compared with the lower moiety *(arrowheads)*.

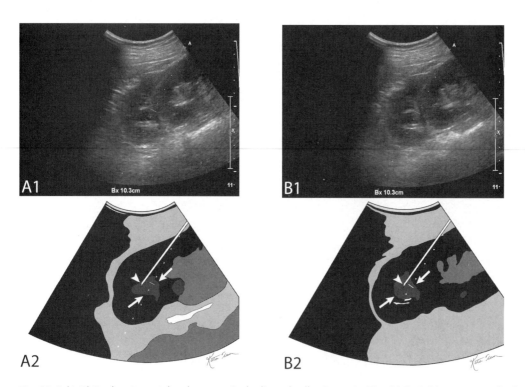

Fig. 11.4 (A,B) Nephrostomy tube placement in duplicated collecting system with upper moiety obstruction. Gray-scale ultrasound images *(top)* and schematic sketches *(bottom)* of the same duplicated system as in **Fig. 11.3**. A 21-gauge needle *(arrowhead at needle tip)* has been passed under real-time ultrasound guidance into the upper pole collecting system *(between arrows)*.

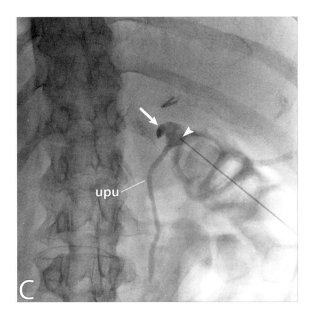

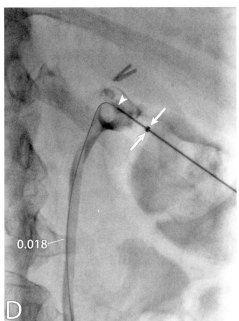

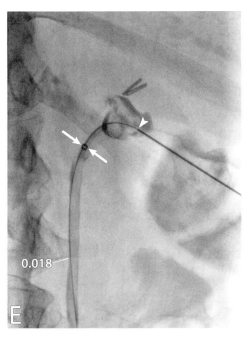

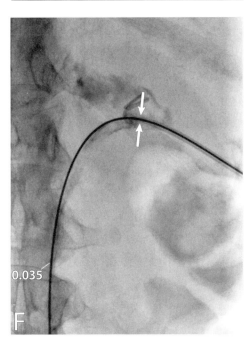

Fig. 11.4 *(Continued)* **(C)** Fluoroscopic image during the initial antegrade pyelogram after the 21-gauge needle (*arrowhead at needle tip*) has been passed under real-time ultrasound guidance into the upper pole collecting system (*arrow*). As can be seen, the upper pole collecting system is small (nondominant), which is typical, and leads to the independent (totally separated upper pole ureter: upu). **(D,E)** Fluoroscopic images obtained after a 0.018-inch wire (0.018) has been passed coaxially through the 21-gauge access needle. The 21-gauge needle has been removed and replaced with an AccuStick (Boston Scientific, Natick, MA) dilator system over the 0.018-inch wire. The arrowhead does not point to the access needle tip (the needle has been removed), but it points to the tip of the inner metal stiffener of the AccuStick system. The outer dilator of the AccuStick system has a radiopaque ring/marker (*between arrows*). The tip of the metal stiffener (*arrowhead*) is stopped short of the 0.018-inch wire turn (metal does not go around corners). At this time **(Fig. 11.4D)**, the operator passed the plastic/dilator portion of the AccuStick system over the wire and metal stiffener to enter the distal renal pelvis/proximal ureter (**Fig. 11.4E**). Notice the filling defects in the collecting system and ureter (compare it with **Fig. 11.4C**): this is blood in the collecting system, which is not uncommon in difficult nephrostomy tube placements. **(F)** Fluoroscopic image obtained after the 0.018-inch wire has been exchanged for a 0.035-inch wire (0.035). The AccuStick system has also been removed. It has done its designed job, which is primarily to upsize the 0.018-inch platform (wire system) to a 0.035- or 0.038-inch wire system, and secondarily, to dilate the tract to up to 6.5-French. The AccuStick system has been replaced with an 8-French fascial dilator to dilate the retroperitoneal tract in preparation for an 8-French nephrostomy drain placement (*arrows at tip of 8-French dilator*). *(Continued on page 134)*

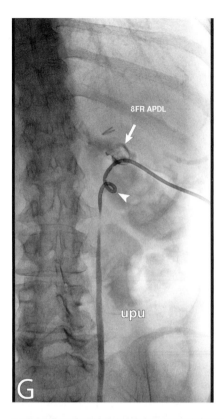

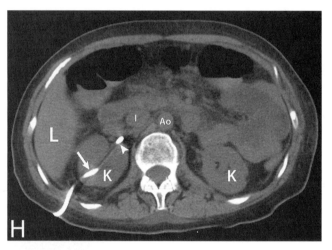

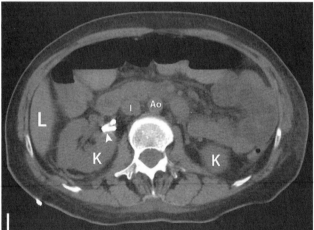

Fig. 11.4 *(Continued)* **(G)** Fluoroscopic image obtained after an 8-French nephrostomy drain has been placed (8-French all purpose draining locking (APDL) catheter). Because the collecting system is duplicated and the less dominant upper pole moiety is not significantly hydronephrotic, there is little room to place a wide (more than 2-cm diameter) pigtail catheter. The 2-cm pigtail catheter is formed/deformed partly in the proximal ureter *(arrowhead)* and partly, unraveled in the small upper pole collecting system *(arrow)*. **(H,I)** Unenhanced axial CT images of the midabdomen at the level of the renal pelvis. The *arrowhead* and *arrow* correlate with the *arrowhead* and *arrow* in the fluoroscopic image of **Fig. 11.4G**, respectively (K, kidney; I, inferior vena cava; Ao, aorta; L, liver).

- Activated partial thromboplastin time (aPTT): ≤50 seconds
  ○ Serum creatinine
    - A prenephrostomy is important as it serves as a baseline to evaluate for improving renal function, if any, after the nephrostomy drain placement.
    - Is important with operators who utilize intravenous (IV) contrast to visualize the renal collecting system for fluoroscopic-guided nephrostomy tube placement.

Obtain Informed Consent

- Indications
  ○ See indications above
  ○ Technical success in acquiring an antegrade pyelogram with nephrostomy tube placement in the renal collecting system is 90–100%.
  ○ Overall clinical success in managing the above indications is probably 85–90%; however, it is less in patients with renal calculi (75–85%).

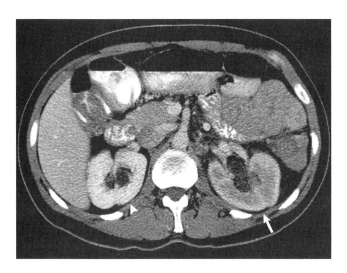

Fig. 11.5 Obstruction of the kidney with delayed nephrogram (obstructive nephropathy). Contrast-enhanced axial CT image through the midportions of the kidneys. The left kidney is obstructed by a stone in the ureter (*not shown*). The acute obstruction has not yet developed into significant hydronephrosis; however, it has caused a delayed nephrogram in the left kidney (*arrow*). As can be seen, the left kidney is in an early nephrogram phase with corticomedullary differentiation. However, the right kidney (*arrowhead*) is in a later nephrogram phase without corticomedullary differentiation.

- Alternatives
  - To refuse the procedure
  - Surgical relief of obstruction (cystoscopy/ureteroscopy). This alternative is usually contraindicated in the setting of urosepsis.
- Procedural risks
  - Infection (see **Table 11.1**)

- This complication occurs in 1–3% overall. Cases of pyonephrosis are reported as high as 7–9%.
- In cases of pyonephrosis and/or documented urinary infection, patients should receive prophylactic antibiotics such as ciprofloxacin 500 mg IV.
  - Bleeding (**Table 11.1**)
    - The most common presentation of bleeding is hematuria.
    - It may present as pain and/or hypotension and a computed tomography (CT) scan may show subcapsular hematoma, dissecting retroperitoneal hematoma, or active extravasation in the few cases were CT IV contrast is used.
    - Bleeding may be transient with or without a blood transfusion.
    - In rare cases, bleeding may require an intervention such as transcatheter hepatic arterial embolization or exploratory surgery with or without nephrectomy (0.1–0.9%).
  - Injury to surrounding organs and/or structures (**Table 11.1**)
    - Pleura (pneumo- and hemothorax)
    - Bowel

Equipment

Ultrasound Guidance

- Multiarray 4–5 MHz ultrasound transducer
- Transducer guide bracket
- Sterile transducer cover

Table 11.1 Complications of Ultrasound-Guided Nephrostomy Procedures

Complication Major Complications Occur in 5–10%*	Incidence Overall and in Straightforward Nephrostomies	Incidence in High-Risk Procedures and/or Clinical Settings
Sepsis	1–3%	7–9%[†]
Hemorrhage requiring transfusion	1–4.3%	12–14%[‡]
Vascular injury requiring embolization or nephrectomy	0.1–0.9%	
Bowel transgression	0.2%	
Hemo and/or pneumothorax	0.1–0.2%	8.7–12%[§]
Unexpected increase in level of care: ICU, surgery, extended hospital stay	4–7%	
30-day mortality (all causes of death/death related to procedure)	(3.1%/Rare)	

*Incidences in percentage are when these complications are mentioned. Not all studies mention all complications.

[†]In the setting of pyonephrosis.

[‡]The higher incidence is in more invasive nephrostomy procedures such as percutaneous nephrolithotripsy (PCNL).

[§]The higher incidence is in more invasive nephrostomy procedures such as percutaneous nephrolithotripsy (PCNL). In addition, and more importantly, PCNL may require entry into upper pole calyces, which increase the risk transgressing the pleural lining.

Abbreviations: ICU, intensive care unit

Standard Surgical Preparation and Draping

- Chlorhexidine skin preparation/cleansing fluid
- Fenestrated drape

Local Infiltrative Analgesia Administration

- 21-gauge infiltration needle
- 10–20 mL 1% lidocaine syringe

Sharp Access Devices

- 11-blade incision scalpel
- 18- to 19-gauge diamond tip needle allows a 0.035-inch wire. If the needle is placed in the intended target calyx, there is no need to upsize wires and a nephrostomy tube can be placed (my preference) (**Figs. 11.6, 11.7, 11.8, and 11.9**).
- 21- or 22-gauge needle allows a 0.018-inch wire. If the needle is placed in the intended target calyx, upsizing the wire to a 0.035-inch wire (additional step) is usually required prior to nephrostomy tube placement.
  - An additional upsizing step requires a Neph-set (Cook Corp., Bloomington, IN) or AccuStick (Boston Scientific, Natick, MA) system, which is a telescoped dilator system with a metal stiffener that goes over a 0.018-inch wire. Once in, the 0.018-inch wire can be removed and exchanged for a 0.035-inch wire.
- A 22-gauge needle may also be flimsy and may deflect away from the intended target calyx by the time it traverses the retroperitoneum and into the renal parenchyma.

Tubular Access Devices

- Telescoped graduate dilation system with metal stiffener (Neph-set or AccuStick); upsize 0.018-inch wire to 0.035-inch wire if a 21- to 22-gauge needle is used for initial definitive calyceal access (see above).
- An 8-French fascial dilator that can be passed over a 0.035-inch guidewire may be used.
- An 8-French self-retaining (string-locking) pigtail drainage catheter, which is the definitive nephrostomy tube to be placed last (final product of the procedure) (**Figs. 11.4 and 11.7**).

Technique

Intravenous Access and Medication

- Required for moderate sedation and fluid replenishment/resuscitation

- Required for IV prophylactic antibiotics such as 500 mg ciprofloxacin

Prebiopsy Ultrasound Exam

- Determine easiest visibility of target calyx (usually lower pole calyx) (**Figs. 11.7, 11.8, and 11.9**)
- Assess renal mobility with breathing and the patient's ability to fixate kidney by breath holding.
- Correlate and triangulate the access site (at skin) and the lower pole renal calyx (target calyx) to choose and mark the skin access site.
  - Ideally for the needle trajectory, a 20- to 22-degree angle from midline is desired to reduce bleeding complications. There is an avascular plane of the kidney that is traversed to access the posterior lower pole calyx. This plane lies between the ventral two-thirds of the kidney and the dorsal one-third of the kidney. This bloodless plain is known as *the Brödel bloodless line of incision* and is created by the main division of the renal artery into a ventral branch and a dorsal branch.
  - Ideally, a distance greater than four finger breadths from the midline (spinous processes) is desired.
    - If too medial, the nephrostomy drain will pass through skeletal muscles including psoas, which is painful and may limit drainage of urine and may increase the risk of bleeding.
    - If too lateral, the risk of colon transgression and splenic injury increases, especially if the spleen is enlarged.
- Make sure that the retroperitoneum to the target calyx is clear of viscera, bowel, and/or organs
- Make sure that the parenchymal tract to the target calyx is clear of renal cysts or tumors
- Manipulation of the transducer (along with the bracketed needle guide) is used to choose and triangulate the skin entry site, the target calyx, and the needle trajectory to achieve the above points. The traditional/common transducer orientation is longitudinal on the target kidney; however, transverse or an orientation in-between can be adopted to achieve the above triangulation aim as well as to acquire the adequate calyceal access (see the Fluoroscopic-Guided Wire and Tube Access section below).

Standard Surgical Preparation and Draping

- Skin preparation/cleansing in the region that was chosen as an ultrasound imaging portal and a needle access portal
- Place a fenestrated drape at the chosen and prepared skin region

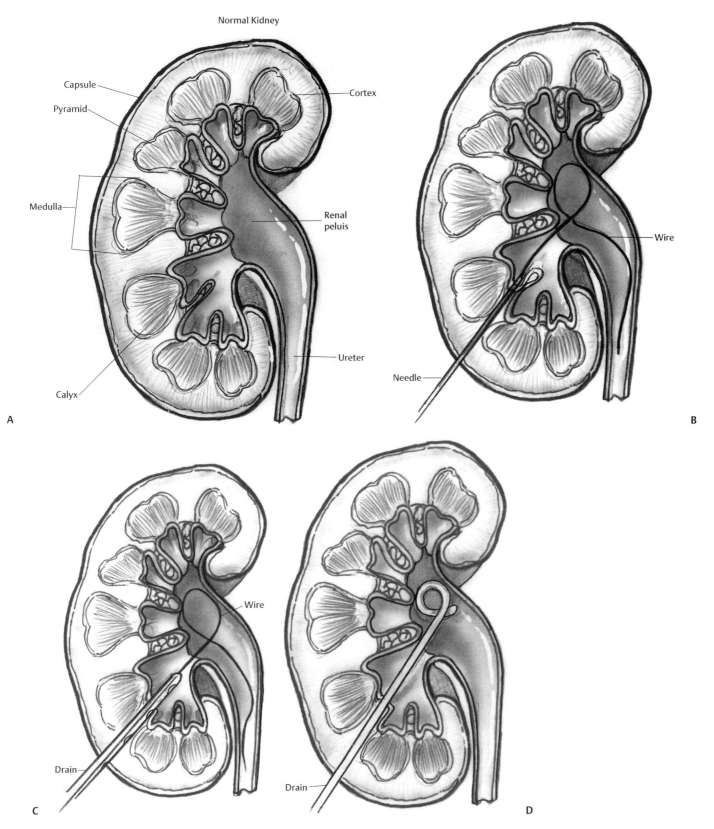

Fig. 11.6 Step-by-step nephrostomy tube placement; **(A)** schematic of the right kidney with an anatomic coronal cut through it. It shows a mildly dilated pelvicalyceal system. **(B)** Schematic of the right kidney with an anatomic coronal cut through it. It shows needle access through one of its lower pole calyces with wire passage into and coiling in the pelvicalyceal system. **(C)** Schematic of the right kidney with an anatomic coronal cut through it. It shows the advancement of the nephrostomy drain over the wire into the pelvicalyceal system. **(D)** Schematic of the right kidney with an anatomic coronal cut through it. It shows the final endpoint (result) of the procedure with the pigtail nephrostomy drain in the renal pelvis.

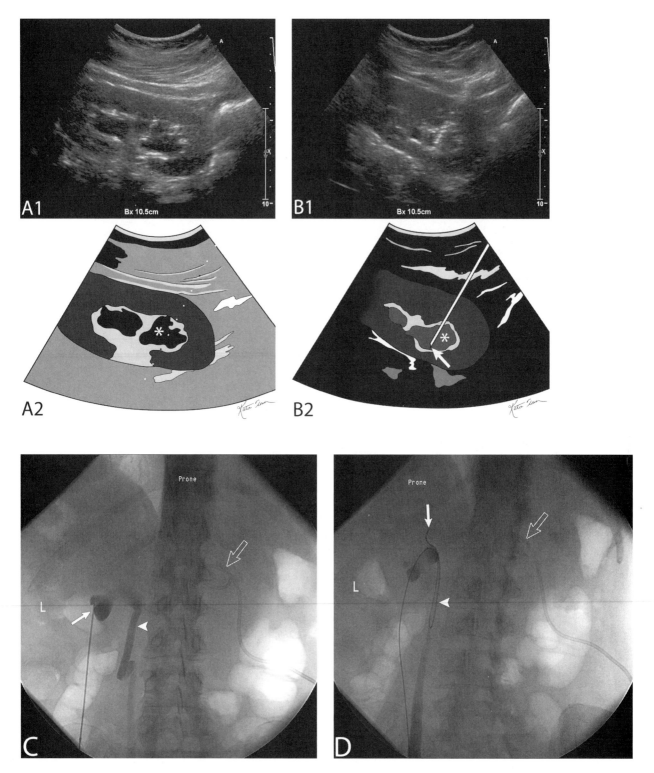

Fig. 11.7 Nephrostomy tube placement in left native kidney. **(A)** Gray-scale ultrasound image (*top*) and schematic sketch (*bottom*) of the left kidney. The operator has his or her sights (*dotted line:* ultrasound guide) at the lower pole calyx (*asterisk*). **(B)** Gray-scale ultrasound image (*top*) and schematic sketch (*bottom*) of the left kidney. The operator has passed an 18-gauge needle (*arrow at needle tip*) into the lower pole calyx (*asterisk*). **(C)** Fluoroscopic image during the initial antegrade pyelogram after the 18-gauge needle (*solid arrow at needle tip*) has been passed under real-time ultrasound guidance into the left lower pole calyx (patient is prone). Contrast is seen opacifying the left ureter (*arrowhead*). Incidentally noted is a prior nephrostomy tube coiled in the right kidney (*hollow arrow*). **(D)** Fluoroscopic image after passage of an 0.035-inch wire through the needle and into the left pelvicalyceal collecting system. The wire is seen doubled back in the proximal ureter (*arrowhead*). The wire tip is at the solid arrow. The operator is ready at this point to dilate the retroperitoneal tract and then place the nephrostomy tube over the wire. Incidentally noted is a prior nephrostomy tube coiled in the right kidney (*hollow arrow*).

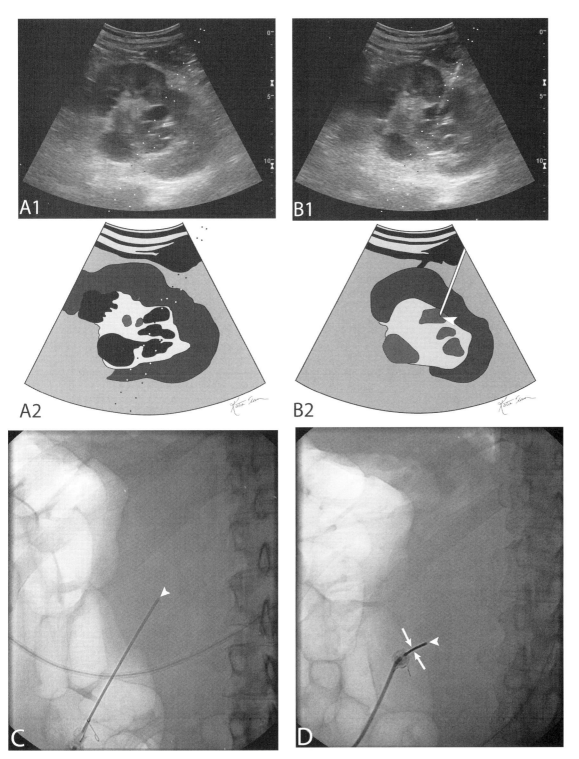

Fig. 11.8 Nephrostomy tube placement in left native kidney. **(A)** Gray-scale ultrasound image (*top*) and schematic sketch (*bottom*) of the left kidney. The operator has his or her sights (*between dotted lines*: ultrasound guide) at the lower pole calyx. **(B)** Gray-scale ultrasound image (*top*) and schematic sketch (*bottom*) of the left kidney. The operator has passed an 18-gauge needle (*arrowhead at needle tip*) into the lower pole calyx. At this moment in time, the procedure is converted into fluoroscopic guidance. **(C)** Fluoroscopic spot image just after the needle tip has been seen entering the lower pole calyx by real-time ultrasound (**Fig. 11.7B**) (*arrowhead at needle tip*). **(D)** Fluoroscopic spot image with the image intensifier angled so that it almost looks down the long axis (shaft) of the needle (left posterior oblique and slight caudad direction). The operator has done this to confirm that he or she has not transgressed the left hemicolon. The *arrowhead* points at the needle tip and the *arrows* point to the medial wall of the left hemicolon (the patient is prone). At this time, the operator removes the inner stylette of the 18-gauge needle and aspirates using a connecting tube and syringe. Once there is a urine return, contrast can be injected to perform the initial antegrade pyelogram. *(Continued on page 140)*

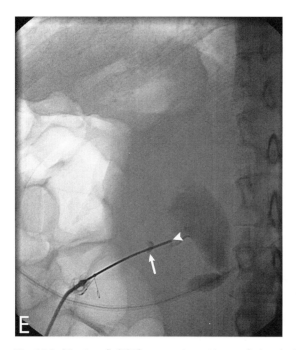
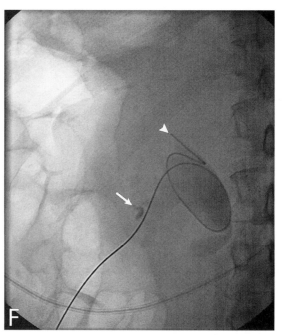

Fig. 11.8 *(Continued)* **(E)** Fluoroscopic spot image during the initial antegrade pyelogram by injecting contrast through the 18-gauge needle (*arrowhead at needle tip*). The *arrow* points to the calyx entry site, which is stained with contrast (calyceal wall puncture/injury). **(F)** Fluoroscopic image after passage of a 0.035-inch wire through the needle and into the left pelvicalyceal collecting system. The wire is seen coiled in the renal pelvis with its tip (*arrowhead*) in an upper pole calyx. The *arrow* points to the calyx entry site, which is stained with contrast (calyceal wall puncture/injury). The operator is ready at this point to dilate the retroperitoneal tract and then place the nephrostomy tube over the wire.

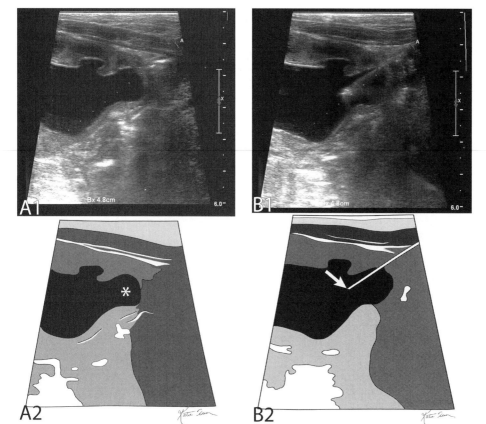

Fig. 11.9 Nephrostomy tube placement in a neonatal kidney with significant hydronephrosis. **(A)** Gray-scale ultrasound image (*top*) and schematic sketch (*bottom*) of the left kidney. The operator has his or her sights (*dotted line*: ultrasound guide in real-time gray-scale ultrasound image) at the lower pole calyx (*asterisk in schematic*). **(B)** Gray-scale ultrasound image (*top*) and schematic sketch (*bottom*) of the kidney. The operator has passed a 21-gauge needle (*arrow at needle tip*) into the lower pole calyx.

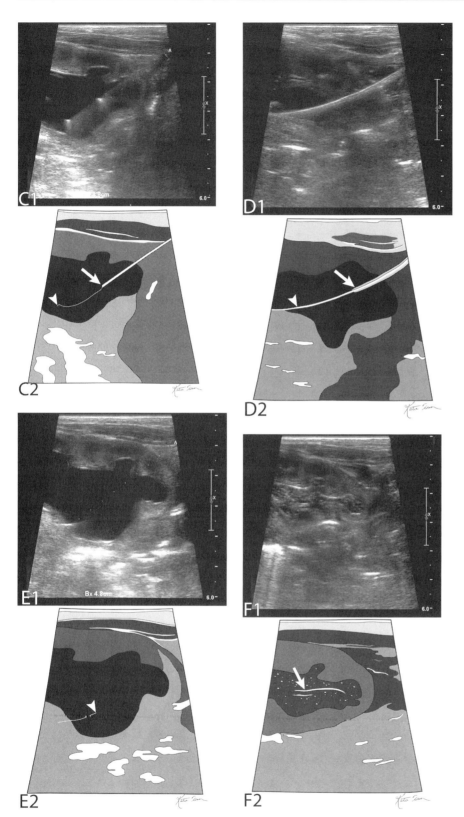

Fig. 11.9 *(Continued)* **(C)** Gray-scale ultrasound image (*top*) and schematic sketch (*bottom*) of the kidney. The operator has passed a 0.035-inch wire (*arrowhead*) under ultrasound through the 21-gauge needle (*arrow at needle tip*) into the renal pelvis. **(D)** Gray-scale ultrasound image (*top*) and schematic sketch (*bottom*) of the kidney. The operator is passing an 8-French nephrostomy drain (*arrow*) over the 0.035-inch wire (*arrowhead*). **(E)** Gray-scale ultrasound image (*top*) and schematic sketch (*bottom*) of the kidney. The operator has removed the needle over the 0.035-inch wire (*arrowhead*). **(F)** Gray-scale ultrasound image (*top*) and schematic sketch (*bottom*) of the kidney. The 8-French drain (*tubular structure, arrow*) is in the renal pelvis.

Local Infiltrative Analgesia Administration

- Utilizing a 21-gauge (by at least a 3.7-cm-long) infiltration needle, 1% lidocaine infiltration is performed. Infiltrating down to the renal capsule is not necessary. The renal capsule is not as sensitive as the liver capsule and is deeper (a higher risk for no or little benefit).

Ultrasound-Guided Sharp Access

- An incision is made utilizing an 11-blade scalpel usually by a 3-mm-depth stab of the 11-blade.
- An 18- to 21-gauge coaxial diamond-tip access needle is passed through the guide (ultrasound needle guide bracket) and into the target calyx (**Figs. 11.4, 11.7, 11.8, 11.9, and 11.10**).
  - The calyx is visualized and the projected needle path is delineated by the ultrasound machine (*dotted line*, **Figs. 11.4, 11.7, and 11.8**).
  - A single pass of the needle is made with conviction (no hesitation). Hesitating or making small jerky movements at a time may not help to see the needle tip at these depths. In addition, hesitation with the needle allows time to inadvertently or intentionally move the ultrasound probe. Moving the probe once the needle

has been passed for some distance (more than 2- to 3-cm depth) makes it impossible to see the needle and may make the needle deflect and miss the target.

- Some operators use ultrasound guidance (real-time or site marking) to make a vertical (posteroanterior) 22-gauge needle access of the renal pelvis. Once in the renal pelvis, contrast with or without air is injected to visualize the entire collecting system and then the definitive calyceal access is performed using a "second stick" or needle pass under real-time fluoroscopy. This technique is somewhat of a cross between single-stick ultrasound guidance (described above) and the traditional double-stick all-fluoroscopic-guidance technique. There is no difference in technical success or procedural complications between the single-stick and the double-stick technique.
- One should not write-off the placement of the definitive access needle under fluoroscopy (with or without the use of ultrasound for the access of the renal pelvis) as "old school." Acquiring fluoroscopic-guidance skill sets is important, particularly in decompressed collecting systems and/or staghorn renal calculi (collecting systems with little room for access and/or catheter wire manipulation).
- Occasionally, the access needle falls short of the target calyx. In this case, the ultrasound probe needle guide

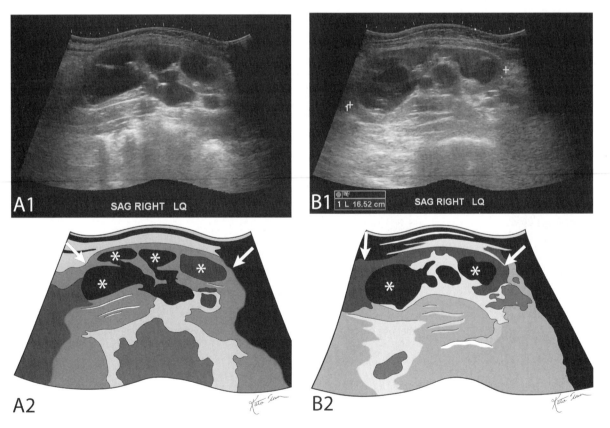

Fig. 11.10 Nephroureteral tube placement in transplanted kidney. **(A,B)** Gray-scale ultrasound images (*top*) and schematic sketches (*bottom*) of a right lower quadrant transplanted kidney with hydronephrosis. The kidney (*arrows*) is superficial and shows dilated calyces (*asterisks*).

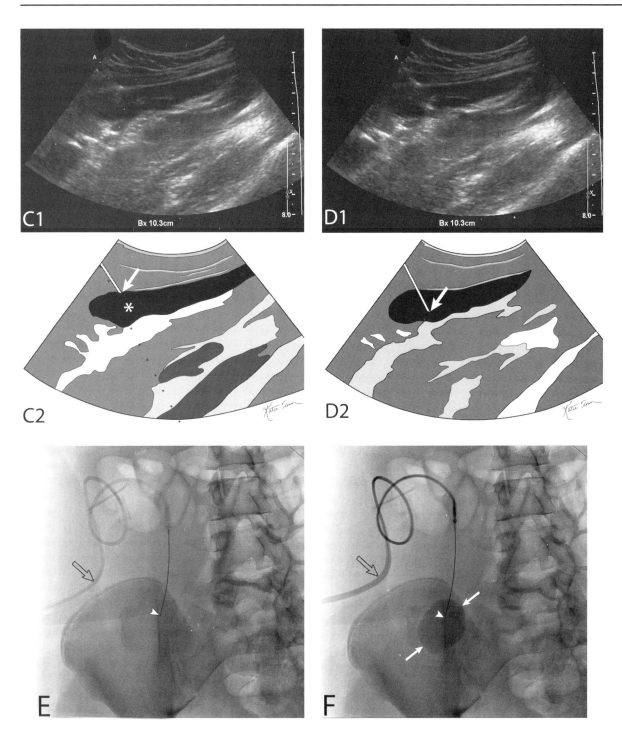

Fig. 11.10 *(Continued)* **(C)** Gray-scale ultrasound image *(top)* and schematic sketch *(bottom)* of the transplanted kidney. The operator has passed a 21-gauge needle *(arrow at needle tip)* to the border of a lateral superficial calyx *(asterisk)*. **(D)** Gray-scale ultrasound image *(top)* and schematic sketch *(bottom)* of the transplanted kidney. The operator has passed a 21-gauge needle *(head at needle tip)* into the lateral superficial calyx. At this moment in time, the procedure is converted from real-time ultrasound to real-time fluoroscopy. **(E)** Fluoroscopic spot image just after the needle tip has been seen entering the lower pole calyx by real-time ultrasound (**Fig. 11.11D**) *(arrowhead at needle tip)*. Through a connecting tube *(hollow arrow)* suction is applied to the needle to aspirate urine to confirm adequate placement of the needle into the collecting system. **(F)** Fluoroscopic spot image during the initial antegrade pyelogram by injecting contrast through the 21-gauge needle *(arrowhead at needle tip)* via the connector tube *(hollow arrow)*. The accessed calyx *(between solid arrows)* is opacified first.   *(Continued on page 144)*

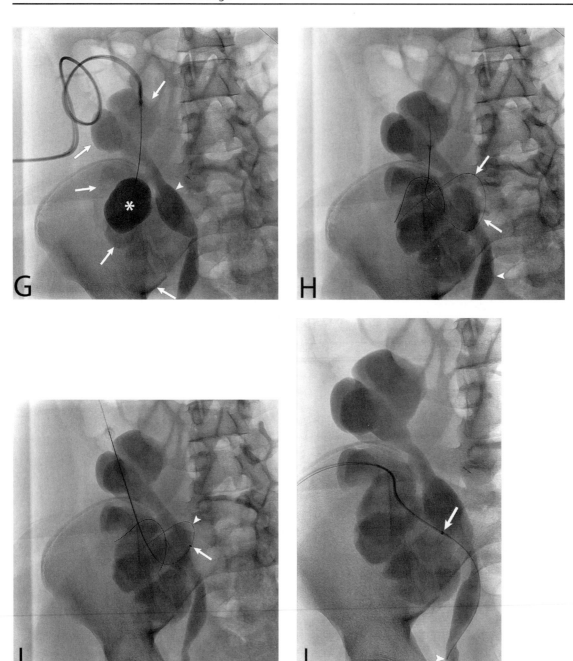

Fig. 11.10 *(Continued)* **(G)** Fluoroscopic spot image during the initial antegrade pyelogram. The accessed calyx *(asterisk)* is opacified most and now the remainder of the pelvicalyceal system is seen *(arrows)*. The renal pelvis is also seen *(arrowhead)*. **(H)** Fluoroscopic image after passage of a 0.018-inch wire through the needle and into the pelvicalyceal collecting system. The wire is seen coiled in the renal pelvis with its tip *(arrows)*. The *arrowhead* points to the proximal ureter. **(I)** Fluoroscopic image after passage of an AccuStick (Boston Scientific, Natick, MA) system dilator *(arrow at radiopaque tip)* over the coiled 0.018-inch wire *(arrowhead)*. The AccuStick system allows the operator to upsize from a 0.018-inch platform to a 0.035- or 0.038-inch wire system (platform). The inner diameter of the outer 6.5-French dilator of the AccuStick system allows the passage of a 4-French catheter, and not a 5-French catheter. **(J)** Fluoroscopic image after passage of a 4-French catheter coaxially through the AccuStick system dilator *(arrow at radiopaque tip of AccuStick)*. The AccuStick dilator has been pulled back and using a 0.035-inch glidewire the catheter has been redirected down into the proximal ureter *(arrowhead at the tip of 0.035-inch glidewire)*.

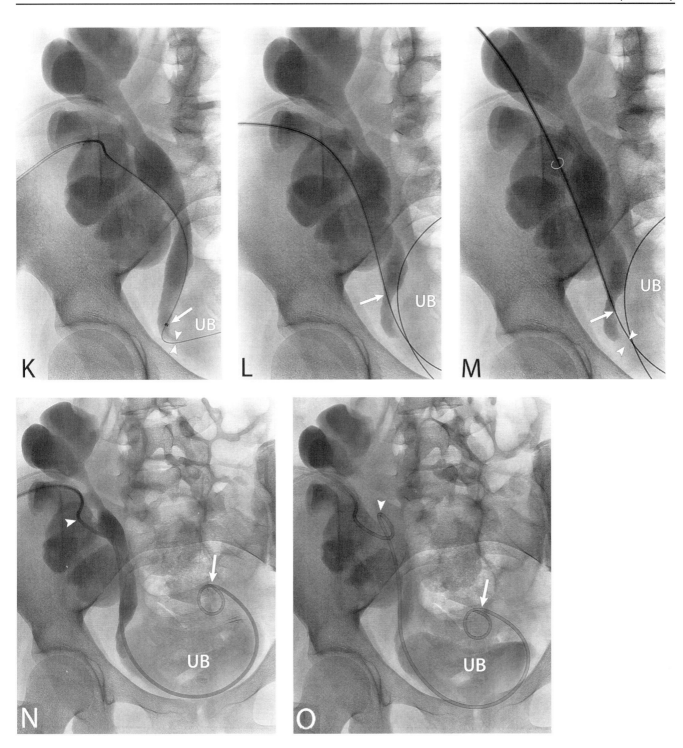

Fig. 11.10 *(Continued)* **(K)** Fluoroscopic image after passage of the 0.035-inch glidewire through the distal ureteric stricture (*between arrowheads*) and into the urinary bladder (UB). The AccuStick system has been advanced into the distal ureter (*arrow at AccuStick tip*). **(L)** Fluoroscopic image after passage of an 8-French dilator over the 0.035-inch wire (*arrow at dilator tip*) to make way for the nephroureteral stent. The glidewire is coiled in the urinary bladder (UB). **(M)** Fluoroscopic image during passage of an 8-French nephroureteral stent over the 0.035-inch wire (*arrow at tip of nephroureteral stent in distal ureter*). The *arrowheads* point to the level of the distal ureteric stricture (at/near the anastomosis with the urinary bladder, UB). The incomplete white circle delineates the calyceal entry site at which the needle and now the nephroureteral stent enter the pelvicalyceal system of the transplanted kidney. **(N)** Fluoroscopic image after passage of the 8-French nephroureteral stent over the 0.035-inch wire and into the urinary bladder (UB). The arrow points to the distal pigtail of the stent, which forms by itself once without constraint in the urinary bladder (UB). The *arrowhead* points to the proximal (pelvicalyceal) loop of the nephroureteral stent, which has not been formed yet. This loop forms by pulling on a string. **(O)** Fluoroscopic image after forming the proximal (pelvicalyceal) loop of the nephroureteral stent by pulling on a string (*arrowhead*). The distal loop (*arrow*) still remains in the urinary bladder (UB). This is the endpoint of the procedure.

bracket is dismantled around the needle. This gives 3 to 4 cm extra on the needle. The operator then can push the needle in deeper with his or her thumb.

- Once the needle is placed, the stylet is removed and the operator aspirates as the needle is pulled back slowly. Getting a return of urine (could be sanguinous urine) is indicative that the needle tip is in the collecting system. At this time, the procedure is converted to real-time fluoroscopy.

Fluoroscopic-Guided Wire and Tube Access

- Contrast is injected through the needle and into the collecting system to confirm the needle location is in an adequate calyx.
- Adequate needle placement
  - Posterior calyx in the lower pole of the kidney if no special access is required – posterior to minimize parenchymal and/or collecting system traversal to reduce complications
  - A particular calyx (not necessarily lower pole) for access to a stone that requires lithotripsy. This calyx can be in the middle of the kidney or even in the upper pole (**Fig. 11.11**).
  - If ureteric interventions are to be subsequently sought, the operator must take into account the angle that is made between the transretroperitoneal

tract (needle trajectory) and the ureter through the pelvicalyceal system. Too acute an angle, especially with a soft thick/obese backside/flank may hinder "up-and-over" efforts to pass sheaths or balloons or even endoscopes into the upper ureters. To increase this angle the operators can

- Target a higher renal calyx (midportion to upper pole)
- Choose a steeper angle ultrasound guide needle bracket if feasible
- Choose a different skin site by revolving or panning the ultrasound transducer and needle bracket to a transverse location (transverse on the kidney or semitransverse instead of the traditional longitudinal approach)

- Fluoroscopic images at multiple obliquities visualizing the colon can be obtained down the shaft (down the barrel-/gun-site technique) to rule out transgression of the colon (**Fig. 11.8**).
- If the calyx accessed is not ideal:
  - A second attempt at accessing the desired calyx can be made utilizing real-time ultrasound guidance from the start again once the first pass needle is removed.
  - An alternative is to utilize real-time fluoroscopy with a gun-site technique at the target calyx.

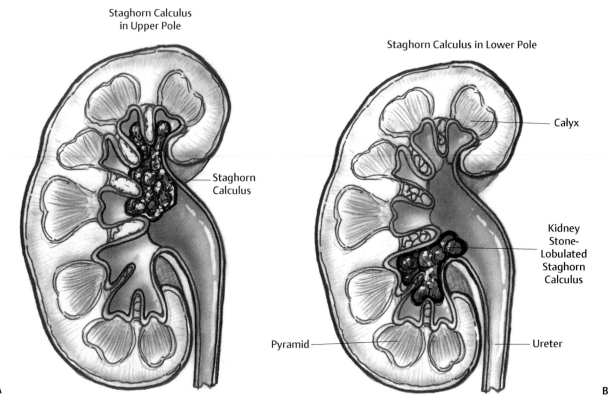

Fig. 11.11 Staghorn calculi. **(A)** Schematic of the right kidney with an anatomic coronal cut through it. It shows a mildly dilated pelvicalyceal system with a staghorn calculus occupying the mid- to upper calyces.

(B) Schematic of the right kidney with an anatomic coronal cut through it. It shows a mildly dilated pelvicalyceal system with a staghorn calculus occupying the lower calyces.

- To differentiate anterior from posterior calyx by fluoroscopy, air can be injected through the needle. Air rises (goes to the least dependant calyx, the posterior calyx) and urine/contrast goes to the dependent calyx (anterior calyx). Obviously, the patient has to be prone to make this air/fluid level differentiation. It cannot be performed accurately when the patient is in an oblique position or a lateral position.
- If the desired calyx is accessed and its position confirmed, a 0.035- to 0.038-inch wire is passed through a 19- to 18-gauge needle or 0.018-inch wire is passed through a 21- to 22-gauge needle (see above).
- A 0.018-inch wire requires it to be upsized to a 0.035- or 0.038-inch wire utilizing an AccuStick system (telescoped and stiffened dilator, see above).
- When utilizing a 0.035-inch wire, a nonglide (hydrophilic wire) can be used particularly in a dilated collecting system. However, some operators utilize a 0.035-inch glidewire in cases of decompressed collecting systems or in the presence of a staghorn calculus occupying the calyx/collecting system.
  - Utilizing the glidewire and a catheter the collecting system can be negotiated and the catheter and wire can be passed through the infundibulum and into the renal pelvis.
  - The problem with hydrophilic glidewires is that they can dissect along the renal collecting system wall and surrounding tissue and not be in the collecting system lumen. This adds trauma to the kidney. Experience is required to avoid this and/or realize peripelvic dissection early on.
- Once the 0.035-inch wire is coiled in the renal pelvis, an 8-French fascial dilator is passed to create a retroperitoneal tract. It is then replaced by a small-bore nephrostomy drain (usually 8–10 French). This drain is usually a self-retaining string locking pigtail catheter. The pigtail is placed and secured ("Coped") in the renal pelvis (**Figs. 11.4 and 11.7**).
- In the absence of infection, and if the nephrostomy needle and wire access has gone smoothly and without event, then an operator may pass a nephroureteral stent that ends in the urinary bladder. This is particularly true when there is ureteral disease (stricture, leaks) that can be traversed easily (**Fig. 11.10**).
- The nephrostomy drain is then secured to the skin utilizing sutures and left to gravity bag drainage.

Postnephrostomy Imaging

- Immediate postnephrostomy imaging is for documentation that the pigtail end of the drain (nephrostomy catheter) is in the renal pelvis.
- Visualizing contrast around the collecting system and occasionally tracking down around the ureter occurs in difficult nephrostomies with decompressed collecting systems and/or multiple initial needle passes. This will resolve usually within 24 hours and should not be a concern.
- New filling defects within the collecting system are most likely the result of clotted hematuria (blood). Heightened observation by the operator and ancillary staff to watch the output of the nephrostomy drain and the patient's hematocrit and/or vital statistics should be made.

Endpoints

- The endpoint of the procedure is a pigtail catheter in the renal pelvis through the intended calyx with urine draining from the catheter without complications.
- Success occurs in 90–100% of cases. Technical failures are more common with staghorn calculi or decompressed collecting systems.
- Urine is not infrequently sanguineous. Remember this is an invasive procedure. However, the urine should not be frank blood (see below).

Postprocedural Evaluation and Management

Percutaneous nephrostomy should not be performed on an outpatient basis. Patients should be admitted for observation for 23 hours. Rarely, a patient can be discharged if an easy, uneventful nephrostomy was performed with at least 8–12 hours of observation afterward. Strict instructions to return to the hospital in case of complications should be given.

Postnephrostomy Observation Period

- Routine admission should be the standard of practice. Deviation from this is rare.
- The nephrostomy drain should be set to gravity drainage.
- Chek on the patient and monitor vital signs.
- Observe the urine output for volume and character
  - Thick pus blocking the drain (rare) requires the drain to be flushed with ~5–7 mL of sterile saline.
  - It is not uncommon to have sanguineous urine. The blood tinge should clear with time.
  - Urine that steadily increases in blood tinge and frank blood should be concerning (see below for management).

Intravenous Fluid and Diet

- IV access should be kept until just prior to hospital discharge.

- Institutions that practice moderate sedation start with a clear liquid diet and advance it as tolerated. This helps to offset patients' nausea and vomiting.
- Some institutions start clear liquid diet immediately and advance it as tolerated. Other institutions/operators commence a clear liquid diet after a period of abstinence of oral intake. This period could be one hour, for example.
- Give IV fluid until oral intake is adequate

Activity

- Bed rest for 4–6 hours
- The nephrostomy drain/bag uses gravity drainage.
- Patients should be instructed on how to maneuver with the nephrostomy drains and to be reminded that they are tethered to a collecting bag.

Pain Management

- Narcotics are usually not required postnephrostomy. Occasionally, some patients require oral narcotic analgesics such as acetaminophen and hydrocodone combination medication. Rarely does a patient require IV narcotics such as fentanyl.
- Continued pain, especially if accompanied with a drop in pressure, should be concerning for a growing retroperitoneal hematoma. A noncontrast CT can be performed to evaluate for this.
- On discharge, patients usually tolerate the procedure well and do not require analgesics more potent than over-the-counter medications.

Monitoring Vital Signs

- Vital sign monitoring includes blood pressure and heart rate. Occasionally, oxygen saturation monitoring is required in cases of shortness of breath and/or chest pain.
- Institutions/operators that practice conscious sedation may record a softer blood pressure than a patient's baseline blood pressure after the biopsy. This is most likely due to sedation with or without dehydration. The patient usually responds in time with hydration, particularly as the sedatives wear off.
- Continued hypotension and, more importantly, a rise in heart rate are concerning for hypovolemia (bleeding). If signs of hypovolemia occur, an IV volume bolus is given and a noncontrast CT exam is performed to confirm the clinical suspicion of bleeding.

Complications and Their Management

As can be seen in **Table 11.1**, the most common specific complication is bleeding. If bleeding that does not require blood transfusion is added (not included in the table) it probably would exceed all other complications. Please see **Table 11.1** for the list of types of complications and their incidence following percutaneous nephrostomies.

Management of Pain and Pain-Related Morbidity

- Continued or increasing pain requires further clinical and possibly imaging evaluation.
- Occasionally operators respond to continued pain by performing a diagnostic imaging exam.
  - A limited ultrasound examination at the site to evaluate for a renal capsular hematoma
  - Possibly a more global exam such as a noncontrast abdominal CT exam. Remember, ultimately the decisive factor for significant bleeding is the patient's stability (vitals) – not what is seen on the images
- If there is no bleeding and the patient is stable, but the patient requires narcotic analgesics for pain, the patient can be admitted for pain management.

Management of Bleeding Complications

- This is the most common complication especially when including frank hematuria not requiring blood transfusion (not included in **Table 11.1**).
- Bleeding postnephrostomy can take several forms.
  - Hematuria (most common)
  - Subcapsular hematoma
  - Extracapsular retroperitoneal hematoma
  - External/site bleeding (rule out a skin bleed first)
  - Hemothorax (rare, see below)
- Frank hematuria should be managed locally by capping the nephrostomy drain to somewhat tamponade the bleed. Do not provide the bleeding a path of least resistance.
- Significant bleeding affecting vital signs and patient stability should be managed by
  - Fluid resuscitation starting with crystalloid fluid bolus
  - Type and cross
  - Repeat hematocrit to compare with baseline
  - Blood transfusion to maintain hematocrit at or above 30%
  - Surgical/urology consult

Management of Pleural/Thoracic Complications

- This is not common – <0.2%.
- Complications are least common in lower pole calyx nephrostomies. However, they are more commonly encountered in upper pole calyx approaches, which are more likely required for percutaneous access for nephrolithotomies.

- If chest pain with or without reduced oxygen saturation is encountered, a chest x-ray should be obtained to rule out pneumothorax or hemothorax.
- Clinically significant hemo- and/or pneumothorax require chest tube placement, increased nasal cannula oxygenation, and fluid resuscitation/bleeding management in the case of the former (see above).

Management of Puncture of Adjacent Organs

- This is rare – <0.3%.
- The organs that may be injured include the colon and spleen in native kidney transplants and the small bowel in renal transplants.
- When transgression of bowel occurs by the drain, the drain should be left in place for the tract to mature. This allows
  - The patient to recover from the acute situation of a procedure, renal failure, and/or sepsis.

- The risk of leaving the drain is a chronic/persistent nephrocolonic fistula, which is not common.
  - A later management of the fistula, if it occurs, can be performed in an elective setting.

Sepsis

- Prophylactic antibiotics should be used in cases of urinary infection, sepsis, or pyonephrosis.
- Operators should not overdistend the collecting system with contrast when there is suspicion of urinary infection.
- In cases of postoperative fever, operators should continue with intravenous antibiotics and should check the culture and sensitivity of the urine sample obtained from the nephrostomy.
- Sepsis requires fluid resuscitation and even vasopressors with admission of the patient to the intensive care unit (ICU).

Further Reading

Dyer RB, Regan JD, Kavanagh PV, Khatod EG, Chen MY, Zagoria RJ. Percutaneous nephrostomy with extensions of the technique: step by step. Radiographics 2002;22(3):503–525

Farrell TA, Hicks ME. A review of radiologically guided percutaneous nephrostomies in 303 patients. J Vasc Interv Radiol 1997;8(5): 769–774

Funaki B, Vatakencherry G. Comparison of single-stick and double-stick techniques for percutaneous nephrostomy. Cardiovasc Intervent Radiol 2004;27(1):35–37

Ramchandani P, Cardella JF, Grassi CJ, et al; Society of Interventional Radiology Standards of Practice Committee. Quality improvement guidelines for percutaneous nephrostomy. J Vasc Interv Radiol 2003;14(9 Pt 2):S277–S281

12 Percutaneous Transhepatic Biliary Drainage

Wael E.A. Saad

Indications

The indications of ultrasound-guided percutaneous transhepatic cholangiography (PTC) with or without subsequent percutaneous biliary drainage (PBD) are usually directed at the left hepatic lobe where the left biliary ducts lie. Right-side PTC with or without PBD is almost always performed under fluoroscopy. The focus of this chapter is on ultrasound-guided left bile duct access with or without drainage. **Table 12.1** lists the advantages and disadvantages of right versus left PTC and PBD.

The following are indications of PTC and PBD placement whether right sided or left sided:

- Drainage of an obstructed biliary tract
  - Cholangitis
  - Pruritus
  - High bilirubin with a patient who is a chemotherapy candidate
  - Diagnostic evaluation of obstructive jaundice (**Table 12.2**)
- Providing a portal (percutaneous access) for minimally invasive biliary interventions
  - For percutaneous removal of biliary stones
    - Transhepatic fluoroscopic-guided stone removal
    - Combined endoscopic retrograde cholangiopancreatogram (ERCP) and transhepatic fluoroscopic stone removal (rendezvous procedure)
    - Transhepatic endoscopic and fluoroscopic stone removal

- For biliary interventions
  - Balloon dilation of biliary strictures
  - Traversal of transected bile ducts (bile leaks/injury)
  - Brush biopsy/sampling for diagnosis of cause of obstruction
  - For placement of brachytherapy
- Bile diversion
  - Biliary leaks/fistulas

Contraindications

Relative Contraindication

- Uncorrected coagulopathy. Relative versus absolute contraindication depends on the degree of coagulopathy, the clinical setting, and the degree of urgency of the PBD procedure.

Preprocedural Evaluation

Evaluate Prior Cross-Sectional Imaging

Preprocedural imaging evaluation is focused on the left hepatic lobe and bile ducts.

- Evaluate
  - The size and orientation of the left hepatic lobe. Is it large enough to be worth draining in the case of relieving malignant obstruction for patients who will undergo chemotherapy.

Table 12.1 Advantages and Disadvantages of Right- and Left-Side Percutaneous Transhepatic Cholangitis (PTC) and Percutaneous Biliary Drain (PBD)

	Left PTC/PBD	Right PTC/PBD
Advantages	Less painful Less contrast intravascular if ultrasound used Less procedure time PBD less likely to dislodge* Lower risk of bleeding* Better care and tending by patient (in front of his/her eyes)	Wider application Less radiation to operators' hands, but more fluoroscopy time in general
Disadvantages	Cannot be applied to all comers (limited application) Increased radiation dose to operators' hands (reduced by ultrasound guidance)	More painful Higher bleeding risk* More likely to dislodge and be tended improperly by patient

*Anecdotal and not evidence-based (unpublished data).

Table 12.2 Diagnostic Indications of Percutaneous Transhepatic Cholangiography and Subsequent Potential Biliary Drainage

Classification of Disease		Detailed Diagnosis
Obstructive disease	Define level, degree, and type of obstruction	Malignant stricture
		Benign stricture
		Biliary stones (choledocholithiasis)
		External compression
	Evaluate for suspected bile duct inflammatory disorders	Primary sclerosing cholangitis
		Secondary sclerosing cholangitis
	Evaluate for potential biliary findings to help diagnose the cause of increased LFTs in liver transplant recipients	Ischemic changes • Ischemic strictures • Biliary necrosis • Biliary breakdown and biloma formation • Biliary leaks
Biliary leak	Define level, degree, and possible cause of bile leak	Recurrent primary sclerosing cholangitis
		Ductopenia (rejection)
		Bliary ischemia
		Anastomotic breakdown (dehiscence)
		Liver cut-surface leak
		Iatrogenic injury (laparoscopy)

○ Which side (right versus left bile ducts) is more prominently dilated. If the right is more prominently dilated, it might be prudent to access and drain the right bile ducts and not the left lobe bile ducts. If both are equally dilated and there are no special features to let the operator choose which side to access, it is left to operator preference.

○ The extent of left-sided biliary duct dilation. Ducts that are not dilated are technically more to access by ultrasound because they may not be seen clearly and even if seen, they may be difficult to target by ultrasound guidance.

○ If there are left lobe liver lesions such as tumors or cysts that may hinder a left-sided PTC/PBD

○ The entire liver to attempt to glean any information to answer the anatomic and pathologic aspects of biliary disease listed in the Indications section and in **Table 12.1**

• Look for adjacent organs that can be inadvertently traversed

○ This may make the operator consider approaching the bile ducts from the right and not the left, if there is close proximity of viscera or if the left lobe is very high up in the chest and covered by the rib cage, particularly costal cartilage.

○ This helps plan the needle trajectory for the PTC/PBD.

○ This can help reduce transgression of adjacent organs with subsequent potential major complication.

○ Particular organs that may be traversed include the colon, heart, stomach, and diaphragm/lung.

Evaluate Preprocedure Laboratory Values

• Laboratory value evaluation mostly revolves around ruling out coagulopathy.
○ Suggested coagulopathy thresholds are
• International normalized ratio (INR): ≤ 1.4
• Platelets (PLT): $\geq 50,000 - 70,000$
• Activated partial thromboplastin time (aPTT): ≤ 50 seconds
○ Serum creatinine
• This is more important in decompressed biliary systems when approaching from the intercostal approach (right side) utilizing fluoroscopy only. In this situation, large volumes of contrast may be inadvertently injected intravenously (in the hepatic and/or portal veins) in an attempt to opacify the decompressed bile ducts. Intravascular contrast injection may have a toll on the kidney, especially with a poor baseline renal function.
• Utilizing ultrasound for access guidance for the left biliary system requires minimal contrast, and if ultrasound-guided left biliary access is successful, there will be no inadvertent contrast injection into the circulation.

Obtain Informed Consent

• Indications
○ See indications above.
○ Technical success in acquiring a PTC (including all PTC techniques: right versus left, fluoroscopy versus

Table 12.3 Technical Success of Percutaneous Transhepatic Cholangiography and Percutaneous Biliary Drainage

	PTC (Opacify Bile Ducts)		Cannulation of Opacified Duct		Internalization of PBD	
	Indiv. Succ.	Cumul. Succ.	Indiv. Succ.	Cumul. Succ.	Indiv. Succ.	Cumul. Succ.
Dilated bile ducts	95%	N/A	95%	90%	90%	81%
Decompressed bile ducts	65%	N/A	70%	45%	90%	40%

Abbreviations: PTC, percutaneous transhepatic cholangiography; PBD: percutaneous biliary drain; Indiv. Succ., individual success of the particular technical stage of the procedure; Cumul. Succ., cumulative success of that particular stage of the procedure and the stage(s) prior to it.

ultrasound guidance) depends on the degree of bile duct dilation (**Table 12.3**). The more dilated the ducts the easier they are to opacify. This is particularly true for ultrasound guidance. Do not try to perform an ultrasound-guided PTC in the absence of significant bile duct dilation.

- ○ **Table 12.3** shows the effect of duct dilation on technical success at every stage of PBD placement including dilation. As can be seen, the cumulative success of opacifying the ducts (successful PTC), followed by cannulating the duct, and subsequently internalizing the PBD is twice as successful in dilated ducts (81%) compared with decompressed ducts (40%).
- Alternatives
  - ○ To refuse the procedure
  - ○ ERCP is the first line of therapy. PTC/PBD is reserved as the second line of therapy. **Table 12.4** lists the indications for PTC/PBD following ERCP or where ERCP is a forgone failure.
- Procedural risks
  - ○ Infection (**Table 12.5**)

Table 12.4 Indications for Percutaneous Transhepatic Cholangiography Relative to Endoscopic Retrograde Cholangiopancreatography

Indications for PTC/PBD in Relation to ERCP
1. Failed ERCP attempt
2. Gastric outlet obstruction
3. Status post gastrointestinal surgery: • Whipple procedure   • Hepaticojejunostomy   • Gastric bypass
4. Cause of obstruction is known intrahepatic (high) significant obstruction such as intrahepatic stricture(s).
5. Liver transplantation (many liver transplant patients have at least one of points 3 or 4 mentioned above.

Abbreviations: PTC, percutaneous transhepatic cholangiography; PBD, percutaneous biliary drain; ERCP, endoscopic retrograde cholangiopancreatography

- This complication in its broader definition occurs in more than 3% of cases.
- Infection can be divided into cholangitis (most common), biliary sepsis (most serious), or perihepatic abscess (least common).
- Patients should receive prophylactic antibiotics prior to any transhepatic biliary procedure. Intravenous antibiotics used include Zosyn (Wyeth Pharmaceuticals, Madison, NJ): 3.375 g intravenously (IV; primary antibiotic used by the authors) and ciprofloxacin: 400 mg IV.
  - ○ Bleeding (**Table 12.5**)
    - Most common presentation of bleeding is bleeding from the biliary drain (hemobilia/upper gastro-intestinal bleeding).
    - It may present as pain and/or hypotension and a computed tomography (CT) scan may show
      - ○ Subcapsular hematoma
      - ○ Active extravasation in the few cases where CT IV contrast is used
    - Bleeding may be transient with or without blood transfusion.
    - In rare cases, bleeding may require intervention such as transcatheter hepatic arterial embolization or exploratory surgery.
  - ○ Injury to surrounding organs and/or structures (**Table 12.5**)
    - Pleura (pneumo- and hemothorax)

Equipment

Ultrasound Guidance

- Multiarray 4–5 MHz ultrasound transducer
- Doppler capabilities to differentiate bile ducts from blood vessels
- Transducer guide bracket
- Sterile transducer cover

Standard Surgical Preparation and Draping

- Chlorhexidine skin preparation/cleansing fluid
- Fenestrated drape

Table 12.5   Complications of Percutaneous Transhepatic Cholangiography and Percutaneous Biliary Drainage (PBD)

Complication	Incidence*
Cholangitis	>3%
Sepsis	2–3%
Hemorrhage requiring transfusion &/or embolization	2–3%
Abscess formation, peritonitis, or pancreatitis	1.2%
Hemo- and/or pneumothorax[†]	0.5%
Death	<2%

*Incidences in percentage are when these complications are mentioned. Not all studies mention all complications.

[†]This is mostly a complication of right-sided PBD and less likely of left-sided PBD.

Local Infiltrative Analgesia Administration

- 21-gauge infiltration needle
- 10 to 20 mL 1% lidocaine syringe

Sharp Access Devices

- 11-blade incision scalpel
- 21- to 22-gauge needle allows a 0.018-inch wire. If the needle is placed in the intended target calyx, upsizing the wire to a 0.035-inch wire (additional step) is usually required prior to nephrostomy tube placement.
  - The needle can be a diamond tip 21-gauge needle.
  - The needle can be a 15-cm 22-gauge Chiba needle.

Tubular Access Devices

- Telescoped graduate dilation system with metal stiffener (Neph-set [Cook Corp., Bloomington, IN] or AccuStick [Boston Scientific, Natick, MA]) to upsize 0.018-inch wire to 0.035-inch wire.
- An 8-French fascial dilator that can be passed over a 0.035-inch guidewire may be used (see below).
- An 8-French self-retaining (string-locking) pigtail drainage catheter, which is the definitive biliary tube/drain to be placed last (final product of the procedure).

Technique

Intravenous Access and Medication

- Required for moderate sedation and fluid replenishment/resuscitation
- Required for IV prophylactic antibiotics such as
  - Zosyn 3.375 g
  - Ciprofloxacin 500 mg

Preaccess Ultrasound Exam

- Determine easiest visibility of left lobe intrahepatic bile ducts
- Place Doppler ultrasound near the target bile ducts to differentiate them from blood vessels. False-positives would be thrombosed blood vessels that are not common.
- Assess left hepatic lobe mobility with breathing and the patient's ability to fixate the visualized bile ducts by breath holding
- Correlate and triangulate the access site (at skin) and the target bile ducts to choose and mark the skin access site
  - Avoid the rib cage. Make sure the needle trajectory does not cross costal cartilage or ribs.
  - It is preferable that the needle skin entry site be 1.5 to 2.0 cm from the subcostal margin to reduce postprocedural chest wall pain complications.
  - Make sure the base of the heart is clear from the needle trajectory
- Make sure that the hepatic parenchymal tract to the target bile duct is clear of hepatic cysts or tumors (preferable, but not a must)
- The transducer (along with the bracketed needle guide) is used to choose and triangulate the skin entry site, the target bile duct, and the needle trajectory to achieve the above points. The traditional/common transducer orientation is transverse to the patient's abdomen/spine and longitudinal along the long axis of the left hepatic lobe. However, a slight panning toward the xyphoid/chest can also be adopted.
- The operator must not only think of successfully "hitting" the target duct, but also of using an ideal angle as well, so that a wire can be passed from lateral to medial to cannulate the left biliary system and be able to internalize the biliary drain if need be.

Standard Surgical Preparation and Draping

- Skin preparation/cleansing in the region that was chosen as an ultrasound imaging portal and a needle access needle portal
- Place a fenestrated drape at the chosen and prepared skin region

Local Infiltrative Analgesia Administration

- Utilizing a 21-gauge (by at least a 3.7-cm-long) infiltration needle, 1% lidocaine infiltration is performed, infiltrating down to the sensitive hepatic capsule.

Ultrasound-Guided Sharp Access

- An incision is made utilizing an 11-blade scalpel usually by a 3-mm-depth stab of the 11-blade.

- A 21-gauge diamond tip access needle or a 22-gauge Chiba needle is passed through the guide (ultrasound needle guide bracket) and into the target bile duct.
  - The bile duct is visualized and the projected needle path is delineated by the ultrasound machine (**Figs. 12.1 and 12.2**). A single pass of the needle is made with conviction (no hesitation). Hesitating or making small jerky movements at a time may not help to see the needle tip at these depths. In addition, hesitation with the needle allows time to inadvertently or intentionally move the ultrasound probe. Moving the probe once the needle has been passed for some distance (more than 2- to 3-cm depth) makes it impossible to see the needle and may make the needle deflect and miss the target.
- Once the needle is placed, the stylet is removed and the procedure is converted to real-time fluoroscopy (**Fig. 12.2**).

Fluoroscopic-Guided Wire and Tube Access

- Contrast is injected very gently through the needle under maximum fluoroscopic magnification to confirm the needle location is in the biliary system. A vessel may be visualized (portal vein or hepatic vein), which may mean
  - The operator was targeting the vessel and not a bile duct.
  - The needle passed through the bile duct target and into the vessel.
  - The needle veered off its target and struck a vessel.
- Hoping that it is the second scenario, the needle is pulled back very gently as contrast is gently injected to visualize the bile duct.
- Adequate needle placement
  - The needle should be in a peripheral bile duct.
  - The needle should be at a trajectory from lateral to medial (pointing centrally) so that a 0.018-inch wire can be passed into the central bile ducts (left main hepatic bile duct, common hepatic duct, and common bile duct).
- If the bile duct accessed is not ideal (too central, needle-duct angle not favorable for wire passage centrally) (**Figs. 12.3 and 12.4**):
  - A second attempt at accessing a more peripheral duct at a more favorable angle can be made utilizing a second needle under real-time fluoroscopic guidance while maintaining the first needle in its place for continued contrast injection to keep the left bile ducts opacified.
  - A second de novo attempt utilizing real-time ultrasound can be made to access the bile ducts more peripherally.

- If the desired calyx is accessed and its position confirmed, a 0.018-inch wire is passed through the 21- to 22-gauge needle (see above).
- A 0.018-inch wire requires it to be upsized to a 0.035 or 0.038-inch wire utilizing an AccuStick system (telescoped and stiffened dilator, see above).
- Once the outer caliber AccuStick system dilator is in the bile duct, a 0.035-inch glidewire and a 4-French catheter are passed coaxially in the bile duct and are used to obtain more central access all the way down to the bowel.
- Once the 0.035-inch wire is in the small bowel, an 8-French fascial dilator is passed to dilate the anterior wall and transhepatic tract. It is then replaced by a biliary internal/external drain (usually 10–12 French). This drain is usually a self-retaining string-locking pigtail catheter. The pigtail is placed and secured ("Coped") in the small bowel.
- The nephrostomy drain is then secured to the skin with sutures and left to gravity bag drainage.

Postpercutaneous Biliary Drainage Imaging

- Immediate postnephrostomy imaging is for documentation that the pigtail end of the drain is in the small bowel and that the side holes traverse the bile ducts and do not traverse the transhepatic tract or anterior abdominal wall.
- New filling defects within the collecting system are most likely the result by clotted hemobilia (blood). Heightened observation by the operator and ancillary staff to watch the output of the biliary drain and the patient's hematocrit and/or vital statistics should be made.

Endpoints

- The endpoint of a diagnostic PTC only is opacification and visualization of the biliary tract to rule out biliary disease (obstruction or bile leak and their etiology) (**Table 12.2**).
  - Success occurs in 65–95% of cases.
  - Technical failures are more common with decompressed biliary systems (65%).
- The endpoint of an internal/external biliary drain placement is a pigtail catheter in the small bowel through the intended bile ducts with bile draining from the catheter without complications.
  - Success occurs in >80% of cases.
  - Technical failures are more common with decompressed biliary systems (as low as 40%).

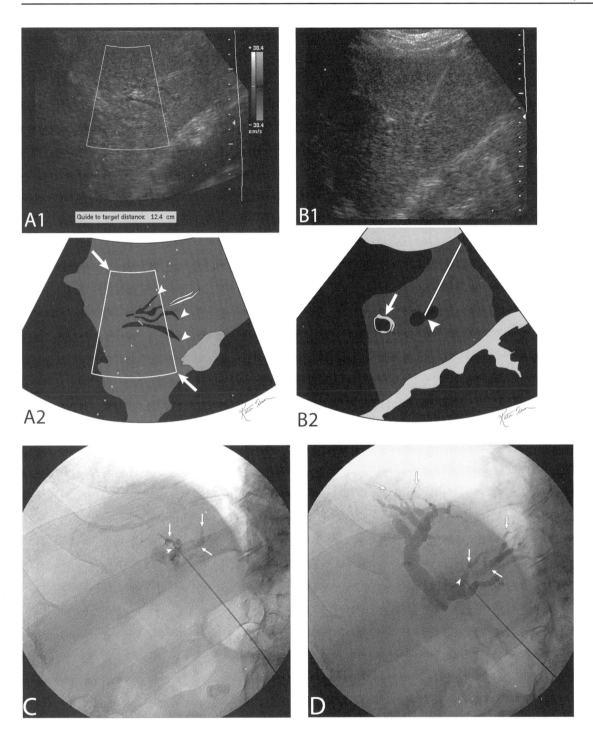

Fig. 12.1 Ultrasound-guided left-sided percutaneous transhepatic cholangiogram. **(A)** Focused gray-scale ultrasound image of the left hepatic lobe with a Doppler ultrasound scan (*between arrows*) focused over target "vessels/bile ducts" within the left lobe (*top*) and schematic sketch of it (*bottom*). The left-sided biliary ducts (*arrowheads*) do not color with Doppler, making them more likely ducts and less likely accompanying vessels. **(B)** Gray-scale ultrasound image of the left hepatic lobe (*top*) and schematic sketch of it (*bottom*). A 21-gauge diamond-tip needle has been passed into one of the peripheral left-sided bile ducts (*arrowhead at needle tip*). The *arrow* point to an adjacent hepatic vessel. **(C)** Single fluoroscopic image as contrast is injected through the 21-gauge needle (*arrowhead at needle tip*). The peripheral bile ducts are visualized immediately (*arrows*). **(D)** Single fluoroscopic image as more contrast is injected through the 21-gauge needle (*arrowhead at needle tip*). The peripheral bile ducts are again visualized (*arrows*) and are dilated due to a left-sided biliary ductal system obstruction.

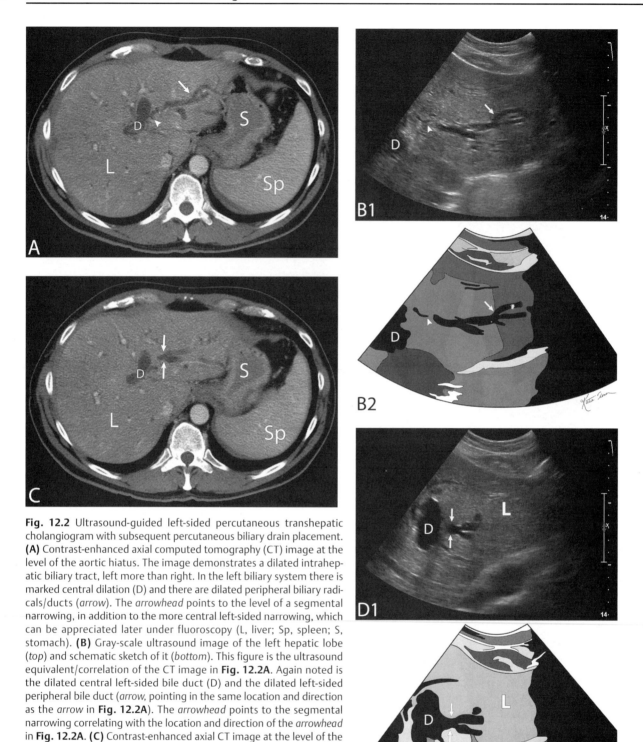

Fig. 12.2 Ultrasound-guided left-sided percutaneous transhepatic cholangiogram with subsequent percutaneous biliary drain placement. **(A)** Contrast-enhanced axial computed tomography (CT) image at the level of the aortic hiatus. The image demonstrates a dilated intrahepatic biliary tract, left more than right. In the left biliary system there is marked central dilation (D) and there are dilated peripheral biliary radicals/ducts (*arrow*). The *arrowhead* points to the level of a segmental narrowing, in addition to the more central left-sided narrowing, which can be appreciated later under fluoroscopy (L, liver; Sp, spleen; S, stomach). **(B)** Gray-scale ultrasound image of the left hepatic lobe (*top*) and schematic sketch of it (*bottom*). This figure is the ultrasound equivalent/correlation of the CT image in **Fig. 12.2A**. Again noted is the dilated central left-sided bile duct (D) and the dilated left-sided peripheral bile duct (*arrow*, pointing in the same location and direction as the *arrow* in **Fig. 12.2A**). The *arrowhead* points to the segmental narrowing correlating with the location and direction of the *arrowhead* in **Fig. 12.2A**. **(C)** Contrast-enhanced axial CT image at the level of the aortic hiatus. The image again demonstrates the dilated intrahepatic biliary tract, left more than right. In the left biliary system, there is marked central dilation (D) and there are dilated peripheral biliary radicals/ducts. Between the *arrows* is the level of a segmental narrowing, which can be appreciated later under fluoroscopy (L, liver; Sp, spleen; S, stomach). **(D)** Gray-scale ultrasound image of the left hepatic lobe (L) (*top*) and schematic sketch of it (*bottom*). This figure is the ultrasound equivalent/correlation of the CT image in **Fig. 12.2C**. Again, noted is the dilated central left-sided bile duct (D) and the dilated left-sided peripheral bile duct. The *arrows* point to the segmental narrowing correlating with the location between the *arrows* in **Fig. 12.2C**.

(E) Gray-scale ultrasound image of the left hepatic lobe (L) (*top*) and schematic sketch of it (*bottom*). A 21-gauge access needle has been passed under ultrasound guidance down to one of the peripheral bile ducts. The needle tip (*arrow*) is pushing up against the peripheral bile duct. Again, noted is the more central dilated bile duct (D).

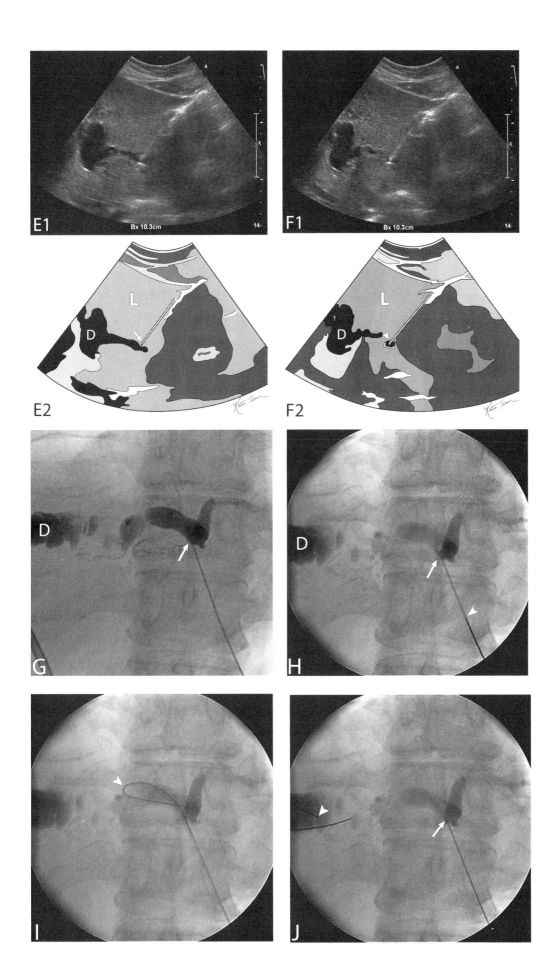

(Continued on page 158)

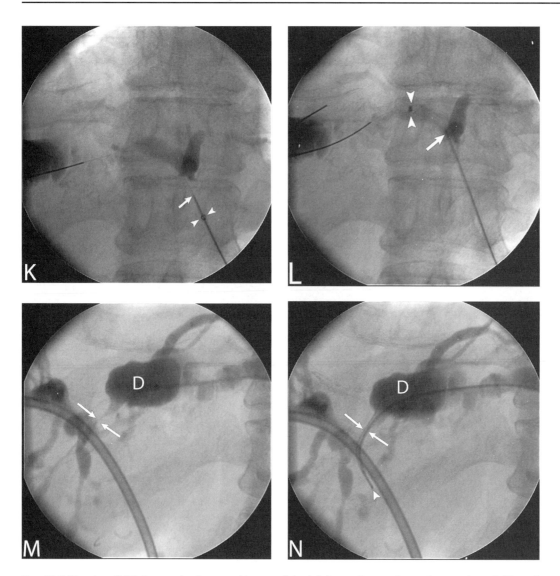

Fig. 12.2 *(Continued)* **(F)** Gray-scale ultrasound image of the left he-patic lobe (L) *(top)* and schematic sketch of it *(bottom)*. The 21-gauge diamond tip access needle has impaled one of the peripheral bile ducts. The needle tip *(arrowhead)* is in the peripheral bile duct. Again, noted is the more central dilated bile duct (D). At this time, the proce-dure is converted from real-time ultrasound guidance to real-time fluoroscopic guidance. **(G)** Single fluoroscopic image as contrast is injected through the 21-gauge needle *(arrow at needle tip)*. The periph-eral bile ducts are visualized immediately. The more central bile duct is dilated (D) correlating with **Figs. 12.2A–12.2D. (H)** Single fluoroscopic image after the inner stylet of the 21-gauge needle has been removed *(arrow at needle tip)*. A 0.018-inch guidewire is being passed down the 21-gauge needle *(arrowhead)*. The more central bile duct is dilated (D) correlating with **Figs. 12.2A–12.2D. (I)** Single fluoroscopic image after the 0.018-inch guidewire has been passed down the 21-gauge needle. The 0.018-inch guidewire is being passed looped as it is being advanced into the peripheral bile duct *(arrowhead)*. **(J)** Single fluoro-scopic image as the 0.018-inch guidewire (arrowhead) is being advanced more centrally through the 21-gauge needle. *Arrow* is at the needle tip. **(K)** Single fluoroscopic image captured as an AccuStick

(Boston Scientific, Natick, MA) dilator *(arrow and arrowheads)* is being passed down the 0.018-inch guidewire. The AccuStick system has three parts to it. The first (most innerpart) is a metal stiffener *(arrow at tip of it)*. The second most inner is a 3-French dilator tapered lead point (not seen, not radiopaque). The outermost part is a 6.5-French dilator that takes a 4-French inner lumen catheter. This outermost component has a radiopaque ring just short of its tip *(arrow)*. The pur-pose of the AccuStick system is to establish a long (deep) access with a metal stiffener to aid in depth support and ultimately allow the opera-tor to upsize from a 0.018-inch wire to a 0.035-inch wire. **(L)** Single flu-oroscopic image captured as the outer AccuStick dilator *(arrowheads at radiopaque marker)* is being passed down the 0.018-inch guidewire and over the metal stiffener *(arrow at tip of metal stiffener)*. **(M)** Single fluoroscopic image captured after contrast is injected through the outer AccuStick dilator. This demonstrates a dilated bile duct (D) and just distal to it a tight stricture *(between arrows)*. **(N)** Single fluoro-scopic image captured as a 0.035-inch glidewire *(arrowhead)* is used to traverse the tight stricture *(between arrows)*. Again, noted is the dilated bile duct more proximally (D).

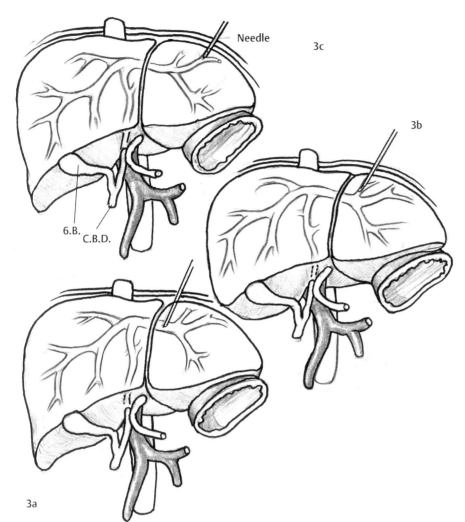

Fig. 12.3 Planning left-side percutaneous biliary drain (PBD) placement. **(A)** Schematic of the liver demonstrating a centrally placed needle in the left main bile duct. This may be acceptable for a percutaneous transhepatic cholangiogram, but it is not acceptable for a definitive access for a PBD placement for two reasons: (1) passing a drain centrally has a higher risk of injuring the central hepatic vessels, and (2) there is little "running room" for adequate drain placement. In other words, there is not enough room for side holes for the drain placement to adequately drain the left-sided biliary system. **(B)** Schematic of the liver demonstrating a segmentally placed needle. This is satisfactory for PBD placement. A more peripheral access is better; however, this segmental access is still acceptable especially if the PBD placement is being performed emergently (cholangitis with sepsis, for example). **(C)** Schematic of the liver demonstrating a peripherally placed needle. This is appropriate for PBD placement. Notice that all the needles in **Figs 12.3A–12.3C** point centrally. This is the trajectory at which the needle should access the biliary system. This allows the wire to be passed centrally toward the direction of the central bile ducts and subsequently the bowel. The images in **Figs. 12.1 and 12.2** demonstrate needle placement toward the central bile ducts (adequate placement). The image in **Fig. 12.4** demonstrates a central bile duct access directed toward the peripheral bile ducts (inadequate definitive needle access placement).

Postprocedural Evaluation and Management

Percutaneous transhepatic cholangiography with biliary drain placement should not be performed on an outpatient basis. Patients should be admitted for observation for 23 hours.

Postpercutaneous Biliary Drainage Observation Period

- Routine admission should be the standard of practice.
- If the PBD is internal/external: The PBD should be set to gravity drainage for at least 24–48 hours even if it is an internal external drain. Ideally, the internal external biliary drain is left until a major step down in external biliary drainage occurs. At this time, an overnight capping of the external component of the PBD is performed. This tests the ability of the internal drainage component of the PBD to drain the obstructed

bile. If the patient passes the "capping test" with no fever or pain, then the patient can be discharged home safely.
- If the PBD is external (failed internalization): The PBD should always be set to gravity drainage without capping and with adequate hydration (see below).
- Check on the patient and monitor vital signs
- Observe the biliary output including volume output and character
  - Thick bile blocking the drain requires the drain to be flushed with ~5–7 mL of sterile saline. A practice that is performed routinely in some institutions (institutions acquainted with native livers and malignant biliary obstruction) and less frequently in other institutions (acquainted with transplanted livers).
  - It is not uncommon to have sanguineous bile discharge. The blood tinge should clear with time.
  - Bile output that steadily increases in blood tinge and frank blood should be a concern (see below for management).

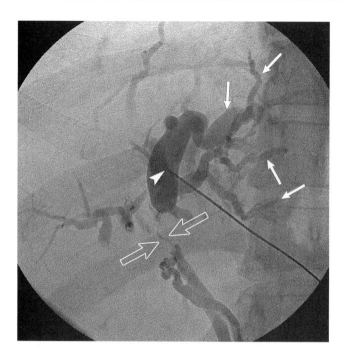

Fig. 12.4 Percutaneous transhepatic cholangiogram after ultrasound-guided needle placement. Single fluoroscopic image after contrast is injected through the 21-gauge needle (*arrowhead at needle tip*). The needle tip is directed toward the peripheral bile ducts (*arrows*) and away from the more central bile duct stricture, which needs to be traversed for adequate percutaneous biliary drain placement and thus adequate biliary drainage. See the discussion in the legend for **Fig. 12.3C**.

Intravenous Fluid and Diet

- IV access should be kept until just prior to hospital discharge.
- IV fluid should be given until oral intake is adequate. This is particularly true in the first 24–48 hours of an internal/external PBD and always in an external PBD. Fluid and electrolyte loss can be considerable from PBD.
- The ideal IV fluid for a biliary patient being drained is lactated Ringers' solution to replace serum potassium loss, in particular.
- Institutions that practice moderate sedation start with a clear liquid diet and advance it as tolerated. This helps to offset patient's nausea and vomiting.
- Start clear liquid diet immediately and advance it as tolerated. Other institutions/operators commence a clear liquid diet after a period of abstinence of oral intake. This period could be one hour, for example.

Activity

- Bed rest for 4 hours
- The biliary drain/bag uses gravity drainage.

- Patients should be instructed on how to maneuver with the biliary drains and to be reminded that they are tethered to a collecting bag.

Pain Management

- Narcotics may be required post-PBD and usually not after PTC only. Some patients require oral narcotic analgesics such as acetaminophen and hydrocodone combination medication. Rarely does a patient require IV narcotics such as fentanyl.
- Continued pain, especially if accompanied with a drop in pressure, should be concerning for a pericapsular hematoma. A noncontrast CT can be performed to evaluate for this.

Monitoring Vital Signs

- Vital sign monitoring includes blood pressure and heart rate. Occasionally, oxygen saturation monitoring is required in cases of shortness of breath and/or chest pain.
- In cases of shortness of breath, one must be able to differentiate between splinting due to pain and pleural complications (pneumothorax or hemothorax). Clinical exam and a chest x-ray would help differentiate between the two.
- Institutions/operators that practice conscious sedation may record a softer blood pressure than a patient's baseline blood pressure after the biopsy. This is the most likely due to sedation with or without dehydration. The patient usually responds in time with hydration, particularly as the sedatives wear off.
- Continued hypotension and more importantly a rise in heart rate are concerning for hypovolemia (bleeding). If signs of hypovolemia occur, an IV volume bolus is given and a noncontrast CT exam is performed to confirm the clinical suspicion of bleeding.

Complications and Their Management

As can be seen in **Table 12.5**, the most common specific complication is cholangitis with or without biliary sepsis. Please see **Table 12.5** for the list of types of complications and their incidence following percutaneous biliary cholangiography and drain placement.

Management of Pain and Pain-Related Morbidity

- It is not uncommon for patients with a freshly placed PBD to have chest pain and splinting from the procedure.

This pain may increase with respiration. The operator must differentiate this pain from a pneumo- or hemothorax (this is mostly a problem of right-sided PBD and less likely of left-sided PBD).

- Chest-wall pain and splinting due to rubbing of the PBD against intercostal nerves is a problem of right-sided PBD and not left-sided PBD. Nevertheless, the pain usually subsides over the next 24–72 hours. Continuous pain may require a change in the transhepatic tracts.
- Continued or increasing pain requires further clinical and possibly imaging evaluation.
- Occasionally operators respond to continued pain by performing a diagnostic imaging exam.
  - A limited ultrasound examination at the site to evaluate for a hepatic capsular hematoma
  - Possibly a more global exam such as a noncontrast abdominal CT exam. Remember, ultimately the decisive factor for significant bleeding is the patient's stability (vitals) – not what is seen in the images

Management of Bleeding Complications

- Bleeding post-PBD can take several forms.
  - Hemobilia (most common)
  - Subcapsular hematoma
  - Extracapsular peritoneal hemorrhage
  - External/site bleeding (rule out a skin bleed first)
  - Hemothorax (rare, see below)
- Frank hemobilia should be managed locally by capping the PBD to tamponade the bleed. Do not provide the bleeding a path of least resistance.
- Significant bleeding affecting vital signs and patient stability should be managed by
  - Fluid resuscitation starting with crystalloid fluid bolus
  - Type and cross
  - Repeat hematocrit to compare with baseline
  - Blood transfusion to maintain hematocrit at or above 30%
  - Surgical/interventional radiology consult
- Interventional radiology can provide the following options in the order given when managing uncontrolled bleeding (**Fig. 12.5**):
  - Removal of PBD over a wire and performing a transhepatic tract sinogram to identify the traversing vessel (portal vein usually) + upsizing the transhepatic tract to tamponade the bleeding
  - Obtain an hepatic angiogram to identify an arterial injury – if identified, then perform a super-selective arterial embolization

  - If a specific arterial injury is not identified, a regional/global arterial Gelfoam (Pfizer Pharmaceuticals, New York, NY) embolization can be performed (not in patients with liver cirrhosis and not in liver transplant recipients).

Management of Pleural/Thoracic Complications

- This is not common; <0.5% in all PBD procedures and is rare in left-sided ultrasound-guided biliary drain placement.
- If chest pain with or without reduced oxygen saturation is encountered, a chest x-ray should be obtained to rule out pneumothorax or hemothorax.
- Clinically significant hemo- and/or pneumothorax require chest tube placement, increased nasal cannula oxygenation, and fluid resuscitation/bleeding management in case of the former (see above).
- If bile accumulates in the pleural space, a chest tube is required as well as diversion of the transhepatic tract to attempt to reduce further bile leak into the pleural space.

Management of Puncture of Adjacent Organs

- This is rare.
- If transgression of bowel occurs by the drain, the drain should be left in place for the tract to mature. This allows
  - The patient to recover from the acute situation of a procedure, renal failure, and/or sepsis
  - Management of the fistula; if one occurs, can be performed in an elective setting.

Sepsis

- Prophylactic antibiotics should be used in all cases.
- Operators should not overdistend the biliary tract with contrast.
- Rigors only without fever can respond to 25–50 mg of Demerol (Sanofi Aventis Pharmaceuticals, Paris, France) administered intramuscularly.
- In cases of postoperative fever (cholangitis), operators should continue with IV antibiotics and should check the culture and sensitivity of the bile sample obtained from the PBD.
- Sepsis requires fluid resuscitation and even vasopressors with admission of the patient to the intensive care unit (ICU).

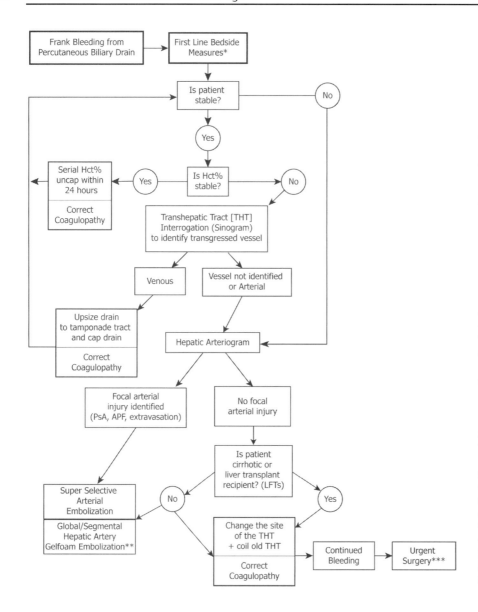

Fig. 12.5 Flowchart demonstrating a suggested algorithm for managing postpercutaneous transhepatic cholangiography and biliary drainage. The intent of this flowchart is to convey a thought process of management, not to dictate a protocol. *First-line bedside measures include (1) assess consciousness and stability by checking vital signs (compare with baseline); (2) type and cross at least 2 units of packed red blood cells; (3) cap percutaneous biliary drain (PBD); and (4) take down soiled dressing and examine site of bleeding (HCT%, Hematocrit [red blood cell concentration in blood]; THT, transhepatic tract; PsA, pseudoaneurysm; APF, arterioportal fistula; LFTs, liver function tests). **Global/segmental Gelfoam (Pfizer Pharmaceuticals, New York, NY) embolization (not with patients who have liver transplants or advanced liver cirrhosis): Global or segmental embolization of the hepatic artery using Gelfoam is an attempt to reduce the perfusion of the liver or the segment of the liver where the PBD passes through. This is a rare scenario and should be considered as a last-line procedure. It is rare because it is very difficult to have a hemorrhagic PBD complication that forces an operator's hand to perform a therapeutic procedure without being able to identify a vascular injury. Nevertheless, the option can be entertained in this rare situation. ***Urgent Surgery: Rarely resorted to nowadays. This is because most PBD bleeding does not warrant this difficult surgery or, if significant, the bleeding can be dealt with decisively via transhepatic and/or endoluminal means. Nevertheless, these surgical procedures have been described (particularly for arterioportal fistula) historically. They are difficult and often bloody surgeries because the injury is often deep and with little vicinity landmarks. These surgeries include hepatic segmentectomies and arterial ligations.

Further Reading

Burke DR, Lewis CA, Cardella JF, et al; Society of Interventional Radiology Standards of Practice Committee. Quality improvement guidelines for percutaneous transhepatic cholangiography and biliary drainage. J Vasc Interv Radiol 2003;14(9 Pt 2):S243–S246

Lorenz JM, Leef JA, Chou CH, Funaki B, Straus CM, Rosenblum JD. Sonographic needle guidance in cholangiography in children. J Vasc Interv Radiol 2001;12(3):342–346

13 Percutaneous Cholecystostomy
Wael E.A. Saad

Indications

Ultrasound-guided percutaneous cholecystostomy was described first in 1979. It is a management alternative to cholecystectomy, mostly for nonsurgical candidates. Overall, cholecystectomy is the first-line treatment and percutaneous cholecystostomy is the second-line treatment. As a result, a contraindication to cholecystectomy (poor surgical candidate) should accompany the indications listed below for percutaneous cholecystectomy to be indicated fully. A soft indication is a patient who is a borderline nonsurgical candidate, who in the acute setting has high surgical morbidity. In this setting, cholecystostomy may be contemplated to resolve the acute situation (cholecystitis among other possible acute medical conditions) and plan for a subsequent elective procedure (cholecystectomy) under stable conditions.

The following are indications of percutaneous cholecystostomy.

Gallbladder Indications (More Common Indications)

- Drainage of the gallbladder
  ○ Calcular cholecystitis
  ○ Acalcular cholecystitis
  ○ Iatrogenic/traumatic gallbladder perforation (bile leak)
- Providing a portal (percutaneous access) for minimal invasive interventions
  ○ For percutaneous removal of biliary stones (cholelithiasis)
    • Fluoroscopic-guided stone removal
    • Percutaneous endoscopic and fluoroscopic stone removal and/or lithotripsy

Bile Duct Indications (Less Common Indications)

- Drainage of the biliary ducts through a patent cystic duct and through the cholecystostomy drain.
- Providing a portal (percutaneous access) for minimally invasive interventions for the common bile duct. An internal/external transcholecystic biliary drain can be placed to drain the gallbladder and the common bile duct.

- Diagnostic opacification of the biliary tract including decompressed intrahepatic bile ducts after failed percutaneous transhepatic cholangiography to opacify the ducts. This makes it possible for a more precise and more selective percutaneous transhepatic biliary drain placement (**Fig. 13.1**).

Contraindications

Relative Contraindication

- Uncorrected coagulopathy. Relative versus absolute contraindication depends on the degree of coagulopathy, the clinical setting, and the degree of urgency of the percutaneous cholecystostomy procedure.

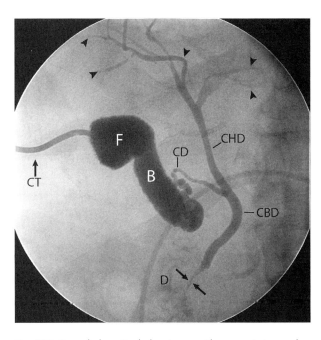

Fig. 13.1 Transcholecystic cholangiogram. Fluoroscopic image demonstrating a cholangiogram through a cholecystostomy tube and a patent cystic duct. Details of the biliary tract including peripheral/intrahepatic bile ducts are seen (*arrowheads*). Notice the mamillated appearance of the fundus of the gallbladder (F, fundus of gallbladder; B, body of gallbladder; CD, cystic duct; CT, cholecystostomy tube; CHD, common hepatic duct; CBD, common bile duct; D, duodenum). (*Arrows*, level of sphincter of Oddi).

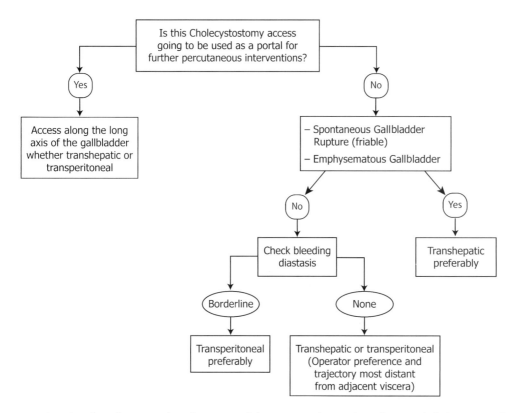

Fig. 13.2 Flowchart illustrating thought process of choosing transhepatic versus transperitoneal access to the gallbladder. Further transcholecystic percutaneous interventions include gallbladder stone extraction (transhepatic choledoscopy, or fluoroscopy), choledocholithiasis stone extraction (transhepatic choledoscopy, or fluoroscopy), and transcholecystic biliary drainage.

Preprocedural Evaluation

The gallbladder can be accessed percutaneously from a strict transperitoneal approach or from a transhepatic approach (crossing a segment of liver to the gallbladder). The details of which and when an approach is better will be discussed in detail in the Technique section below (**Fig. 13.2**).

Evaluate Prior Cross-Sectional Imaging

Look for collaborative evidence of cholecystitis such as a thick gallbladder wall (>3 mm) or gallbladder stones (cholelithiasis) (**Figs. 13.3 and 13.4**).

- It helps to see prior images and see if the gallbladder wall thickening is new (**Fig.13.3**).
- Remember that a thick gallbladder wall is sensitive, but not specific (several causes besides cholecystitis).
- Causes of thick gallbladder wall
  - Cholecystitis
    - Acute versus chronic cholecystitis
    - Calcular versus acalcular cholecystitis
  - Adjacent inflammation/infection
    - Hepatitis

- Pancreatitis
- Diverticulitis
  - Adjacent fluid/edema, causes of fluid overload
    - Ascites
    - Anasarca
    - Renal failure, nephritic syndrome
    - Liver failure, cirrhosis
    - Severe heart failure
    - Protein deficiency (malnutrition, liver disease, etc.)
  - Focal > diffuse wall thickening
    - Adenomyomatosis
    - Gallbladder adenoma/adenocarcinoma
    - Adherent stone(s)

Look for access routes (access planning) (**Figs. 13.5, 13.6, 13.7, and 13.8**)

- Evaluate the size and orientation of the gallbladder
- Evaluate the percutaneous window to the gallbladder
  - Is there a transperitoneal (nonhepatic) window?
  - Is there a transhepatic window?
  - Is there both a transperitoneal and a transhepatic option for the gallbladder?

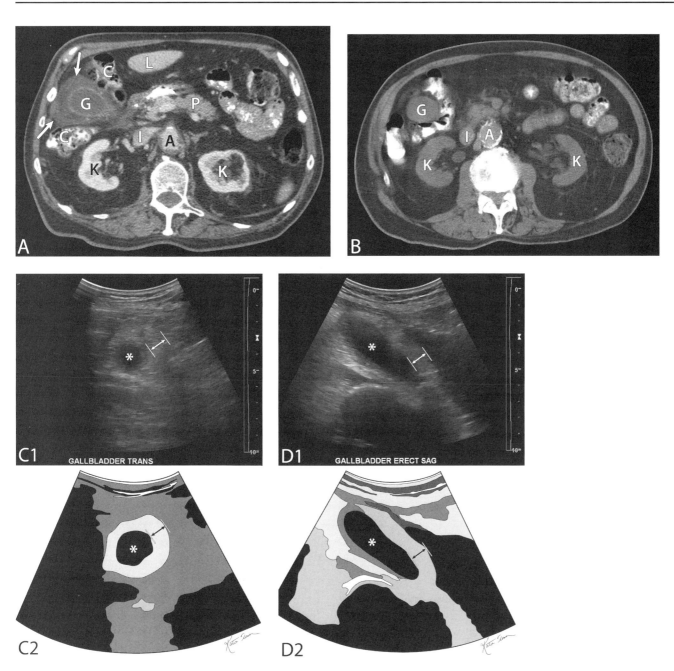

Fig. 13.3 Collaborative evidence of cholecystitis. **(A)** Contrast-enhanced axial computed tomography (CT) image of the abdomen just below the liver demonstrating a very thick gallbladder wall (*arrows*). Compare with the unenhanced CT of the same patient 3 months earlier in **Fig. 13.3B** (K, kidneys; L, liver; C, colon; P, pancreas; A, aorta; I, inferior vena cava [IVC]; G, gallbladder). **(B)** Nonenhanced axial CT image of the abdomen just below the liver of the same patient as **Fig. 13.3A**, however, 3 months earlier demonstrating a gallbladder with imperceptible walls (G). Compare with the contrast-enhanced CT of the same patient 3 months later (K, kidneys; A, aorta; I, IVC; G, gallbladder).

(C) Gray-scale ultrasound image of the gallbladder (transverse on gallbladder) of the patient with the thick gallbladder wall in **Figs. 13.3A and 13.3B** (*top*) and schematic sketch of it (*bottom*). Again, noted is the thick gallbladder wall (*two-way arrow*) surrounding the gallbladder lumen (*). **(D)** Gray-scale ultrasound image of the gallbladder (long on gallbladder) of the patient with the thick gallbladder wall in **Figs. 13.3A, 13.3B, and 13.3C** (*top*) and schematic sketch of it (*bottom*). Again, noted is the thick gallbladder wall (*two-way arrow*) surrounding the gallbladder lumen (*).

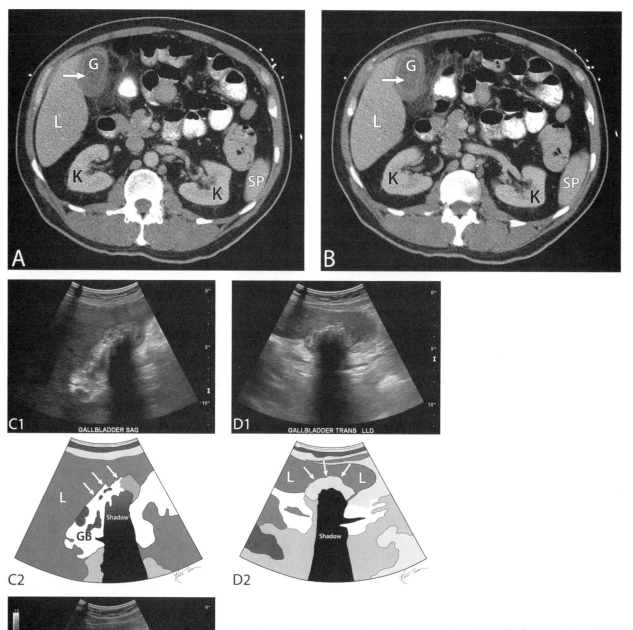

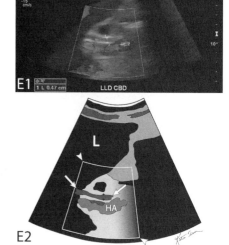

Fig. 13.4 Collaborative evidence of cholecystitis: cholelithiasis. **(A)** Contrast-enhanced axial computed tomography (CT) image of the abdomen at the lower aspect of the liver demonstrating a thick gallbladder wall and what appears to be one or two stones (*arrow*) within the gallbladder (K, kidneys; L, kiver; G, gallbladder; Sp, spleen). **(B)** Contrast-enhanced axial CT image (adjacent to the slice of **Fig. 13.4A**) of the abdomen at the lower aspect of the liver demonstrating a thick gallbladder wall and what appears to be one or two stones (*arrow*) within the gallbladder (K, kidneys; L, liver; G, gallbladder; Sp, spleen). **(C)** Gray-scale ultrasound image of the gallbladder (long on gallbladder) of the patient with the gallbladder stones in **Figs. 13.4A and 13.4B** (*top*) and schematic sketch of it (*bottom*). The ultrasound image (ultrasound is more sensitive at detecting stones than CT) demonstrates numerous stones filling the gallbladder (*arrows*), which cause shadowing. The CT has underestimated the amount of stones, which in this case are numerous and are impacting the gallbladder (L, liver; GB, gallbladder). **(D)** Gray-scale ultrasound image of the gallbladder (transverse on gallbladder) of the patient with the gallbladder stones in **Figs. 13.4A, 13.4B, and 13.4C** (*top*) and schematic sketch of it (*bottom*). The ultrasound image (ultrasound is more sensitive at detecting stones than CT) demonstrates numerous stones filling the gallbladder (*arrows*), which cause shadowing. The CT has underestimated the amount of stones, which in this case are numerous and are impacting the gallbladder (L, Liver). **(E)** Doppler ultrasound image of the hepatic hilum of the patient in **Figs. 13.4A–13.4D** (*top*) and schematic sketch of it (*bottom*). The ultrasound image demonstrate the common bile duct (*between arrows*), which measures 4.7 mm in diameter anterior to the hepatic artery (HA). The Doppler "box" is between the *arrowheads* (L, liver).

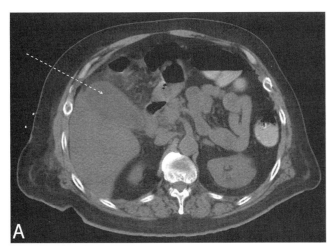

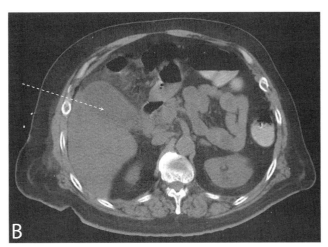

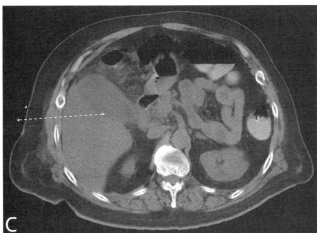

Fig. 13.5 Transperitoneal and transhepatic accesses into the gallbladder. **(A)** Unenhanced axial computed tomography (CT) image of the abdomen at the lower aspect of the liver. The *dashed line* indicates the access trajectory going along the long axis of the gallbladder through a direct transperitoneal approach, through the gallbladder fundus, and without transgressing the liver. **(B)** Unenhanced axial CT image of the abdomen at the lower aspect of the liver. The *dashed line* indicates the access trajectory transgressing a small part of the liver and entering the gallbladder at the lateral one-third of its wall. This access is transhepatic; however, it most likely is also transperitoneal because it does not pass through the bare area of the gallbladder. **(C)** Unenhanced axial CT image of the abdomen at the lower aspect of the liver. The dashed line indicates the transhepatic access trajectory transgressing the liver and entering the gallbladder at the medial one-third of its wall. This access is transhepatic, and most likely (but not definitely) passes through the bare area of the gallbladder.

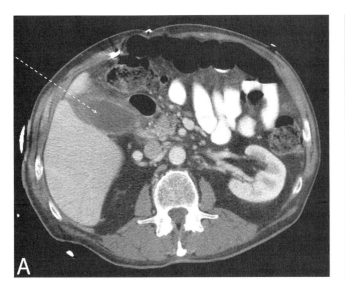

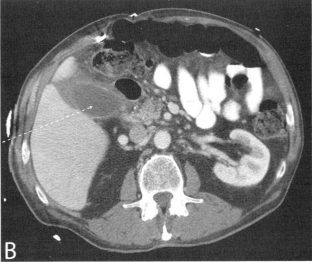

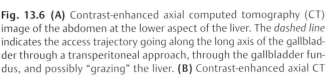

Fig. 13.6 (A) Contrast-enhanced axial computed tomography (CT) image of the abdomen at the lower aspect of the liver. The *dashed line* indicates the access trajectory going along the long axis of the gallbladder through a transperitoneal approach, through the gallbladder fundus, and possibly "grazing" the liver. **(B)** Contrast-enhanced axial CT image of the abdomen at the lower aspect of the liver. The *dashed line* indicates the transhepatic access trajectory transgressing the liver and entering the gallbladder at the medial one-third of its wall. This access is transhepatic, and most likely (but not definitely) passes through the bare area of the gallbladder. *(Continued on page 168)*

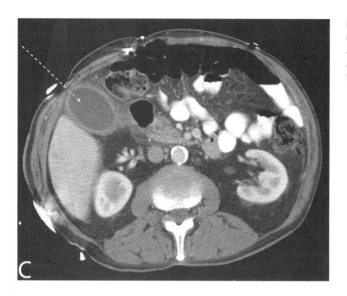

Fig. 13.6 *(Continued)* **(C)** Contrast-enhanced axial CT image of the abdomen at the lower aspect of the liver. The *dashed line* indicates the access trajectory to the gallbladder through a direct transperitoneal approach, through the gallbladder fundus, and without transgressing the liver.

- Evaluate if there is focal wall thickening or associated masses to the gallbladder. Can this mass be avoided?
- Evaluate the hepatic segment that may be traversed by the cholecystostomy drain and make sure it is free of cysts and/or masses

Look for adjacent organs that can be inadvertently traversed (**Figs. 13.7 and 13.8**)

- The right colon is the organ that may be traversed.
- This can help reduce transgression of adjacent organs with subsequent potential major complications.

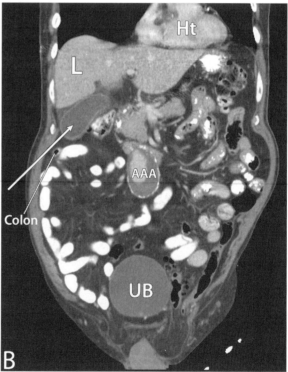

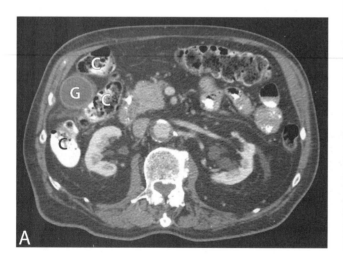

Fig. 13.7 Computed tomography (CT) images demonstrating proximity of structures to the gallbladder fundus. **(A)** Contrast-enhanced axial CT image of the abdomen below the liver. The fundus of the gallbladder (G) is surrounded by colon (C). Whenever contemplating transperitoneal gallbladder fundus access, the colon is usually in close proximity.

(B) Contrast-enhanced coronal CT reconstruction of the patient in **Fig. 13.7A**. The *solid line* indicates the transperitoneal access trajectory entering the gallbladder along its long axis. Again, noted is the close proximity of bowel to the gallbladder fundus (Ht, heart; L, liver; AAA, abdominal aortic aneurysm; UB, urinary bladder).

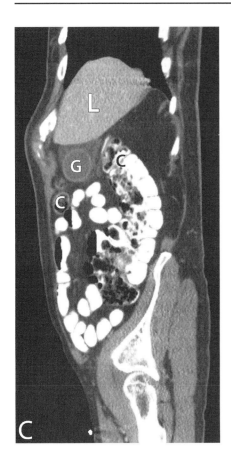

Fig. 13.7 *(Continued)* **(C)** Contrast-enhanced sagittal CT reconstruction of the patient in **Fig. 13.7A**. Again, noted is the close proximity of bowel to the gallbladder fundus (G; L, liver; C, colon).

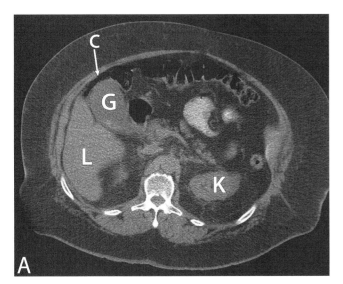

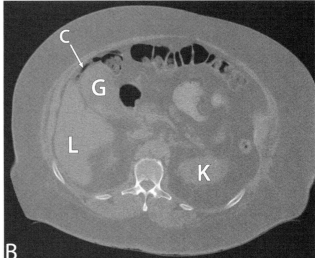

Fig. 13.8 (A) Unenhanced axial computed tomography (CT) image of the abdomen below the liver (soft tissue window). The fundus of the gallbladder (G) is surrounded by colon (C). Whenever contemplating transperitoneal gallbladder fundus access, the colon is usually in close proximity (L, liver; K, kidney). **(B)** Unenhanced axial CT image of the abdomen below the liver (bone window). The fundus of the gallbladder (G) is surrounded by colon (C). Whenever contemplating transperitoneal gallbladder fundus access, the colon is usually in close proximity (L, liver; K, kidney).

- This helps plan the needle trajectory for the cholecystostomy.
- This may make the operator consider approaching the gallbladder transhepatically, if there is close proximity of the colon to the fundus of the gallbladder and a transperitoneal approach is proposed.

Evaluate Prior Hepatobiliary Nuclear Scan

- Look for proof of cholecystitis (**Fig. 13.9**).
- Nonvisualization of the gallbladder despite administration of morphine is the greatest indication along with the clinical symptoms of cholecystitis (the most common indication).
- Remember the classic clinical presentation may be masked: intensive care unit (ICU) patients may be on narcotic analgesic and even sedatives.

Evaluate Preprocedure Laboratory Values

- Laboratory value evaluation mostly revolves around ruling out coagulopathy.
  ○ Suggested coagulopathy thresholds for a transhepatic approach are
    - International normalized ratio (INR): ≤1.4
    - Platelets (PLT): ≥50,000–70,000
    - Activated partial thromboplastin time (aPTT): ≤50 seconds
  ○ Suggested coagulopathy thresholds for an emergent transperitoneal (no hepatic transgression) approach are
    - INR: ≤1.7–1.8
    - PLT: ≥40,000
    - aPTT: ≤65 seconds

Obtain Informed Consent

- Indications
  ○ See indications above
  ○ Technical success in placing a drain in the gallbladder is high (95–100%).
  ○ The clinical success (resolving the presenting symptoms) rate ranges from 56–100%.
- Alternatives
  ○ To refuse the procedure. The patient takes antibiotics only.
  ○ Surgical cholecystectomy – usually contraindicated – why cholecystostomy is proposed
  ○ Future elective cholecystectomy may be the long-term plan under more stable (nonacute) conditions.
- Procedural risks
  ○ Major complications occur in 3–8% of patients.
  ○ Bile leak and biliary peritonitis causing extreme pain (2.5%)

○ Infection (**Table 13.1**)
  - This complication in its broader definition occurs in more than 3% of cases.
  - Infection can be divided into
    ○ Cholangitis (most common)
    ○ Biliary sepsis (most serious)
    ○ Biloma/abscess formation (least common)
  - Patients should receive prophylactic antibiotics prior to any biliary procedure. Intravenous antibiotics used include Zosyn (Wyeth Pharmaceuticals, Madison, NJ): 3.375 g intravenously (IV; primary antibiotic used by the authors), and ciprofloxacin: 400 mg IV.
○ Bleeding (**Table 13.1**)
  - Most common presentation of bleeding is bleeding from the biliary drain (hemobilia/upper gastrointestinal bleeding).
  - It may present as pain and/or hypotension and a computed tomography (CT) scan may show subcapsular hematoma or active extravasation in the few cases where CT IV contrast is used.
  - Bleeding may be transient with or without blood transfusion.
  - In rare cases, bleeding may require intervention such as transcatheter hepatic arterial embolization or exploratory surgery.
○ Injury to surrounding organs and/or structures (**Table 13.1**)
  - Pleura (pneumo- and hemothorax)
  - Colon

Equipment

Ultrasound Guidance

- Multiarray 4–5 MHz ultrasound transducer
- Transducer guide bracket (not necessary)
- Sterile transducer cover

Standard Surgical Preparation and Draping

- Chlorhexidine skin preparation/cleansing fluid
- Fenestrated drape

Local Infiltrative Analgesia Administration

- 21-gauge infiltration needle
- 10 to 20 mL 1% lidocaine syringe

Sharp Access Devices

- 11-blade incision scalpel
  ○ 8-gauge needle that allows a 0.035-inch or 0.038-inch wire

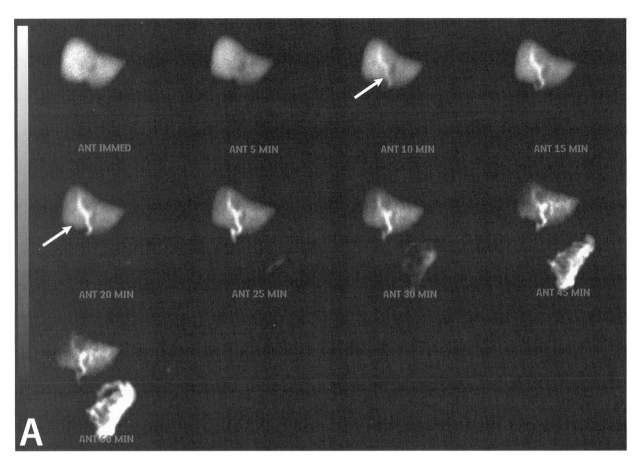

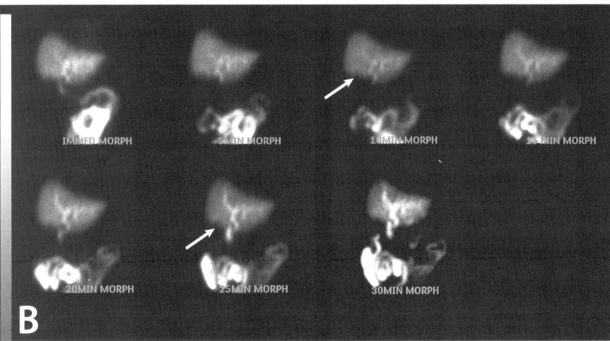

Fig. 13.9 **(A)** Hepatobiliary scan over 60 minutes without morphine administration. There is prompt uptake of the radiotracer at time-zero. At 10 minutes, radiotracer is excreted into the intrahepatic biliary tract. Radiotracer is seen in the small bowel from 25–60 minutes. The gallbladder is not visualized in the entire series (*arrows*). **(B)** Hepatobiliary scan after administering morphine. Again, the gallbladder is not visualized in the entire series (*arrows*). These findings are consistent with cholecystitis.

Table 13.1 Complications of Percutaneous Cholecystostomy

Complication	Incidence*
Cholangitis/sepsis	Not uncommon†
Hemorrhage requiring transfusion &/or embolization	1.6–2.2%
Biliary leak and peritonitis	2.4–4.4%
Hemo- and/or pneumothorax	Rare
30-day mortality (not related to procedure)‡	0–25%

*Incidences in percentage are when these complications are mentioned. Not all studies mention all complications.

†Not necessarily due to procedure. Usually present prior to and during the procedure (part of the indications of cholecystostomy). As a result it is difficult to assess after the cholecystostomy procedure.

‡The wide range in mortality depends on how morbid the patient population is.

Tubular Access Devices

- An 8-French fascial dilator that can be passed over a 0.035-inch guidewire may be used (see below).
- An 8-French self-retaining (string-locking) pigtail drainage catheter, which is the definitive cholecystostomy tube/drain to be placed last (final product of the procedure)

Technique

There are two approaches to access the gallbladder: (1) a transhepatic access, and (2) an extrahepatic transperitoneal access. Some operators religiously utilize the transhepatic approach with the belief that this technique allows the drain to pass the bare area of the gallbladder, thus preventing any bile leak from extending into the peritoneum (uncontained bile leak), which may lead to biloma and/or pain. However, the bare area cannot be reliably imaged or traversed; hence, over 50% of presumed transhepatic cholecystostomies aiming for the bare area of the gallbladder miss the bare area and are actually transperitoneal (**Table 13.2; Figs. 13.10, 13.11, and 13.12**). Either of

these approaches may be used dependent on the circumstances. Details of how and when to use each approach are given in **Fig. 13.2**.

Intravenous Access and Medication

- Required for moderate sedation and fluid replenishment/resuscitation
- Required for IV prophylactic antibiotics such as
  - Zosyn 3.375 g
  - Ciprofloxacin 500 mg

Preprocedure Ultrasound Exam

- Identify the gallbladder
- Identify the long axis of the gallbladder if the cholecystostomy will be a portal for further percutaneous interventions. In addition, identify if there are viscera in the way of the long axis trajectory. A common anatomic scenario is colon in the way of the transperitoneal long axis of the gallbladder (**Fig. 13.8**).
- Identify whether the liver has to be crossed; if so, determine if there is a bleeding diathesis
- Correlate and triangulate the access site (at skin) and the gallbladder to choose and mark the skin access site
  - Be away from the rib cage; make sure the needle trajectory does not cross costal cartilage or ribs
  - The preferred needle skin entry site is 1.5–2.0 cm from the subcostal margin to reduce postprocedural chest wall pain complications.
- Make sure that the hepatic parenchymal tract (if a transhepatic tract is chosen) to the target gallbladder is clear of hepatic cysts or tumors.
- Manipulating the transducer (along with the bracketed needle guide) is used to choose and triangulate the skin entry site, the target gallbladder site, and the needle trajectory to achieve the above points.

Standard Surgical Preparation and Draping

- Skin preparation/cleansing in the region that was chosen as an ultrasound imaging portal and a needle access needle portal

Table 13.2 Advantages and Disadvantages of Transhepatic versus Transperitoneal Cholecystostomy

	Transhepatic	Transperitoneal
Advantages	Better support to drain placement especially in ascites May prevent bile leaking into peritoneum (painful)	Higher levels of coagulopathy can be tolerated
Disadvantages	Coagulopathy not tolerated (authors' experience) 58% of cases are actually transperitoneal (partly a myth)	Can be extremely painful if bile leaks and touches the peritoneal lining (bile/chemical peritonitis); however, 58% of so-called transhepatic cholecystostomies are actually transperitoneal

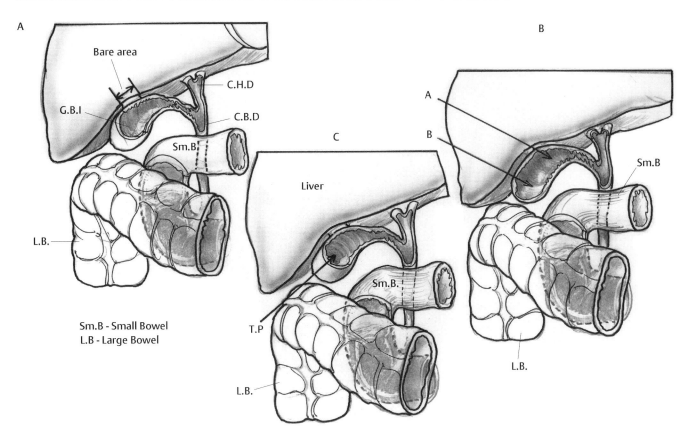

Fig. 13.10 Anatomy of the gallbladder and potential access trajectories. **(A)** Schematic drawing of the right upper quadrant of the abdomen. The bare area is a reflection of the peritoneum where the gallbladder is "adherent" to the liver without an intervening peritoneal lining (CHD, common hepatic duct; CBD, common bile duct; SmB, small bowel; LB, large bowel). **(B)** Schematic drawing of the right upper quadrant of the abdomen demonstrating two hypothetical transhepatic access needle trajectories (A and B). Trajectory A traverses the bare area of the gallbladder and does not transgress any peritoneal linings (schematic equivalent of **Fig. 13.5C**). Any leakage from the gallbladder will most likely be extraperitoneal. Trajectory B, despite traversing liver, transgresses the peritoneal lining at two places (at the undersurface of the right hepatic lobe and at the supralateral surface of the gallbladder) (schematic equivalent of **Fig. 13.5B**). Leakage from this access most likely will be intraperitoneal. Unfortunately, imaging (CT and ultrasound) does not clearly identify the bare area of the gallbladder. As a result, transhepatic access does not necessarily ensure traversal of the gallbladder via its bare area (extraperitoneal). Actually, there is almost a 50–50 chance that a transhepatic cholecystostomy access will be actually extraperitoneal (via the bare area) (SmB, small bowel; LB, large bowel). **(C)** Schematic drawing of the right upper quadrant of the abdomen. A strictly transperitoneal (TP) access needle trajectory is drawn going down the long axis of the gallbladder and intentionally avoiding the liver altogether. This is the schematic equivalent of **Figs. 13.5A, 13.6C, and 13.7B**.

- Place a fenestrated drape at the chosen and prepared skin region

Local Infiltrative Analgesia Administration

- Utilizing a 21-gauge (by at least a 3.7-cm-long) infiltration needle, 1% lidocaine infiltration is performed, infiltrating down to the sensitive hepatic capsule and even gallbladder wall (**Fig. 13.13**).

Ultrasound-Guided Sharp Access

- Free-hand ultrasound guidance and an 18-gauge hypodermic needle (no stylet) connected to a 20-mL syringe half filled with radiographic contrast via connector/extension tubing
  - Once the needle traverses the skin into the subcutaneous tissue suction is applied (operator aspirates using syringe) as the needle is advanced further.
  - The connector tubing allows the operator to have flexibility in manipulating the needle free-hand.
  - Needle tip entry (seen by real-time ultrasound) into the lumen of the gallbladder should correlate with an abrupt return of bile into the syringe (**Figs. 13.13 and 13.14**).
  - Once a bile sample is obtained, radiographic contrast is injected under fluoroscopy to confirm adequate placement of the needle into the gallbladder.

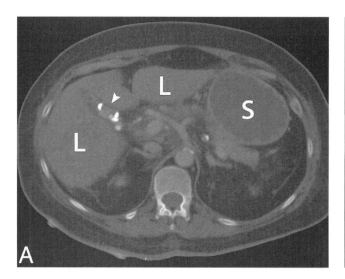

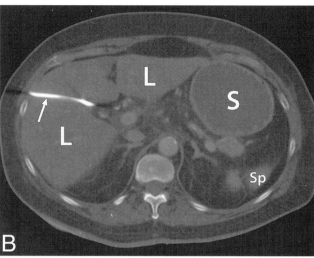

Fig. 13.11 **(A)** Unenhanced axial computed tomography (CT) image of the upper abdomen in a patient with an indwelling transhepatic cholecystostomy drain. The cholecystostomy tube is seen coiled in this image within a decompressed gallbladder (*arrowhead*) (L, liver; S, stomach). **(B)**

Unenhanced axial CT image of the upper abdomen (more cephalad cut than **Fig. 13.11A**) in a patient with an indwelling transhepatic cholecystostomy drain (*arrow*) (Sp, spleen; L, liver; S, stomach).

- Alternatives to the above technique include the use of a 21- to 18-gauge needle with or without the use of a needle guide (ultrasound needle guide bracket).
  - Once the needle is placed, the stylet is removed and the procedure is converted to real-time fluoroscopy (**Figs. 13.13** and **13.15**).

Fluoroscopic-Guided Wire and Tube Access

- Once the needle is in place, contrast is injected to confirm adequate placement of the needle (**Figs. 13.13** and **13.15**).
- An 0.018-inch wire is passed through the 21- to 22-gauge needle or a 0.035-inch wire is passed through a

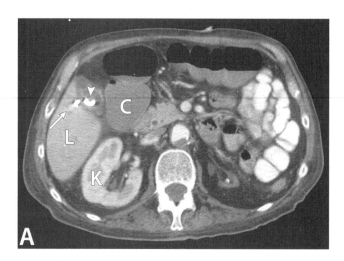

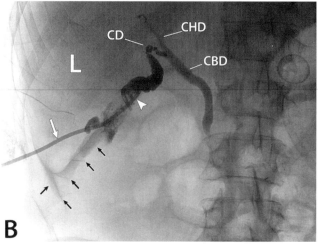

Fig. 13.12 Transhepatic access that is also transperitoneal. **(A)** Contrast-enhanced axial computed tomography (CT) image of the upper abdomen in a patient with an indwelling transhepatic cholecystostomy drain. The cholecystostomy tube is seen in this image traversing a short and peripheral segment of the liver (*arrow*) and ending coiled within the gallbladder (*arrowhead*) (L, liver; K, kidney; C, colon). **(B)** Fluoroscopic image during a cholecystogram through the cholecystostomy tube seen in **Fig. 13.12A**. The cholecystostomy drain is seen traversing a short and

peripheral segment of the liver (*white arrow*, also the equivalent to the *arrow* in **Fig. 13.12A**) and ending coiled within the gallbladder (*arrowhead*, the equivalent to the *arrowhead* in **Fig. 13.12A**). A contrast leak is noted (immature tract); it is clearly leaking into the peritoneum outlining the lower aspect of the right hepatic lobe (*black arrows*). This fluoroscopic image is reminiscent to Trajectory B in the schematic drawn in **Fig. 13.10B** (L, liver; CD, cystic duct; CHD, common hepatic duct; CBD, common bile duct).

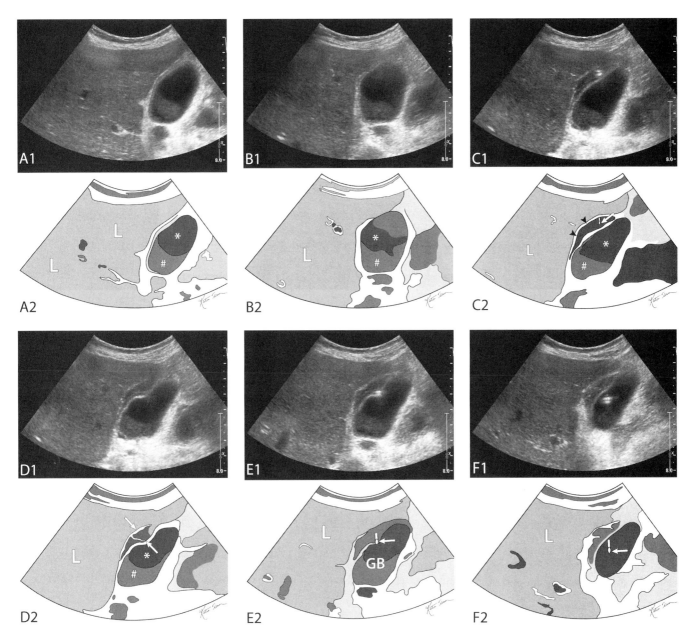

Fig. 13.13 Cholecystostomy tube placement, step-by-step. **(A)** Gray-scale ultrasound image of right upper quadrant of the abdomen (*top*) and schematic sketch of it (*bottom*). The image is oblique on the gallbladder (almost long). The gallbladder is seen "hugged" by the liver (L). In the dependent portion of the gallbladder, inspissated bile/sludge is seen layering (#). Above it is hypoechoic (less dense) bile (*). Both the # and * represent the gallbladder lumen. **(B)** Gray-scale ultrasound image of right upper quadrant of the abdomen (*top*) and schematic sketch of it (*bottom*). The image is more transverse on the gallbladder. Again, the gallbladder is seen "hugged" by the liver (L). Again, in the dependent portion of the gallbladder, inspissated bile/sludge is seen layering (#). Above it is hypoechoic (less dense) bile (*). Both the # and * represent the gallbladder lumen. **(C)** Gray-scale ultrasound image of right upper quadrant of the abdomen (*top*) and schematic sketch of it (*bottom*). A 21-gauge lidocaine infiltrative needle has been advanced (*arrow*). Lidocaine is injected and infiltrates between the gallbladder and liver (*arrowheads*). Again, in the dependent portion of the gallbladder, inspissated bile/sludge is seen

layering (#). Above it is hypoechoic (less dense) bile (*). Both the # and * represent the gallbladder lumen. **(D)** Gray-scale ultrasound image of right upper quadrant of the abdomen (*top*) and schematic sketch of it (*bottom*). The 21-gauge lidocaine infiltrative needle has been removed. The effect of lidocaine infiltration is seen with the infiltrative space created between the gallbladder and the liver (*between arrows*). In the dependent portion of the gallbladder, inspissated bile/sludge is again seen layering (#). Above it is hypoechoic (less dense) bile (*). Both the # and * represent the gallbladder lumen. **(E)** Gray-scale ultrasound image of right upper quadrant of the abdomen (*top*) and schematic sketch of it (*bottom*). The 18-gauge access needle (*arrow*) has been placed and is right at the hepatic-side wall of the gallbladder (GB; L, liver). **(F)** Gray-scale ultrasound image of right upper quadrant of the abdomen (*top*) and schematic sketch of it (*bottom*). The 18-gauge access needle (*arrow*) has been advanced further and its tip (*arrow*) is now placed in the gallbladder lumen. At this time the procedure is converted to real-time fluoroscopy (L, liver). *(Continued on page 176)*

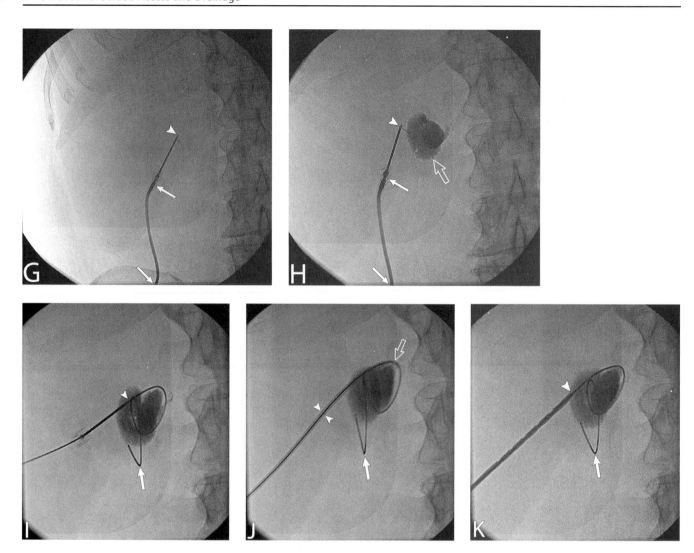

Fig. 13.13 *(Continued)* **(G)** Fluoroscopic image during a cholecystostomy tube placement after the ultrasound-guided procedure steps illustrated in **Figs. 13.13C–13.13F.** The tip of the 18-gauge access needle is in the gallbladder lumen (*arrowhead*) as proven by ultrasound in **Fig. 13.13F.** The 18-gauge access needle is connected to a connector tube (*between arrows*), which is filled with contrast. **(H)** Fluoroscopic image during a cholecystogram during a cholecystostomy tube placement. Contrast is being injected by an 18-gauge access needle with its tip in the gallbladder lumen (*arrowhead*). The 18-gauge access needle is connected to a connector tube (*between arrows*), which is filled with contrast. Contrast is seen staring to fill the gallbladder lumen (*hollow arrow*). Notice the mamillated appearance of the inside of the gallbladder lumen. This is typical and is the result of the mucosal fold or pattern that gives this imprint. This helps the operator identify that the needle is truly in the gallbladder. **(I)** Fluoroscopic image during a cholecystostomy tube placement. A 0.035-inch wire (*arrow*) has been passed through the 18-gauge access needle (*tip of needle at arrowhead*). The 0.035-inch wire is seen coiled in the gallbladder. Again, notice the mamillated appearance of the inside of the gallbladder lumen. This is typical and is the result of the mucosal fold or pattern that gives this imprint. This helps the operator identify that the needle is truly in the gallbladder. **(J)** Fluoroscopic image during a cholecystostomy tube placement. An 8-French dilator (*between arrowheads*) has been passed over the 0.035-inch wire (*solid arrow*). Dilator has been stopped where the wire takes it first sharp turn (*hollow arrow*). **(K)** Fluoroscopic image during a cholecystostomy tube placement. An 8-French cholecystostomy drain has been passed over the 0.035-inch wire (*solid arrow*). The tip of the cholecystostomy tube is just in the gallbladder. At this point, the operator should pass the dilator with controlled conviction and with good counter tension on the wire, while keeping an eye on the gallbladder lumen and making sure it does not distort away from the drain (be pushed away from the drain). If not, the cholecystostomy drain has an inner metal stiffener.

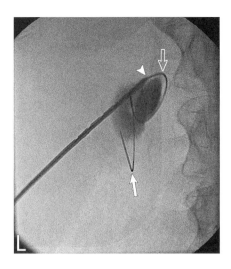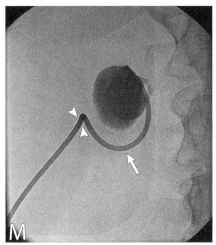

Fig. 13.13 *(Continued)* **(L)** Fluoroscopic image during a cholecystostomy tube placement. The 8-French cholecystostomy drain has been advanced over the 0.035-inch wire (*solid arrow*) with the aid of its inner metal stiffener. The tip of the cholecystostomy tube (*arrowhead*) is in the gallbladder. It stops short of the curve on the 0.035-inch wire (*hollow arrow*). At this point, the dilator is advanced over the wire leaving the metal stiffener behind. Metal does not go around corners. **(M)** Fluoroscopic image during a cholecystostomy tube placement. This is the final image. The 8-French drain enters the gallbladder between the *arrowheads*, loops at the fundus and body of the gallbladder (*arrow*) and ends in the proximal body of the gallbladder where there is contrast.

19- to 18-gauge needle under fluoroscopy. The wire is coiled in the gallbladder lumen.

- An 0.018-inch wire requires it to be upsized to a 0.035 or 0.038-inch wire utilizing an AccuStick (Boston Scientific, Natick, MA) system (telescoped and stiffened dilator, see above).
- Once there is a 0.035-inch wire coiled in the gallbladder, an 8-French fascial dilator is passed to dilate the tract. It is important that the dilator skewers the gallbladder wall and does not just push it away (**Figs. 13.13, 13.15, and 13.16**).
- The dilator is removed and is quickly replaced by a self-retaining string-locking pigtail catheter (8- to 10-French). The pigtail is placed and secured ("Coped") in the gallbladder (**Figs. 13.13, 13.15, and 13.16**). Again, it is important that the stiffened drain skewers the gallbladder wall and does not just push it away (**Figs. 13.13, 13.15, and 13.16**).

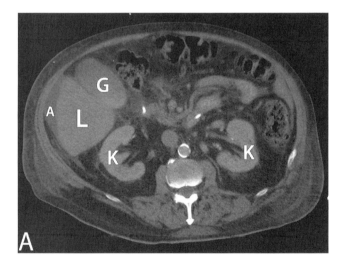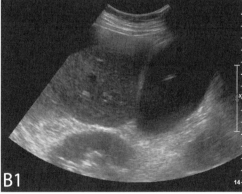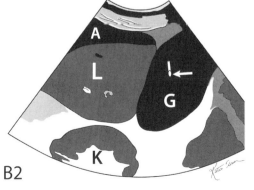

Fig. 13.14 Gallbladder access. **(A)** Unenhanced axial computed tomography (CT) image of the upper abdomen. Perihepatic fluid is seen by CT (A, ascites; G, gallbladder; L, liver; K, kidney). **(B)** Gray-scale ultrasound image of the right upper quadrant (*top*) and schematic sketch of it (*bottom*). Again, noted is the small amount of perihepatic fluid (A). This gray-scale image correlates well with the CT image in **Fig.13.14A**. An 18-gauge access needle has been passed into the gallbladder lumen (*arrow*) (L, liver; G, gallbladder; K, kidney).

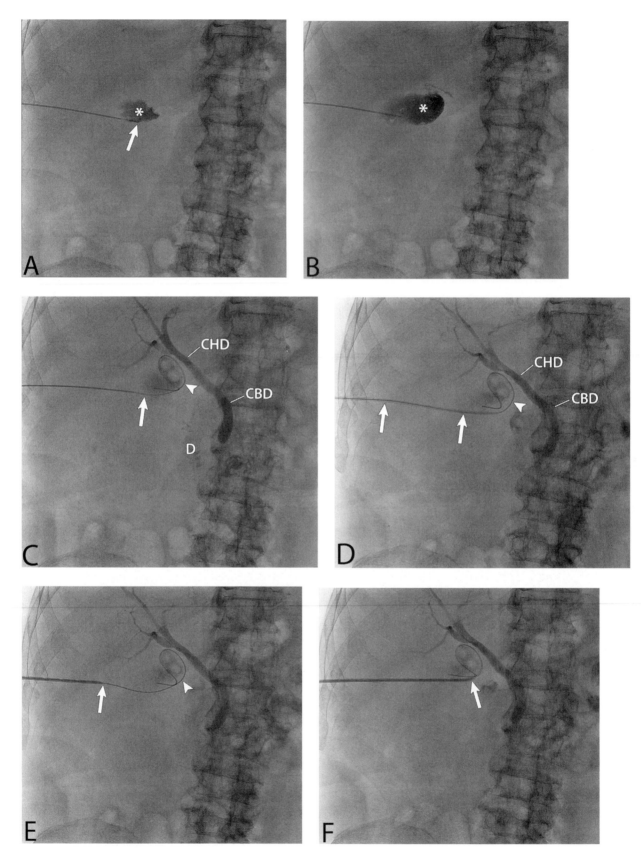

Fig. 13.15 *(Continued)*

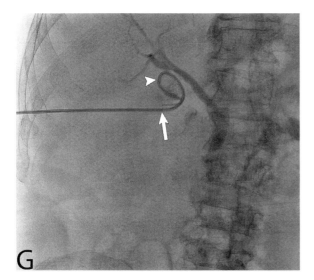

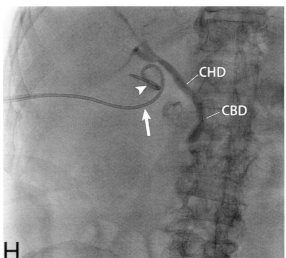

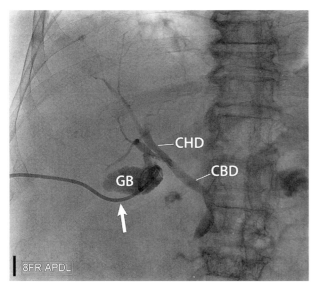

Fig. 13.15 Cholecystostomy tube placement, step-by-step. **(A)** Fluoroscopic image during a cholecystostomy tube placement after the access needle has been placed under ultrasound guidance. The tip of the 18-gauge access needle is in the gallbladder lumen (*arrow at needle tip*). Contrast is seen partly filling (early filling) the gallbladder lumen (*). **(B)** Fluoroscopic image during a cholecystostomy tube placement after the access needle has been placed under ultrasound guidance. More contrast has been injected and is seen partly filling the gallbladder lumen (*). **(C)** Fluoroscopic image during a cholecystostomy tube placement.

A 0.035-inch wire (*arrowhead*) has been passed through the 18-gauge access needle (*tip of needle at arrowhead*). The 0.035-inch wire is seen coiled in the gallbladder (*arrowhead*). Incidentally noted is a cholangiogram due to a patent cystic duct (CHD, common hepatic duct; CBD, common bile duct; D, duodenum). **(D)** Fluoroscopic image during a cholecystostomy tube placement. An 8-French dilator (*arrows*) has been passed over the 0.035-inch wire (*arrowhead*) (CHD, common hepatic duct; CBD, common bile duct). **(E)** Fluoroscopic image during a cholecystostomy tube placement. An 8-French cholecystostomy drain (*tip at arrow*) has been passed over the 0.035-inch wire (*arrowhead*). **(F)** Fluoroscopic image during a cholecystostomy tube placement. The 8-French cholecystostomy drain has been advanced over the 0.035-inch wire with the aid of its inner metal stiffener. The tip of the cholecystostomy tube (*arrow*) is in the gallbladder. It stops short of the curve on the 0.035-inch wire. At this point, the dilator is advanced over the wire leaving the metal stiffener behind. **(G)** Fluoroscopic image during a cholecystostomy tube placement. The 8-French cholecystostomy drain (*arrowhead*) has been advanced over the 0.035-inch wire and beyond the metal stiffener. The pigtail portion of the 8-French drain is coiled in the gallbladder. The tip of the metal stiffener is at the arrow. The inner metal stiffener supports the drain along its entire length into the gallbladder. **(H)** Fluoroscopic image during a cholecystostomy tube placement. The 0.035-inch wire and inner metal stiffener have been removed. The *arrow* points to where the tip of the metal stiffener lies (compare with **Fig. 13.15G**). The pigtail portion of the 8-French drain is coiled in the gallbladder (*arrowhead*). The tip of the metal stiffener is at the arrow. The inner metal stiffener supports the drain along its entire length into the gallbladder. **(I)** Final fluoroscopic image during a cholecystostomy tube placement. The pigtail portion of the 8-French drain is coiled in the gallbladder (GB). Contrast has been injected through the 8-French drain (*arrow*). Visualized is the biliary tree including the intrahepatic bile ducts, the common hepatic duct (CHD) and the common bile duct (CBD).

- The cholecystostomy drain is then secured to the skin utilizing sutures, and left to gravity bag drainage.

Postpercutaneous Biliary Drainage Imaging

- Immediate postcholecystostomy imaging is for documentation that the pigtail end of the drain is in the gallbladder and that the side holes traverse the bile

ducts and do not traverse the transhepatic tract or transperitoneal tract.

Endpoints

- Bacterial culture of bile extracted from percutaneous cholecystostomy is positive in 16–49% of cases.
- The endpoint of a cholecystostomy is a pigtail catheter looped in the gallbladder.

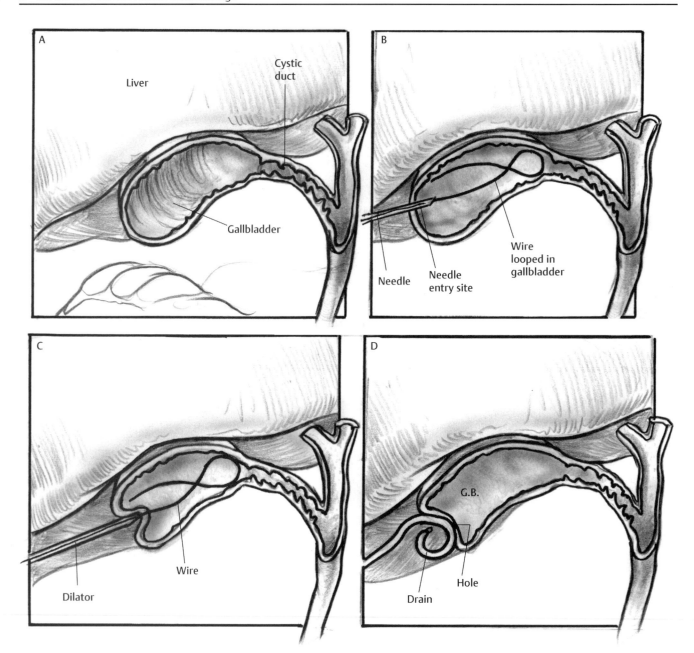

Fig. 13.16 Schematics demonstrating the transperitoneal access of the gallbladder where gallbladder wall displacement can pose a problem in placing a cholecystostomy drain. **(A)** Drawing demonstrating the coronal section of the right upper quadrant through the gallbladder and the right hepatic lobe. **(B)** Drawing demonstrating the transperitoneal needle passage through the fundus of the gallbladder. The wire is looped in a figure of eight in the gallbladder. **(C)** Drawing demonstrating the displacement of the gallbladder fundus away from the access site. The fundus is being pushed away by the dilator. The operator may not notice this, particularly when not using fluoroscopy and occasionally under fluoroscopy with little contrast opacification in the gallbladder. The operator should be aware of this possibility. Good counter-tension on the wire and a forceful but controlled push of the dilator is required to avoid this. **(D)** Drawing demonstrating the final outcome of displacement of the fundus away from the access site. The drain will ultimately be deployed/curled outside the gallbladder leaving the access hole in the fundus, which could possibly leak bile into the peritoneum.

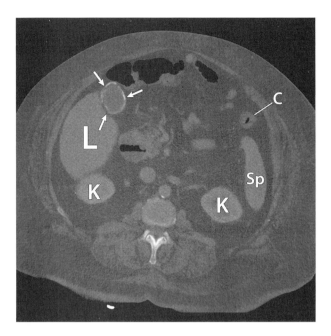

Fig. 13.17 Contrast-enhanced axial computed tomography (CT) image of the abdomen demonstrating a gallbladder with calcifications in its wall (*arrows*). This finding is consistent with a porcelain gallbladder. Porcelain gallbladders have a higher risk of developing adenocarcinoma of the gallbladder. In addition, they have a higher rate of cholecystostomy drain placement failures (L, liver; C, colon; K, kidney; Sp, spleen).

- ○ Technical success occurs in 95–100% of cases.
- ○ Technical failures are more common with
  - Decompressed gallbladder
  - Gallbladder impacted with stones (**Figs. 13.4C, 13.4D**)
  - Porcelain gallbladder (**Fig. 13.17**)
  - Significant gallbladder wall thickening
- Clinical success of cholecystostomy occurs in 56–100% of cases. This depends on inclusion criteria and criteria for success. Criteria for clinical success include
  - ○ Reduction of temperature to less than 37.5°C
  - ○ Reduction of white blood cell count (WBC) by 25% of preprocedure value or a reduction of WBC of less than 10,000/mm³ within 72 hours of the procedure

Postprocedural Evaluation and Management

Percutaneous cholecystostomy is performed on inpatients. Many of whom are patients of the ICU. Outpatient cholecystostomy is not indicated and not applicable.

Postpercutaneous Biliary Drainage Observation Period

- Patients return to their unit (regular floor or ICU).
- Septic patients at baseline or patients who become septic postcholecystostomy (become worse) should be transferred to the ICU for resuscitation and even cardiopulmonary support.
- Check on the patient and monitor vital signs
- Observe the biliary output including volume output and character
  - ○ Thick bile blocking the drain requires the drain to be flushed with ∼5–7 mL of sterile saline.

Intravenous Fluid and Diet

- IV fluid should be given until oral intake is adequate. Oral intake may not be feasible in this particular population because many patients can be septic and/or in the ICU. Once these patients defervesce, oral intake can be contemplated.
- The ideal IV fluid for a biliary patient being drained is lactated Ringers' solution to replace serum potassium loss in particular.

Activity

- Bed rest. Patients are usually not in a condition to ambulate.
- The cholecystostomy drain/bag uses gravity drainage.
- If ambulatory, patients should be instructed on how to maneuver with the biliary drains and to be reminded that they are tethered to a collecting bag.

Pain Management

- Narcotics may be required postcholecystostomy particularly if there is biliary peritonitis, which can be extremely painful.

Monitoring Vital Signs

- Vital sign monitoring includes blood pressure and heart rate. Occasionally, oxygen saturation monitoring is required in cases of shortness of breath and/or chest pain.
- In cases of shortness of breath, one must be able to differentiate between splinting due to pain and pleural complications (pneumo- or hemothorax). Clinical exam and a chest x-ray would help differentiate between the two.
- Hypotension may be a result of sepsis. Careful postprocedural clinical evaluation to differentiate sepsis versus hypovolemia is required.

Table 13.3 Types, Causes, Characteristics, and Management of Postcholecystostomy Pain

Type/Category	Cause	Characteristics & Management
Peritonitis	Bile leak (can be very painful) Bleeding	Severe pain Pain referred to left shoulder May require narcotics
Tube site pain	Soft tissue pain Glisson's capsular pain	Responds to narcotics or even nonnarcotic analgesics Resolves with time
Chest wall pain (chest site pain)	Not common* Intercostal nerve pain	Increases with respiration Associated with splinting and atelectasis
Pleural	Pneumothorax Hemothorax	Increases with respiration Related to desaturation/SOB The only pain that can be life threatening and may require further intervention (chest tube)

* Chest wall pain is uncommon because usually the operator can access the gallbladder without traversing intercostals spaces/chest wall. Chest wall pain and splinting due to rubbing of the cholecystostomy drain against intercostal nerves usually subsides over the next 24–72 hours. Continuous pain may require a change in the cholecystostomy drain tract/site.

Abbreviations: SOB, Shortness of breath.

Complications and Their Management

Please see **Table 13.1** for the list of the most common complications and their incidence following percutaneous cholecystostomy.

Management of Pain and Pain-Related Morbidity

- **Table 13.3** describes the types/causes of pain that may be encountered following cholecystostomy.

Management of Bleeding Complications

- Bleeding postcholecystostomy can take several forms.
  - Hemobilia
  - Intraperitoneal hemorrhage (hemoperitoneum)
  - External/site bleeding (rule out a skin bleed first)
- Significant bleeding affecting vital signs and patient stability should be managed by
  - Fluid resuscitation starting with crystalloid fluid bolus
  - Type and cross
  - Repeat hematocrit to compare with baseline
  - Blood transfusion to maintain hematocrit at or above 30%
  - Surgical/interventional radiology consult
  - Interventional radiology can provide visceral (including hepatic) angiography with super-selective embolization.

Management of Puncture of Adjacent Organs

- This is not common.
- If transgression of bowel occurs by the drain, the drain should be left in place for the tract to mature. This allows
  - The patient to recover from the acute situation of a procedure, renal failure, and/or sepsis
  - A later management of the fistula, if it occurs, can be performed in an elective setting.
- The most common organ to be transgressed is the colon, particularly from an extrahepatic transperitoneal approach.

Sepsis

- Prophylactic antibiotics should be used in all cases.
- Operators should not overdistend the gallbladder with contrast.
- Rigors only without fever can respond to 25–50 mg of meperidine administered intramuscularly.
- In cases of postoperative fever (cholangitis), operators should continue with IV antibiotics and should check the culture and sensitivity of the bile sample obtained from the cholecystostomy.
- Sepsis requires fluid resuscitation and even vasopressors with ICU admission (the patient may already be in the ICU).

Further Reading

Akhan O, Akinci D, Ozmen MN. Percutaneous cholecystostomy. Eur J Radiol 2002;43:229–236

Burke DR, Lewis CA, Cardella JF, et al; Society of Interventional Radiology Standards of Practice Committee. Quality improvement guidelines for percutaneous transhepatic cholangiography and biliary drainage. J Vasc Interv Radiol 2003;14(9 Pt 2): S243–S246

Byrne MF, Suhocki P, Mitchell RM, et al. Percutaneous cholecystostomy in patients with acute cholecystitis: experience of 45 patients at a US referral center. J Am Coll Surg 2003;197(2):206–211

Kubota K, Abe Y, Inamori M, et al. Percutaneous transhepatic gallbladder stenting for recurrent acute acalculous cholecystitis after failed endoscopic attempt. J Hepatobiliary Pancreat Surg 2005; 12(4):286–289

Chopra S, Dodd GD III, Mumbower AL, et al. Treatment of acute cholecystitis in non-critically ill patients at high surgical risk: comparison of clinical outcomes after gallbladder aspiration and after percutaneous cholecystostomy. AJR Am J Roentgenol 2001;176: 1025–1031

Hatzidakis AA, Prassopoulos P, Petinarakis I, et al. Acute cholecystitis in high-risk patients: percutaneous cholecystostomy vs conservative treatment. Eur Radiol 2002;12(7):1778–1784

Spira RM, Nissan A, Zamir O, Cohen T, Fields SI, Freund HR. Percutaneous transhepatic cholecystostomy and delayed laparoscopic cholecystectomy in critically ill patients with acute calculus cholecystitis. Am J Surg 2002;183(1):62–66

14 Percutaneous Suprapubic Cystostomy
Wael E.A. Saad

Indications

The following are indications of suprapubic catheter placement:

- Adults: Bladder outlet obstruction/catheter placement
  - Acute urine retention (AUR)
    - Defined as sudden and painful inability to pass urine
    - By far the most common indication
    - This occurs in 10% of men in their 70s or 80s over any given 5-year period (10% risk of occurrence in a 5-year period in men over 70 years of age)
    - Suprapubic catheterization is considered second in line to transurethral catheterization in cases of AUR in the majority (>85%) of urologists.
  - Posttraumatic avulsion on the urinary bladder from its neck or in cases of posttraumatic bladder leakage with multiple other traumas (a temporizing measure for a less significant and less life-threatening injury: bladder injury) (**Fig. 14.1**).
- Urinary bladder access as a first step for a subsequent intervention in cases where retrograde urethral cannulation has failed (not common)
  - Removing urinary bladder stones
  - Fulgurating superficial premalignant lesions in the urinary bladder
  - Antegrade cannulation of the urethra to help guide retrograde cannulation
- Pediatric: Bladder aspiration for fever workup
  - To obtain a sterile urine sample in fever workup (septic infants)

Contraindications

Relative Contraindication

- Uncorrected coagulopathy. Relative versus absolute contraindication depends on the degree of coagulopathy, the clinical setting, and the degree of urgency of the percutaneous fluid drainage procedure.

Absolute Contraindication

- Status posttotal cystectomy

Preprocedural Evaluation

Evaluate Prior Cross-Sectional Imaging

- Confirm the location of the bladder (central in the pelvis and sits above prostate)
- Confirm that the bladder is central and not pushed off to the side (**Fig. 14.1**).
- Rule out other objects/structures (pathology versus normal structures) that may mimic the bladder in the pelvis by ultrasound
  - Dilated fluid-filled bowel loops
  - Duplication cysts (gastrointestinal duplication cysts)
  - Giant urinary bladder Hutch diverticulum
  - Urachal cysts
  - Lymphoceles
  - Ovarian cysts
  - Cystic tumors (the most confusing tumors are most likely ovarian cystic tumors)
- Evaluate the percutaneous window to the urinary bladder and check that nothing stands between the anterior abdominal wall and the anterior bladder wall
- Look for adjacent organs that can be inadvertently traversed
  - Small bowel and decompressed redundant large bowel
  - This can help reduce transgression of adjacent organs with subsequent potential major complication.

Evaluate Preprocedure Laboratory Values

- Laboratory value evaluation mostly revolves around ruling out coagulopathy
  - Suggested coagulopathy thresholds for a suprapubic urinary bladder catheter
    - International normalized ratio: ≤1.7–1.8
    - Platelets: ≥50,000
    - Activated partial thromboplastin time: ≤50 seconds

Obtain Informed Consent

- Indications
  - See indications above
  - Technical success for urine aspiration in children is high (79–100%).
  - Technical success in placing a suprapubic urinary bladder (>90%)

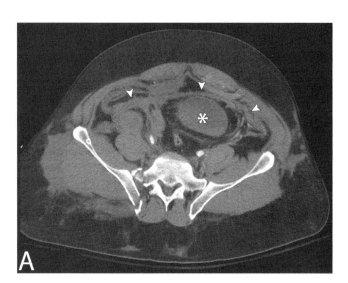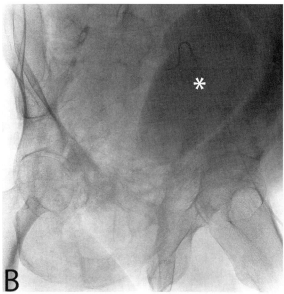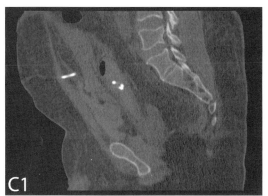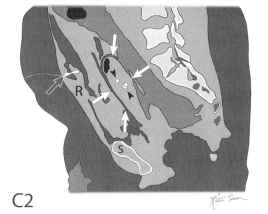

Fig. 14.1 Suprapubic catheter (cystostomy) in a detached urinary bladder. **(A)** Contrast-enhanced axial computed tomography (CT) image of the upper pelvis in a patient status postblunt trauma (car accident). The image demonstrates fluid/blood in the peritoneum from the trauma (*arrowheads*). This blood (*arrowheads*) is most likely blood from pubic rami fractures (*not shown*). The urinary bladder (*) is seen high riding because it has been detached/avulsed from its neck. **(B)** An oblique fluoroscopic image during angiography demonstrating the pear-shaped avulsed urinary bladder (*). The underlying angiographic catheter is in the arteries for pelvic angiography and a subsequent embolization. **(C)** Sagittal reconstruction of an unenhanced CT of the pelvis after a suprapubic catheter has been placed (*top*) and schematic sketch of it (*bottom*). The suprapubic catheter is seen traversing the anterior abdominal wall (*hollow arrow*) and coiled in the urinary bladder (*arrowheads*). The urinary bladder sits between the four solid arrows (R, rectus abdominis; S, symphysis pubis).

- Alternatives
  - To drain the bladder via the urethra (usually the first choice by the majority of urologists)
  - Emergent surgery to resolve bladder outlet obstruction (rarely done)
- Procedural risks
  - Overall complications occur in 18–20% of patients.

- Major complications occur in <1% of patients.
- Infection (**Table 14.1**)
  - This complication in its broader definition (urinary tract infection) occurs in 18% of cases.
  - Epididymoorchitis (rare)
  - Sepsis is rare.
- Bleeding (**Table 14.1**)

Table 14.1 Complications of Percutaneous Suprapubic Cystostomy Compared with Transurethral Catheterization

Complication	Transurethral	Suprapubic
Urinary tract infection	40%	18%
Epididymoorchitis	7%	Rare
Sepsis	3%	Rare
Urethral strictures	17%	0%
Hematuria	Less likely	More likely
Catheter obstruction &/or dislodgment	Less likely	More likely
Urine leaks	More likely	Less likely

- It may present as hematuria (most common) or bleeding outside the bladder in the abdomen.
- In rare cases, bleeding may require intervention such as angiography with transcatheter arterial embolization or exploratory surgery.
  ○ Injury to surrounding organs and/or structures
- Rare

Equipment

Ultrasound Guidance

- Multiarray 4–5 MHz ultrasound transducer
- Transducer guide bracket (if needed)
- Sterile transducer cover

Standard Surgical Preparation and Draping

- Chlorhexidine skin preparation/cleansing fluid
- Fenestrated drape

Local Infiltrative Analgesia Administration

- 21-gauge infiltration needle
- 10 to 20 mL 1% lidocaine syringe

Sharp Access Devices

- 11-blade incision scalpel
- 18-gauge needle that allows a 0.035-inch or 0.038-inch wire
- 21- or 22-gauge needle for aspirating infant urinary bladder

Tubular Access Devices

- An 8- to 12-French self-retaining (string-locking) pigtail drainage catheter, which is the definitive fluid collection drain to be placed last (final product of the procedure)

- Fascial dilators sized to the final size of the percutaneous drain

Technique

The Seldinger technique utilizes a hollow needle with wire passage into the collection. The drain is then placed as a third and last step over the wire, replacing the needle. The technique described below is the Seldinger technique.

Intravenous Access and Medication

- Required for moderate sedation and fluid replenishment/resuscitation

Preprocedure Ultrasound Exam

- Identify the urinary bladder
- Identify if there are viscera in the way of the needle trajectory
- Correlate and triangulate the access site (at skin) and the urinary bladder to choose and mark the skin access site
- The skin site is usually midline at the linea alba (least vascular plain) and the urinary bladder is usually a midline structure.

Standard Surgical Preparation and Draping

- Skin preparation/cleansing in the region that was chosen as an ultrasound imaging portal and a needle access needle portal
- Place a fenestrated drape at the chosen and prepared midline skin region

Local Infiltrative Analgesia Administration

- Utilizing a 21-gauge (by at least a 3.7-cm-long) infiltration needle, 1% lidocaine infiltration is performed, infiltrating down to the sensitive peritoneum (**Fig. 14.2**).

Ultrasound-Guided Sharp Access

- Free-hand ultrasound guidance and an 18-gauge hypodermic needle (no stylet) connected to a 20-mL syringe half filled with radiographic contrast via connector/extension tubing
  ○ Once the needle traverses the skin into the subcutaneous tissue, suction is applied (operator aspirates using syringe) as the needle is advanced further.
  ○ The connector tubing allows the operator to have flexibility in manipulating the needle free-hand.

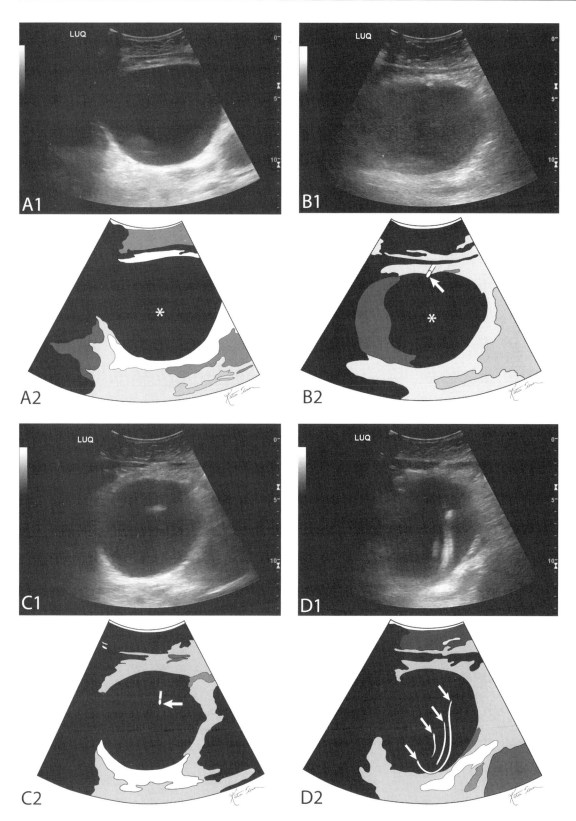

Fig. 14.2 Suprapubic catheter (cystostomy) placement. **(A)** Gray-scale ultrasound image of a distended urinary bladder (*top*) and schematic sketch of it (*bottom*). The asterisk is in the center of the urinary bladder. **(B)** Gray-scale ultrasound image of the urinary bladder (*top*) and schematic sketch of it (*bottom*). The needle tip is at the urinary bladder wall (*arrow*). The asterisk is in the center of the urinary bladder.

(C) Gray-scale ultrasound image of the urinary bladder (*top*) and schematic sketch of it (*bottom*). The needle tip is well within the lumen of the urinary bladder (*arrow*). **(D)** Gray-scale ultrasound image of the urinary bladder (*top*) and schematic sketch of it (*bottom*). A 0.035-inch wire has been passed through the access needle. The 0.035-inch wire is coiled within the lumen of the urinary bladder (*arrows*).

○ Needle tip entry (seen by real-time ultrasound) (**Fig. 14.2**) into the urinary bladder should correlate with an abrupt return of urine into the syringe.
○ Once a urine sample is obtained, radiographic contrast is injected under fluoroscopy to confirm adequate placement of the needle into the urinary bladder.

Fluoroscopic-Guided Wire and Tube Access

- Once the needle is in place, contrast is injected to confirm adequate placement of the needle.
- Once there is a 0.035-inch wire coiled in the collection, fascial dilators are passed sequentially to dilate the tract to an appropriate size drain.
- The operator may find it difficult to penetrate the urinary bladder wall and pass fascial dilators followed by the definitive suprapubic catheter.
  ○ Try to use a stiffer wire and hold adequate countertension on the wire while passing the dilators/suprapubic catheter
  ○ Choose dilators (if in your inventory) with a more tapered and harder lead point
  ○ Try to "stab" the dilators (fast jab) through over the stiff wire in an attempt to "skewer" the urinary bladder. Make sure the wire is stiff and does not get kinked.
  ○ Another technique is to maintain constant forward pressure over a stiff wire while rotating (screwing-in) the dilator.
  ○ If the dilators pass but the definitive suprapubic catheter does not pass into the urinary bladder, try to place a peel-away sheath. If it passes, the catheter is passed through it as the sheath is peeled away.
- The largest dilator fitted to size the suprapubic catheter (8- to 12-French in size) is removed and is quickly replaced by a drainage catheter (8- to 12-French in size). The pigtail is placed and secured ("Coped") in the urinary bladder.
- The suprapubic catheter is then secured to the skin utilizing sutures and left to gravity bag drainage.

Postdrain Placement Imaging

- Immediate postdrainage imaging is usually by fluoroscopy and is to document that the pigtail end of the suprapubic catheters is in the urinary bladder and that it is well formed (well "Coped").

Endpoints

- Aspirate sample (79–100%) in infants for
  ○ Ultrasound improves sample acquisition by more than 2.5-fold compared with blind (nonimage-guided) urinary bladder aspiration attempts (36–60%).

○ Gram stain and a bacterial culture are usually requested.
- The endpoint of a suprapubic urinary bladder is a catheter looped and well positioned in the fluid collection.
  ○ Technical success occurs in >90% of cases.
  ○ Technical failures are more common with thick trabeculated bladder wall, where the operator was able to access the bladder with the needle but found it difficult to pass a drain. This is overcome with a peel-away sheath (see above).
  ○ Narrow windows of sharp access coupled with limited acoustic windows for visualization (rare).
- Clinical success is to be able to void anatomically (through the urethra) usually 1–3 days after the suprapubic catheter placement, which allows a subsequent elective surgery (TURP: transurethral retrograde prostatectomy).
  ○ The success rate of voiding after 1–3 days is ~23–40%.
  ○ 69% of patients who fail voiding require a second catheterization.
  ○ 3% of patients require immediate surgery.
  ○ The advantage of suprapubic catheter over transurethral catheterization is that suprapubic catheter can be clamped to test for the patient's ability to void without losing access or subjecting the patient to another retrograde Foley catheter placement.
  ○ Alpha blockers help reduce outflow obstruction and increase the success rate of voiding.
  ○ Increased risk of failure to void include
    - Patient age >65 years
    - Detrusor pressure <35 cm water
    - Original urinary bladder drainage >1 liter of urine
    - Short period of catheterization

Postprocedural Evaluation and Management

The majority of suprapubic catheters are performed on inpatients. This is primarily due to the nature of the underlying condition (infantile sepsis, adult acute urine retention). Even with transurethral catheters in the setting of adult acute urine retention, up to 80% of urologists admit their patients.

Postdrainage Observation Period

- Patients return to their unit (see above statement).
- Patients who become septic postdrainage (rare for suprapubic catheters) should be transferred to the ICU for resuscitation and even cardiopulmonary support.

- Check on the patient and monitor vital signs
- Observe the drain output including volume output and character. The initial urine output aliquot is a prognostic indicator of whether the patient will be able to void spontaneously in 1–3 days (>1 L is a bad prognostic indicator).
- A standard (standing order) for drain flushes every nurse shift (2–3 times a day) is usually not required. However, if there is gross hematuria, the suprapubic catheter should be flushed/irrigated using normal sterile saline (NS).
  - Nursing staff should be instructed to push the NS steadily and not forcefully and not to draw back (aspirate) after the push the saline flush.

Intravenous Fluid and Diet

- IV fluid should be given until oral intake is adequate.

Activity

- The fluid collection drain/bag uses gravity drainage.
- If ambulatory, patients should be instructed on how to maneuver with the fluid collection drains and to be reminded that they are tethered to a collecting bag.

Pain Management

- Nonnarcotic medication usually is enough to control pain from fluid collection drains. Narcotic medications for pain management may occasionally be required.

Monitoring Vital Signs

- Vital sign monitoring includes blood pressure and heart rate.
- Hypotension may be a result of sepsis. Careful postprocedural clinical evaluation to differentiate sepsis versus hypovolemia is required.

Complications and Their Management

Please see **Table 14.1** for the list of the most common complications and their incidence following percutaneous suprapubic catheter placement.

Management of Pain and Pain-Related Morbidity

- Pain is usually not a problem after suprapubic catheter placement.
- Narcotic medications for pain management may occasionally be required.

Management of Bleeding Complications

- Bleeding postfluid drainage can take several forms
  - Intraperitoneal hemorrhage (hemoperitoneum)
  - Extraperitoneal hemorrhage
  - Hematuria
- Significant bleeding affecting vital signs and patient stability should be managed by
  - Fluid resuscitation starting with crystalloid fluid bolus
  - Type and cross
  - Repeat hematocrit to compare with baseline
  - Blood transfusion to maintain hematocrit at or above 30%
  - Surgical/interventional radiology consult
  - Interventional radiology can provide pelvic angiography with super-selective embolization.

Management of Puncture of Adjacent Organs

- This is not common.
- If transgression of bowel occurs by the drain, the drain should be left in place for the tract to mature. This allows
  - The patient to recover from the acute situation of a procedure, renal failure, and/or sepsis
  - Later management of a fistula, if one occurs, can be performed in an elective setting.

Sepsis

- Rigors only without fever can respond to 25–50 mg of Demerol (Sanofi Aventis Pharmaceuticals, Paris, France) administered intramuscularly.
- In cases of postoperative fever, operators should continue with IV antibiotics and should check the culture and sensitivity of the urine sample obtained from the urinary bladder suprapubic catheter.
- Sepsis requires fluid resuscitation and even vasopressors with ICU admission.

Further Reading

Fitzpatrick JM, Kirby RS. Management of acute urinary retention. BJU Int 2006;97(Suppl 2):16–20, discussion 21–22

Horgan AF, Prasad B, Waldron DJ, O'Sullivan DC. Acute urinary retention. Comparison of suprapubic and urethral catheterisation. Br J Urol 1992;70(2):149–151

Peate I. Patient management following suprapubic catheterization. Br J Nurs 1997;6(10):555–562

Tibbles CD, Porcaro W. Procedural applications of ultrasound. Emerg Med Clin North Am 2004;22(3):797–815

15 Percutaneous Drainage of Fluid Collection

Wael E.A. Saad

Classification

Fluid collections can be classified in many ways.
- By body location
  - Neck
    - Infraplatysmal versus supraplatysmal (deep versus superficial)
    - Carotid sheaths
    - Neck triangles, etc.
  - Thoracic
    - Pleural: empyema, hydrothorax, hemothorax chylothorax, simple effusion
    - Extrapleural (chest wall, mediastinum – anterior, middle, and posterior)
  - Abdominal
    - Intraperitoneal
    - Abdominal wall
    - Retroperitoneal
  - Pelvic
    - Intraperitoneal
    - Extraperitoneal
  - Extremity
- Infected versus potentially infected
  - Infected (abscess, empyema)
  - Potentially infected
    - Hematoma
    - Seroma
    - Lymphocele
    - Bile (biloma)
    - Transudate
    - Exudate
- Visceral or intravisceral versus extravisceral
  - Visceral
    - Intrahepatic
    - Intrarenal
    - Subcapsular (hepatic, renal, etc.)
  - Extravisceral (in spaces, potential spaces, or no spaces at all such as in the abdominal wall)

Extravisceral abdominal fluid collection drainage is the primary focus in this chapter. There are minor variations to what is described here when it comes to other types of fluid collections.

Indications

The following are indications of percutaneous drainage of fluid collections:

- Urgent drainage of fluid collections
  - Fluid collection (potential abscess) with enhancing wall by contrast-enhanced computed tomography (CT) in the setting of sepsis
- Elective drainage of fluid collections (within 24–48 hours of the diagnosis)
  - Fluid collection (potential abscess) with enhancing wall by contrast-enhanced CT with fever (no sepsis)
  - Fluid collection without fever (no sepsis)
  - Fluid collection with pressure symptoms on adjacent organs/viscera and/or pain (**Fig. 15.1**)
  - Fluid collection with suspected leak causing the collection (no sepsis)
  - Postoperative fluid collections (no sepsis)
  - Sampling of fluid for diagnosis (infected or not, malignant or not, etc.)
- Elective drainage of uncontained fluid in potential body spaces (discussed in separate chapters)
  - Peritoneal fluid (ascites): See Chapter 16
  - Pleural fluid: See Chapter 17
  - Sampling of fluid for diagnosis (infected or not, malignant or not, etc.)

When consulting to drain postoperative or posttraumatic hematomas, one must use caution. The clinical indication (symptomatology) directs whether to place a drain or not. This is because solid hematomas do not drain well and require large drains that dwell for extended periods. In addition, a hematoma may not be infected; however, the indwelling drain may introduce an infection (skin or nosocomial fungal and/or bacterial seeding) and convert a benign hematoma into an abscess. The indications for percutaneously accessing (aspiration or drain placement) a hematoma are as follows:

- Pressure symptoms causing pain – placing a drain relieves the pain quickly if the hematoma is the actual cause of the pain

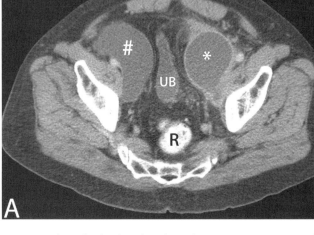
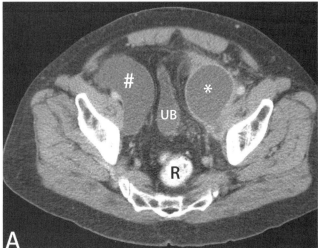

Fig. 15.1 Bilateral pelvic lymphoceles with pressure symptoms on the urinary bladder. **(A)** Contrast-enhanced axial computed tomography (CT) image of the midpelvis of a patient status postradical prostatectomy demonstrating bilateral pelvic fluid collections (* and #). These collections compress the centrally located urinary bladder (UB). The patient was complaining of urgency and frequency in micturating. No compression is appreciated on the rectum (R). These collections, given the clinical history and location, are most likely postoperative lymphoceles as a result of pelvic lymphatic injury and postoperative lymph leakage collecting as lymphoceles. Of note, the right-sided collection (#) has less of a perceptible wall with less stranding around it. The left-sided collection (*) has a thicker enhancing wall with stranding of the surrounding pelvic fat. If one of these lymphoceles is infected the likeli- hood is that the left-sided collection (lymphocele) is more likely to be infected. **(B)** Coronal reconstruction of the contrast-enhanced CT study of **Fig. 15.1A**. Again noted are the bilateral pelvic fluid collections (* and #) which are most likely lymphoceles. These collections compress the centrally located urinary bladder (UB). The patient was complaining of urgency and frequency in micturating. The left-sided collection (*) has a thicker enhancing wall with stranding of the surrounding pelvic fat. If one of these lymphoceles is infected the likeli- hood is that the left-sided collection (lymphocele) is more likely to be infected. Remember that thick enhancing walls are not definite evi- dence of infection especially in the setting of postoperative collections such as hematomas or lymphoceles (L, liver; Ht, heart).

- Pressure symptoms on adjacent structures such as urgency and frequency (bladder), dyspepsia (stomach and bowel), nausea and vomiting (stomach and bowel), etc. – drain placement (**Fig. 15.1**) is required
- Possible infection. Hematomas can cause fever without being infected. Fever can be a result of many postoperative causes. In this case, aspirate for cultures without placing a drain. If the hematoma is solid and fluid cannot be aspirated, a lavage/nonbacteriostatic irrigation through the needle can be used to obtain a microbiology sample. If the microbiology results come back positive for pathologic microbiology, then a percutaneous drain can be placed.

Contraindications

Relative Contraindication

- Uncorrected coagulopathy. A relative versus absolute contraindication depends on the degree of coagulopathy, the clinical setting, and the degree of urgency of the percutaneous fluid drainage procedure.

Absolute Contraindication

- Growing hematomas (as seen on imaging and/or dropping hematocrit) – an angiogram may be warranted, or at least a surgical consult should be obtained.

- Hematomas in the clinical setting and in certain anatomic locations that may be the result of pseudoaneurysms (postoperative vascular anastomosis with infection, or pancreatitis, for example)
- New and contained retroperitoneal hematomas without evidence of infection

Preprocedural Evaluation

Evaluate Prior Cross-Sectional Imaging

- One of the most concerning disease processes that should be ruled out prior to percutaneous drain placement is a necrotic tumor mistaken for an abscess. Placement of a percutaneous drain in a necrotic tumor may lead to tumor seeding along the percutaneous drain tract and the creation of a productive malignant cutaneous fistula that does not heal and carries a high morbidity (poor quality of life).
- Occasionally, an infected necrotic tumor (a tumor that has been seeded by bacteria or a tumor that has eroded into adjacent contaminated viscera such as the gastrointestinal tract) is encountered. Drainage of these infected tumors carries a high risk of chronic malignant cutaneous fistula formation and subsequent poor quality of life. However, if drains are to be placed in these necrotic tumors, the primary service and the patient should be made fully aware of this complication and the patient should be counseled about this chronic complication.
- Rule out other objects/structures (pathology versus normal structures) that may mimic an abscess
  - Neobladder (ileal loop diversion)
  - Dilated bowel loops
  - Bowel diverticulum (duodenal or jejunal diverticula, or giant sigmoid diverticula)
  - Hartman's pouch
  - Duplication cysts (gastrointestinal duplication cysts)
  - Giant urinary bladder Hutch diverticulum
  - Urachal cysts
  - Urinary bladder proper
  - Gallbladder proper
  - Mesenteric cysts
  - Exophytic solid organ cysts such as large exophytic renal or hepatic cysts
  - Large thrombosed saccular aneurysms/pseudoaneurysms – may cause vascular rupture and bleeding
  - Ovarian cysts
  - Cystic tumors (the most confusing tumors are most likely ovarian cystic tumors)
  - Cystic or necrotic sarcoma
- Look for signs of infection
  - Thickened wall by CT/ultrasound
    - Can be seen in abscesses
    - Can be seen in uninfected hematomas, bilomas, and lymphoceles (**Fig. 15.1**)
    - Can be a visceral structure (bowel)
    - Can be a true cyst and cystic tumor
  - Enhancing wall by CT/magnetic resonance imaging (MRI) (**Figs. 15.1, 15.2, 15.3**)
    - Can be seen in abscesses
    - Can be seen in uninfected hematomas, bilomas, and lymphoceles
    - Can be a visceral structure (bowel)
    - Can be a true cyst and cystic tumor
  - Air in the collection – due to gas-forming organisms or communication with bowel, skin, or tracheobronchial tree (**Fig. 15.4**)
- Evaluate the percutaneous window to the collection
  - Is there a transperitoneal (nonhepatic) window?
  - Is there a transvisceral, especially transhepatic window?
  - Is there both a transperitoneal and a transhepatic option for the gallbladder?
  - A transgastric route can be entertained in lesser sac and/or pancreatic collections (pancreatic pseudocysts).
- In certain clinical settings (in the case of pancreatic pseudocysts and in postoperative patients, especially those having vascular surgeries, as well as in collections), a careful evaluation of contrast-enhanced CT or MRI is required to rule out pseudoaneurysms. If intravenous (IV) contrast is contraindicated, a careful Doppler ultrasound evaluation is best near the ultrasound-guided drainage (see below).
- Look for adjacent organs that can be inadvertently traversed
  - Small bowel and decompressed large bowel can be missed by CT, especially in a postoperative abdomen with infections and "dirty" mesenteric fat or retroperitoneal fat.
  - This can help reduce transgression of adjacent organs with subsequent potential major complications.
  - This helps plan the needle trajectory for the abscess drainage.
  - This may make the operator consider approaching the abscess transgastrically or via the retroperitoneum rather than risk traversing an organ or bowel that may be less forgiving. In other words, give in to traversing stomach, for example, and reduce the risk of traversing colon or small bowel.
  - Evaluate for mesentery and mesenteric vessels in the mesentery or engorged vessels in the pelvis. Avoid traversing the mesentery or regions with engorged pelvic and/or mesenteric blood vessels.

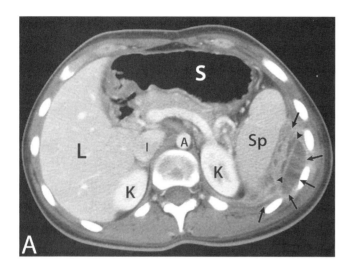

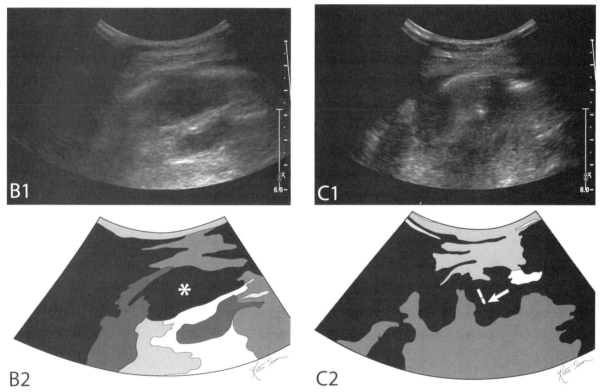

Fig. 15.2 Drain placement of a left-sided chest wall abscess. **(A)** Contrast-enhanced axial computed tomography (CT) image of the abdomen demonstrating a thick enhancing walled abscess (*arrows*). The abscess is multiloculated and septated. A clear septum is seen (*between arrowheads*). The abscess is extrapleural and extraperitoneal (K, kidney; L, liver; A, aorta; I, IVC; S, stomach). **(B)** Gray-scale ultrasound image of the abscess in the patient depicted in **Fig. 15.2A** (*top*) and a schematic sketch of it (*bottom*). The abscess is seen (* *in epicenter of abscess*). The collection is not clearly hypoechoic because of the thick pus and turbid nature of its contents and the numerous fibrin septations with it. **(C)** Gray-scale ultrasound image of the abscess in the patient despicted in **Figs. 15.2A and 15.2B** (*top*) and a schematic sketch of it (*bottom*). An 18-gauge needle has been passed into it (*arrow at needle tip*).   *(Continued on page 194)*

- Look for adjacent organs that can be mistaken for the collection by ultrasound. Identify and characterize them to rule them out by ultrasound during the drainage procedure.
  - Focally dilated small bowel loop
  - Gallbladder
  - Urinary bladder
  - Distended stomach – whole or partial/bypassed
  - Ovaries, fallopian tubes, and uterus (see below)
- Identify the female genital organs in low-lying abdominal and pelvic collections. Do not misdiagnose obstetrics-gynecology (ob-gyn) pathology for plain abscesses (although ob-gyn pathology can be pyogenic – a predrainage diagnosis, if not a differential diagnosis, is best). Do not misdiagnose the following:
  - Torsed ovary
  - A tuboovarian abscess can be drained percutaneously; however, an ob-gyn consult should be obtained prior to drainage.
  - Hydro- or pyosalpinx
  - Hydro- or pyometrium

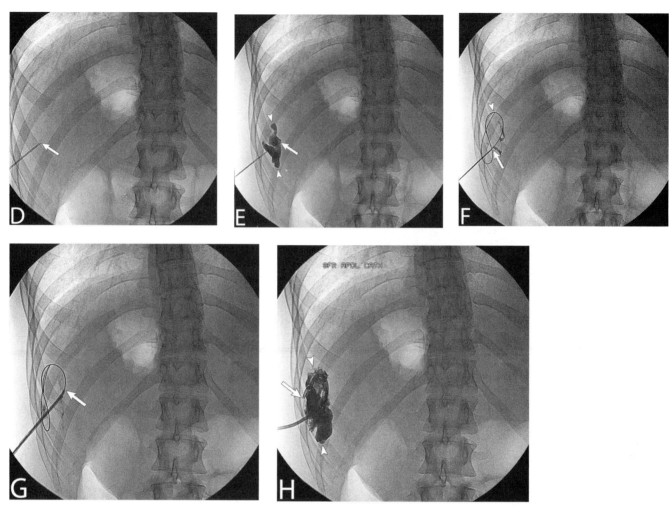

Fig. 15.2 *(Continued)* **(D)** Fluoroscopic image with the 18-gauge access needle (*arrow at needle tip*) in position within the main locule of the abscess. This was confirmed by ultrasound (**Fig. 15.2C**). **(E)** Fluoroscopic image after injecting contrast through the 18-gauge access needle (*arrow at needle tip*). Contrast is seen to fill the abscess (*between arrowheads*). This confirms the findings by CT. The operator should correlate the size, orientation, and location of what is seen by fluoroscopy with the collection on the preprocedural CT. This confirms adequate placement of the collection. **(F)** Fluoroscopic image after passing a 0.035-inch wire (*arrowhead*) through the 18-gauge access needle (*arrow at needle tip*) and coiling it inside the collection (*arrowhead*). Injecting contrast and coiling a wire inside the abscess helps break locules and ultimately helps drainage of the fluid collection/abscess. **(G)** Fluoroscopic image after passing an 8-French drain over the 0.035-inch wire. The drain has an inner metal stiffener, which supports the drain as it is passed through the tissues. The drain is passed over the wire and beyond the metal stiffener just beyond the point marked by the *arrow*. **(H)** Fluoroscopic image after injecting contrast through the 8-French drain, which has been coiled in the collection (*arrow at tip of drain*). The contrast fills the collection (*between the arrowheads*).

Evaluate Prior Operative Reports

- What type of surgery? (Recent surgery or prior/past surgeries)
  - Bowel surgery
    - Abscess can be from a leak (council patient for potential other surgery or prolonged drainage intubation)
    - Where is the bowel anastomosis?
    - Any blind-ending pouches that may be confused with a collection (Hartman's pouch, for example)
  - Pancreatic surgery
    - Abscess can be from a pancreatic leak (council patient for potential chronic intubation and possible cutaneous fistula)
    - Council patient for potential subsequent endoscopic retrograde cholangiopancreatography (ERCP) with stent placement
    - Higher risk of having pseudoaneurysms near the collection/abscess
  - Hepatobiliary surgery
    - Abscess can be from a bile leak (biloma)

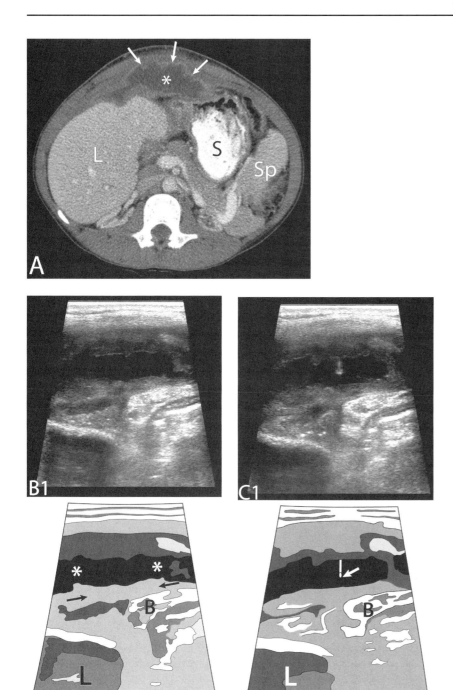

Fig. 15.3 Drain placement of a central anterior abdominal wall abscess. **(A)** Contrast-enhanced axial computed tomography (CT) image of the abdomen demonstrating a thick irregular enhancing walled abscess (*arrows*). The center of the abscess is marked by the asterisk (L, liver; Sp, spleen; S, stomach). **(B)** Gray-scale ultrasound image of the abscess in the patient depicted in **Fig. 15.3A** (*top*) and a schematic sketch of it (*bottom*). The abscess is seen (* *in abscess*) superficial to the peritoneum (*between arrows*). Just deep to the peritoneal plane is echogenic gas-filled bowel (B) and deeper yet the liver (L). **(C)** Gray-scale ultrasound image of the abscess in the patient depicted in **Figs. 15.3A and 15.3B** (*top*) and a schematic sketch of it (*bottom*). An 18-gauge access needle has been passed into the collection (*arrow at needle tip*). At this time in the procedure, the procedure is converted to real-time fluoroscopic guidance (B, bowel; L, liver).   *(Continued on page 196)*

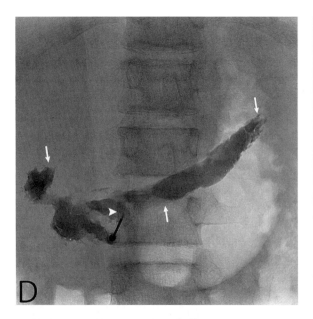

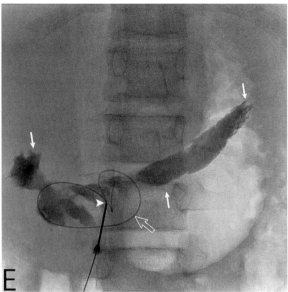

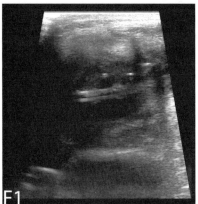

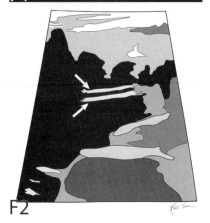

Fig. 15.3 *(Continued)* **(D)** Fluoroscopic image after injecting contrast through the 18-gauge access needle *(arrowhead at needle tip)*. Contrast is seen to fill the abscess *(arrows)*. This confirms the findings by CT. The operator should correlate the size, orientation, and location of what is seen by fluoroscopy with the collection on the preprocedural CT (**Fig. 15.3A**). This confirms adequate placement of the collection. **(E)** Fluoroscopic image after passing a 0.035-inch wire *(hollow arrow)* through the 18-gauge access needle *(arrowhead at needle tip)* and coiling it inside the collection *(arrows)*. Injecting contrast and coiling a wire inside the abscess helps break locules and ultimately helps drainage of the fluid collection/abscess. **(F)** Gray-scale ultrasound image of the abscess after a 10-French drain was placed *(top)* and schematic sketch of it *(bottom)*. The tubular structure *between the arrows* is the 10-French drain. This image is not necessary for the procedure. Confirmation of drain placement should have been already confirmed by fluoroscopy.

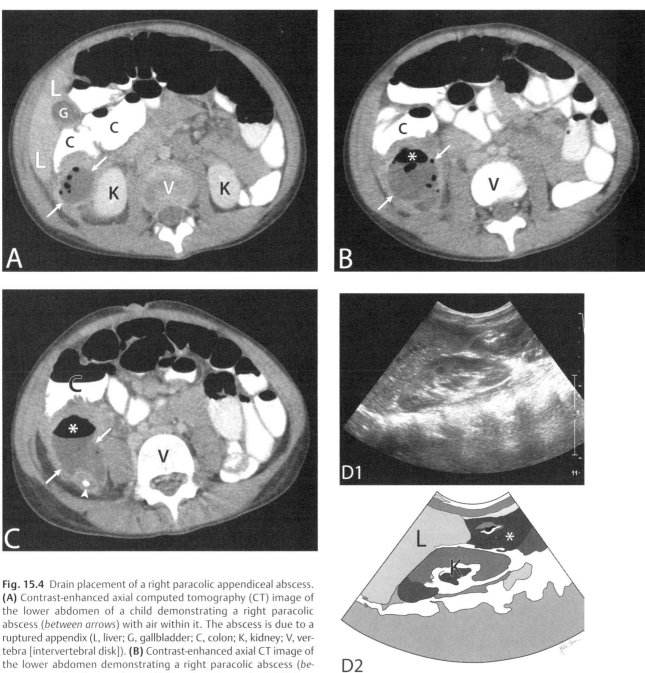

Fig. 15.4 Drain placement of a right paracolic appendiceal abscess. **(A)** Contrast-enhanced axial computed tomography (CT) image of the lower abdomen of a child demonstrating a right paracolic abscess (*between arrows*) with air within it. The abscess is due to a ruptured appendix (L, liver; G, gallbladder; C, colon; K, kidney; V, vertebra [intervertebral disk]). **(B)** Contrast-enhanced axial CT image of the lower abdomen demonstrating a right paracolic abscess (*between arrows*) with air within it (*) (C, colon; V, vertebra). **(C)** Contrast-enhanced axial CT image of the lower abdomen demonstrating a right paracolic abscess (*between arrows*) with air within it (*). An appendicolith is seen adjacent to the abscess (C, colon; V, vertebra). **(D)** Gray-scale ultrasound image of the abscess in the patient depicted in **Figs. 15.4A–15.4C** (*top*) and schematic sketch of it (*bottom*). The abscess is seen (* *in abscess*) superficial to the kidney (K) and inferior to the right hepatic lobe (L, liver).   *(Continued on page 198)*

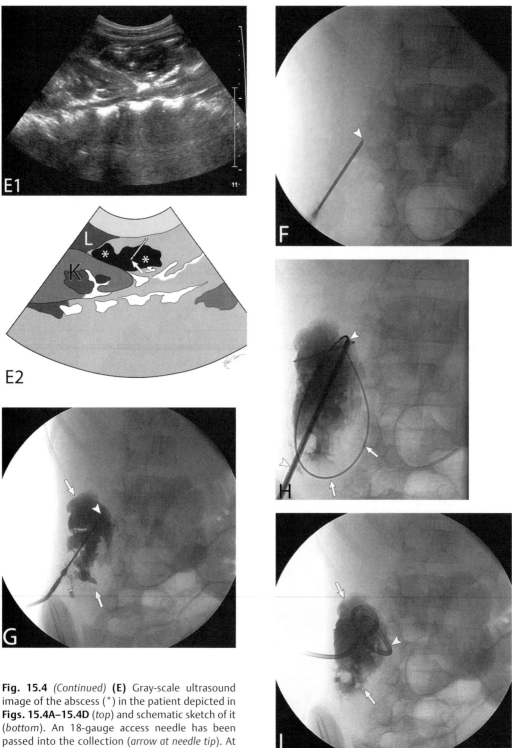

Fig. 15.4 *(Continued)* **(E)** Gray-scale ultrasound image of the abscess (*) in the patient depicted in **Figs. 15.4A–15.4D** *(top)* and schematic sketch of it *(bottom)*. An 18-gauge access needle has been passed into the collection *(arrow at needle tip)*. At this point in the procedure, the procedure is converted into fluoroscopic guidance (K, kidney; L, liver). **(F)** Fluoroscopic image with the 18-gauge access needle *(arrowhead at needle tip)* in the collection. This is confirmed by ultrasound in **Fig.15.4E** and by injecting contrast under fluoroscopy. **(G)** Fluoroscopic image after injecting contrast through the 18-gauge access needle *(arrowhead at needle tip)*. Contrast is seen to fill the abscess *(arrows)*. This

confirms the findings by CT. The operator should correlate the size, orientation, and location of what is seen by fluoroscopy with the collection on the preprocedural CT **(Figs. 15.4A–15.4C)**. This confirms adequate placement of the collection. **(H)** Fluoroscopic image after passing a 0.035-inch wire *(arrows)* through the 18-gauge access needle and coiling it inside the collection *(arrows)*. A 10-French drain *(between arrowheads)* with an inner metal stiffener is being advanced over the wire. **(I)** Fluoroscopic image after injecting contrast through the 10-French drain, which has been coiled in the collection *(arrowhead)*. The contrast fills the collection *(between the arrows)*.

- Council patient for potential subsequent ERCP with stent placement or percutaneous transhepatic cholangiogram (PTC) with transhepatic biliary drain placement
  - Vascular surgery
    - Are vascular anastomoses near or incorporated by the abscess? Higher risk of bleeding, can be life threatening
    - Are bypass grafts (especially synthetic grafts) involved within the abscess? If synthetic grafts are involved, a subsequent surgery is inevitable.
    - Is this collection a pseudoaneurysm?
  - Urology surgery
    - Fluid collection (abscess) can be from a urine leak (urinoma).
    - Fluid collection (abscess) can be from a lymphatic leak (lymphocele) from pelvic surgeries such as radical prostatectomies.
    - Council patient for potential subsequent endoscopic retrograde ureteroscopy with stent placement or percutaneous nephrostomies
    - Council patient for potential subsequent lymphocele recurrence and sclerotherapy (ablative treatment of lymphocele or surgical marsupialization)

Evaluate Preprocedure Laboratory Values

- Laboratory value evaluation mostly revolves around ruling out coagulopathy.
  - Suggested coagulopathy thresholds for an extravisceral abscess drainage are
    - International normalized ratio (INR): ≤1.7–1.8
    - Platelets (PLT): ≥50,000
    - Activated partial thromboplastin time (aPTT): ≤50 seconds
  - Suggested coagulopathy thresholds for a visceral abscess drainage (transhepatic approach, for example) are
    - INR: ≤1.4
    - PLT: ≥ 50,000–70,000
    - aPTT: ≤50 seconds

Obtain Informed Consent

- Indications
  - See indications above
  - Technical success for fluid aspirations is high (95%).
  - Technical success in placing a drain in the abscess is high (90–95%).
  - The clinical success (resolving the presenting symptoms) is probably 80–90%.
  - Abscess recurrence occurs in 5–10% of cases.

- Alternatives
  - To refuse the procedure. The patient takes antibiotics only.
  - Surgical abscess evacuation and peritoneal lavage
  - Future elective surgery may still be needed and would be the long-term plan under more stable (nonacute) conditions to manage the underlying problem, for example, colectomy for diverticulosis after percutaneous drainage of an abscess from diverticulitis.
- Procedural risks
  - Overall complications occur in 10% of patients.
  - Major complications occur in 3–5% of patients.
  - Infection (**Table 15.1**)
    - This complication in its broader definition occurs in 1–5% of cases.
    - Infection can be divided into bacteremia and fever (most common: 2–5%) or sepsis (most serious: 1–2%). Patients usually are on antibiotics prior to the drainage procedure if infection is suspected.
  - Bleeding (**Table 15.1**)
    - It may present as pain and/or hypotension and a CT scan may show
      - Bleeding in the collection (expanding collection with high-density fluid)
      - Bleeding from adjacent viscera – subcapsular hematoma
      - Active extravasation if CT IV contrast is used. The active bleeding could be into the collection or along the path of the needle/drain.
    - Bleeding may be transient with or without blood transfusion
    - In rare cases, bleeding may require intervention such as angiography with transcatheter arterial embolization or exploratory surgery.
  - Injury to surrounding organs and/or structures (**Table 15.1**)
    - Pleura – pneumo- and hemothorax
    - Bowel (1%)

Table 15.1 Complications of Percutaneous Abdominal Fluid Collection Drainage

Complication	Incidence%
Sepsis	1–2
Bacteremia/fever	2–5
Hemorrhage requiring transfusion &/or embolization	1
Bowel transgression requiring intervention	1
Pleural transgression requiring interventions* (Hemothorax, pneumothorax, and/or empyema)	1

*Pleural transgression requiring additional interventions for chest procedures (thoracic drainages) has a risk rate of 2–10%.

Equipment

Ultrasound Guidance

- Multiarray 4–5 MHz ultrasound transducer
- Transducer guide bracket
- Sterile transducer cover

Standard Surgical Preparation and Draping

- Chlorhexidine skin preparation/cleansing fluid
- Fenestrated drape

Local Infiltrative Analgesia Administration

- 21-gauge infiltration needle
- 10 to 20 mL 1% lidocaine syringe

Sharp Access Devices

- 11-blade incision scalpel
- 18-gauge needle that allows a 0.035-inch or 0.038-inch wire
- 21-gauge needle that allows a 0.018-inch wire, which requires an eventual upsizing to a 0.035- to 0.038-inch wire

Tubular Access Devices

- An 8- to 16-French self-retaining (string-locking) pigtail drainage catheter, which is the definitive fluid collection drain to be placed last (final product of the procedure)
- Fascial dilators sized to the final size of the percutaneous drain

Technique

There are two approaches to draining fluid collections. One is a trocar technique, where the drain is placed in one step over a sharp lead-point cannula. The other is with the Seldinger technique utilizing a hollow needle with wire passage into the collection. The drain is then placed as a third and last step over the wire, replacing the needle. The technique described below is the Seldinger technique.

Intravenous Access and Medication

- Required for moderate sedation and fluid replenishment/resuscitation

Preprocedure Ultrasound Exam

- Identify the collection/abscess
- Identify if there are viscera in the way of the needle trajectory

- Correlate and triangulate the access site (at skin) and the fluid collection/abscess to choose and mark the skin access site. Be away from the rib cage if possible. Make sure the needle trajectory does not cross the costal cartilage or ribs.
- By manipulating the transducer (along with the bracketed needle guide), choose and triangulate the skin entry site, the target abscess site, and the needle trajectory to achieve the above points.
- Perform Doppler ultrasound exam to
  - Make sure no vessels are traversed in the proposed needle trajectory
  - Make sure that the target collection does not involve a pseudoaneurysm or is not a pseudoaneurysm itself (this is particularly true in cases of pancreatitis with pancreatic pseudocysts)

Standard Surgical Preparation and Draping

- Skin preparation/cleansing in the region that was chosen as an ultrasound imaging portal and a needle access needle portal
- Place a fenestrated drape at the chosen and prepared skin region

Local Infiltrative Analgesia Administration

- Utilizing a 21-gauge (by at least a 3.7-cm-long) infiltration needle, a 1% lidocaine infiltration is performed, infiltrating down to the sensitive peritoneum.

Ultrasound-Guided Sharp Access

- Use free-hand ultrasound guidance and an 18-gauge hypodermic needle (no stylet) connected to a 20-mL syringe half filled with radiographic contrast via connector/extension tubing
  - Once the needle traverses the skin into the subcutaneous tissue, suction is applied (the operator aspirates using a syringe) as the needle is advanced further.
  - The connector tubing allows the operator to have flexibility in manipulating the needle free-hand.
  - Needle tip entry (seen by real-time ultrasound) (**Figs. 15.2, 15.3, 15.4, and 15.5**) into the fluid collection site/abscess should correlate with an abrupt return of fluid into the syringe. If the fluid is very thick in consistency or particulate (necrotic/liquefied tissue) if may not draw back, especially if using a 21- to 22-gauge needle.
  - If the intention of the procedure is just aspiration microbiology sampling without drain placement and no aspirate (sample) is obtained, a lavage or irrigation

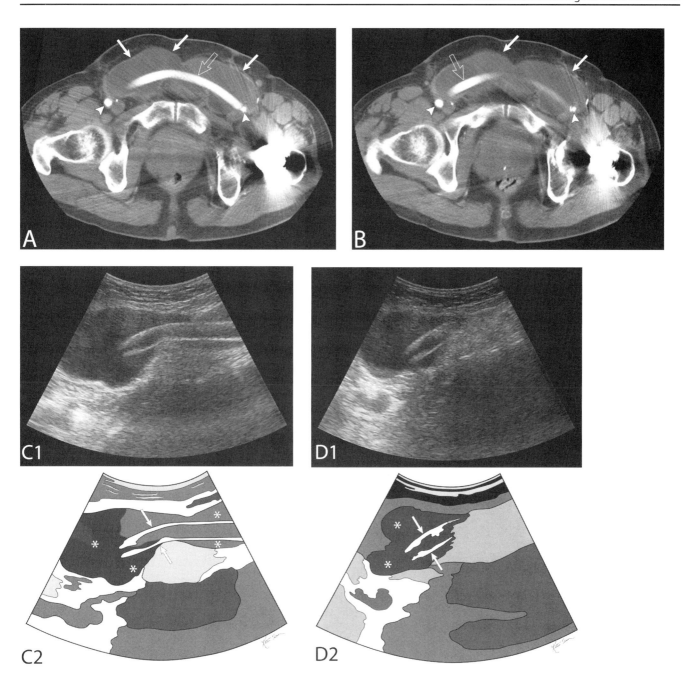

Fig. 15.5 Aspiration of fluid accumulating around a vascular graft. **(A)** Contrast-enhanced axial computed tomography (CT) image of the lower pelvis on a patient who had recently undergone a femoral-to-femoral (fem-fem) bypass (*hollow arrow*). There is a fluid collection (*arrows*) around the fem-fem bypass. The *arrowheads* point to the common femoral arteries. **(B)** Contrast-enhanced axial CT image (one slice below **Fig. 15.5A**) of the lower pelvis on a patient who had recently undergone a fem-fem bypass (*hollow arrow*). There is fluid collection (*arrows*) around the fem-fem bypass. The *arrowheads* point to the common femoral arteries. **(C)** Gray-scale ultrasound image of the anterior abdominal wall in the patient with the fem-fem bypass depicted in **Figs. 15.5A and 15.5B** (*top*) and schematic sketch of it (*bottom*). Again, noted is the fem-fem bypass (*tubular structure between arrows*). Around the bypass is the collection (***). **(D)** Gray-scale ultrasound image of the anterior abdominal wall in the patient with the fem-fem bypass in **Figs. 15.5A and 15.5B** (*top*) and schematic sketch of it (*bottom*). The ultrasound examination is swerved to the right close to the common femoral artery. Again, noted is the fem-fem bypass (*tubular structure between arrows*). Around the bypass is the collection (***). *(Continued on page 202)*

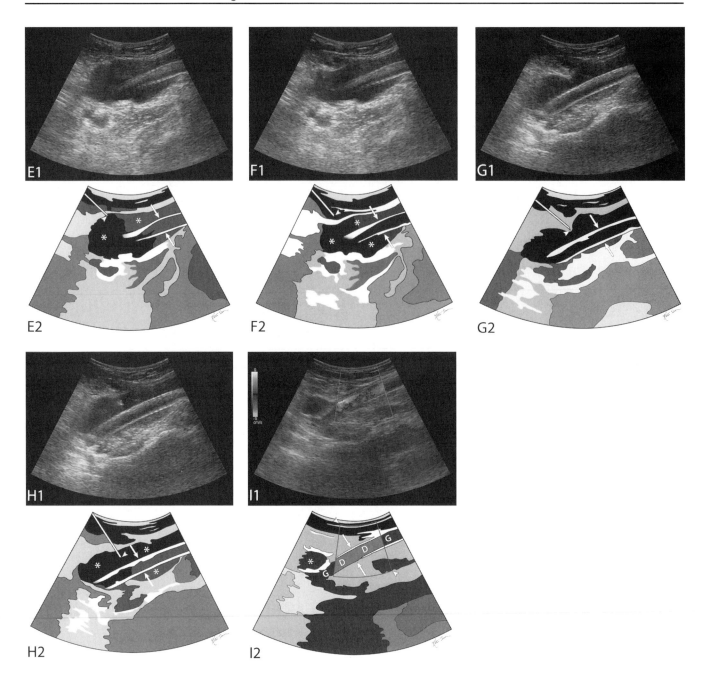

Fig. 15.5 *(Continued)* **(E)** Gray-scale ultrasound image of the anterior abdominal wall in the patient with the fem-fem bypass depicted in **Figs. 15.5A–15.5D** *(top)* and schematic sketch of it *(bottom)*. A lidocaine needle has been passed close to the wall of the collection *(arrowhead at needle tip)*. Again noted is the fem-fem bypass *(tubular structure between arrows)*. Around the bypass is the collection (*). **(F)** Gray-scale ultrasound image of the anterior abdominal wall *(top)* and schematic sketch of it *(bottom)*. Lidocaine infiltration through the needle has been passed, creating a bulge *(arrowhead at needle tip)*. Again, noted is the fem-fem bypass *(tubular structure between arrows)*. Around the bypass is the collection (*). **(G)** Gray-scale ultrasound image of the anterior abdominal wall *(top)* and schematic sketch of it *(bottom)*. An 18-gauge access needle has been passed tenting the superficial wall of the collection *(arrowhead at needle tip)*. Again, noted is

the fem-fem bypass *(tubular structure between arrows)*. **(H)** Gray-scale ultrasound image of the anterior abdominal wall *(top)* and schematic sketch of it *(bottom)*. The 18-gauge access needle *(arrowhead at needle tip)* has been passed into the collection (*). The superficial wall of the collection has recoiled back to its original position. Again, noted is the fem-fem bypass *(tubular structure between arrows)*. **(I)** Doppler ultrasound image over the fem-fem bypass *(top)* and schematic sketch of it *(bottom)*. The Doppler box is *between the arrowheads*. The 18-gauge access needle has been removed from the collection after the majority of the fluid has been aspirated. A residual part of the collection is still seen (*). Again, noted is the fem-fem bypass *(tubular structure between arrows)*. The fem-fem bypass is patent with flow within it (color is marked in this image as "D" and the lumen outside the Doppler box *(between arrowheads)* as "G."

through the needle can be performed. Inject 5 to 10 mm of nonbacteriostatic saline or sterile water into the "fluid collection" and then aspirate the residual back.

○ Once a fluid sample is obtained, radiographic contrast is injected under fluoroscopy to confirm adequate placement of the needle into the collection (**Figs. 15.2, 15.3, and 15.4**). The operator correlates the shape and location of the collection with the predrainage CT findings to confirm that he or she is in the appropriate fluid collection site.

• Alternatives to the above technique include the use of a 21- to 18-gauge needle with or without the use of a needle guide (ultrasound needle guide bracket). This method is used for deeper fluid collections.

○ Once the needle is placed, the stylet is removed and the procedure is converted to real-time fluoroscopy (**Figs. 15.2, 15.3, and 15.4**).

Fluoroscopic-Guided Wire and Tube Access

• Once the needle is in place, contrast is injected to confirm adequate placement of the needle.
• A 0.018-inch wire is passed through the 21- to 22-gauge needle or a 0.035-inch wire is passed through a 19- to 18-gauge needle under fluoroscopy. The wire is coiled in the fluid collection/abscess.
• A 0.018-inch wire requires it to be upsized to a 0.035 or 0.038-inch wire utilizing an AccuStick (Boston Scientific, Natick, MA) system (telescoped and stiffened dilator, see above).
• Once there is a 0.035-inch wire coiled in the collection, fascial dilators are passed sequentially to dilate the tract to an appropriate size drain (**Table 15.2**).

• The largest dilator fitted to size the drain (8- to 16-French in size) is removed and is quickly replaced by a drainage catheter (8- to 16-French in size). The pigtail is placed and secured ("Coped") in the fluid collection/abscess (**Figs. 15.2, 15.3, and 15.4**).
• The drain sizes used based on the collection drained are listed in **Table 15.2**.
• The fluid collection/abscess drain is then secured to the skin utilizing sutures and left to gravity bag drainage.

Postdrain Placement Imaging

• Immediate postdrainage imaging is usually by fluoroscopy and is for documentation that the pigtail end of the drain is in the intended fluid collection and that the side holes do not traverse the percutaneous tract.
• If ultrasound only is used for the drainage (not preferred by the authors), ultrasound scanning of the collection prior to the commencement of drainage may delineate the location of the pigtail catheter end in the collection. However, often the operator cannot clearly see the end of the drain in the collection especially in the following circumstances:

○ Deep collections
○ Thick and particulate fluid/discharge
○ Air in the collection either originally or introduced during the procedure

Endpoints

• Aspirate sample (95%) for
○ Gram stain and bacterial culture
○ Cytology if malignancy is suspected clinically or sanguinous discharge without being a postoperative collection

Table 15.2 Percutaneous Fluid Collection Drain Sizes Appropriate to Type of Collection and Character of Fluid

French Size of Fluid Collection Drain	Type of Fluid Collection	Examples
8-French	Collections in infant and small children	
10-French	Most collections that are not perceived as being thick (not viscid) on the initial aspiration	Seroma Thin infected fluid Simple fluid (transudate)
12- to 16-French	Thick/viscid fluid collections	Liquefying hematoma Purulent discharge
16-French	Smallest drain required for pleurodesis	
>16-French*	Very thick particulate/necrotic tissue	Necrotic tissue (pancreatitis) Large solid hematoma Pancreatic pseudocyst

*Drains above 16-French are not "Cope-loop" string-retaining pigtail catheters. These "nonpigtail" catheters are less secure than pigtail catheters.

- ○ Transudate versus exudate analysis (see Chapter 17)
- ○ Bilirubin if biloma is suspected (status posthepato-biliary surgery with green or gold-brown discharge, for example)
- ○ Amylase and lipase in cases of pancreatic surgery or pancreatitis
- ○ Creatinine to prove urine (status posturology surgery, for example)
- ○ Cell count and differential to evaluate for lymphocele
- The endpoint of a biliary drain is a catheter looped and well positioned in the fluid collection.
  - ○ Technical success occurs in 90–95% of cases.
  - ○ Technical failures are more common with
    - Deep collections
    - Air-filled collections with poor ultrasound visualization
    - Ultrasound characteristics that are similar to surrounding organs and/or structures such as bowel, making the operator less confident about the target. In this setting, thin needles (21- to 22-gauge needles) coupled with contrast and fluoroscopy can be used to confirm adequate placement of the needle in the intended collection (and not bowel, for example) prior to committing to a larger bore catheter/drain.
    - Narrow windows of sharp access coupled with limited acoustic windows for visualization
- Clinical success of fluid collection drainage and either partial or complete improvement in symptoms occurs in 80–90% of the time. This depends on the types of collections studied/drained and their clinical settings as well as inclusion criteria and criteria for success. Criteria for clinical success include
  - ○ Reduction of temperature to <37.5°C
  - ○ Reduction of white blood cell count (WBC) by 25% of preprocurement value or a reduction of WBC of less than 10,000/mm³ within 72 hours of the procedure
  - ○ Reduction of pain
- Abscess recurrence occurs in 5–10% of cases. Recurrence occurs at a greater degree in the following (higher risk of occurrence)/directly attributed to the following:
  - ○ Drain prematurely removed (intentionally or inadvertently)
  - ○ Communication with viscera (fistula) overlooked
  - ○ Underlying problem not resolved (not definitively treated) especially with high recurrence risk diseases.
    - Crohn's disease
    - Pancreatitis
    - Debilitated malnourished patients
    - Fistula formation with distal obstruction
  - ○ A nidus presides in the bed of the collection (infection nidus must be removed).
    - Bullet/projectile

- Bile stone outside the biliary tract (fell out intraoperatively or from ruptured gallbladder, former more common)
- Appendicolith

Postprocedural Evaluation and Management

The vast majority of percutaneous abscess drains are performed on inpatients. This is primarily due to the nature of the underlying disease processes that contribute to the abscess formation. It is uncommon to encounter a request for drainage of a true abscess, large enough to require drainage, on an outpatient basis. Occasionally, drainage of noninfected collections in nonseptic (nontoxic) conditions can be performed. A typical example of this is an outpatient drainage of a pelvic lymphocele.

Postdrainage Observation Period

- Patients return to their unit (regular floor or intensive care unit [ICU]).
- Septic patients at baseline or patients who become septic postdrainage (become worse) should be transferred to the ICU for resuscitation and even cardiopulmonary support.
- Check on the patient and monitor vital signs
- Observe the drain output including volume output and character
- A standard (standing order) for drain flushes every nurse shift (2–3 times a day is usually prudent)
  - ○ The drain flushes are usually performed using sterile normal saline (NS).
  - ○ Nursing staff should be instructed to push the NS steadily and not forcefully and not to draw back (aspirate) after the push of the NS flush.
  - ○ 5–10 mL of NS usually used to flush drains that are 8- to 10-French in diameter.
  - ○ 10–15 mL of NS usually used to flush drains that are 12- to 16-French in diameter.
  - ○ 15–20 mL of NS usually used to flush drains that are larger than 16-French in diameter.
- Output of the drain is important to study the trend of discharge from the collection. Based on the output comes the management of these drains and of these fluid collections (see below) (**Figs. 15.6 and 15.7**).

Intravenous Fluid and Diet

- Intravenous fluid should be given until oral intake is adequate. Oral intake may not be feasible in this particular population because many patients can be septic and/or in the ICU. Once these patients defervesce, oral intake can be contemplated.

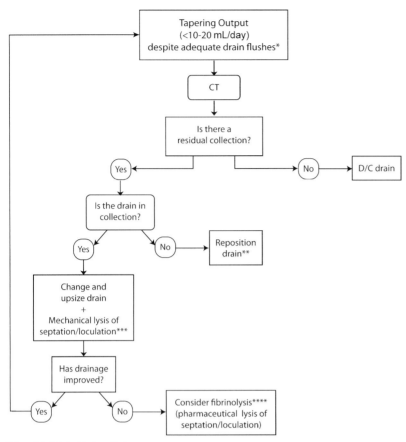

Fig. 15.6 Flowchart illustrating the management of decreasing output from an abscess drain.

*Signs of drain/tube blockage/kinks
– Resistance to flushing
– Drainage around tube

**Repositioning drain can be performed in two ways.
– Reposition intraabdominal draining site under fluoroscopy with catheter and wire manipulation.
– Remove drain and de novo placement of another percutaneous drain.

***Mechanical lysis/breakup of septation/loculation
– Inject contrast under fluoroscopy through the drain and compare the size of the cavity/collection with the CT.
– If smaller, or no cavity, then try to break up wall of cavity around the drain with a catheter and wire.

****1-2 mg tPA in 10-30 mL of normal saline every 12 hours for 2 to 3 times. Must r/o insidious bleeding/pseudo-aneurysm prior to therapy.

Abbreviations: D/C, discontinue; r/o, rule out; tPA, tissue plasminogen activator.

Activity

- Bed rest for the first 1–2 hours. The patient can ambulate (if capable) afterwards.
- The fluid collection drain/bag uses gravity drainage.
- If ambulatory, patients should be instructed on how to maneuver with the fluid collection drains and to be reminded that they are tethered to a collecting bag.

Pain Management

- Nonnarcotic medication usually is enough to control pain from fluid collection drains.

- Narcotic medications for pain management may occasionally be required in
  - Intercostal transhepatic abscess drains
  - Transgluteal drains
    - Usually not performed under ultrasound, but is performed under CT guidance or even fluoroscopic guidance
    - Up to 20% of cases would complain of chronic pain.
    - Less than 5% of cases require narcotics (my estimate).
    - If pain continues despite narcotics or if narcotics are contraindicated (or complicated), remove the drain and place another one with a different traversal tract (can still be transgluteal).

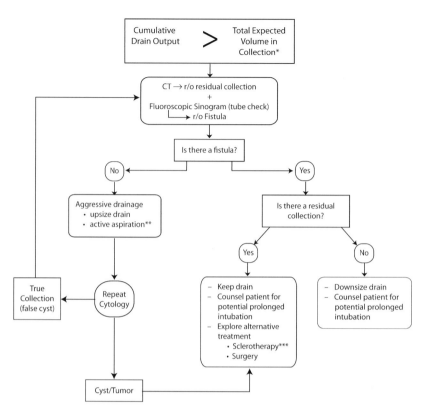

Fig. 15.7 Flowchart illustrating the management of persistent, if not increasing, output from an abscess drain.

r/o = rule out

*Total Expected Volume of Collection (*TEVC*) is the maximum axial dimension on CT ($X \times Y$) multiplied by the craniocaudad dimension (*Z*), multiplied by 0.52 [*TEVC = X × Y × Z × 0.52*].

**Active aspiration refers to intraabdominal vacuum suction using a syringe.

***Sclerotherapy can be performed using doxycycline or absolute alcohol.

Monitoring Vital Signs

- Vital sign monitoring includes blood pressure and heart rate. Occasionally, oxygen saturation monitoring is required in cases of shortness of breath and/or chest pain.
- In cases of shortness of breath, one must be able to differentiate between splinting due to pain and pleural complications (pneumothorax or hemothorax). Clinical exam and a chest x-ray would help differentiate between the two.
- Hypotension may be a result of sepsis. Careful postprocedural clinical evaluation to differentiate sepsis versus hypovolemia is required.

Long-Term Management of Fluid Collection Drains

- It is important to study the output of the drain and the trend of the discharge from the collection. The management of these drains and of these fluid collections is based on the output (**Figs. 15.6, 15.7, 15.8, and 15.9**).
- Pharmaceutical fibrinolysis of loculated/septated fluid collections

  ○ Performed to lyse the fibrin strands (synechia) that occur as part of an inflammatory process (subacute to chronic aseptic inflammation or due to infection) (**Fig. 15.6**)
  ○ Performed also to help liquefy hematomas
  ○ It is contraindicated in (high risks for bleeding)
    • Expanding hematomas and/or dropping hematocrit
    • Active extravasation in the collection/hematoma
    • Concern that there is a pseudoaneurysm associated with the hematoma
    • Concern for insidious bleeding related to or into the collection
    • Traversal of a vascular bypass or anastomosis in the collection
  ○ It is performed using 1–2 mg of tissue plasminogen activator (tPA) diluted in 10–30 mL of NS and injected through the drain. The drain is clamped for 30–60 minutes, then unclamped for gravity drainage. This administration is repeated every 12 hours for 2–3 times (total 12- to 24-hour period for the fibrinolysis therapy).

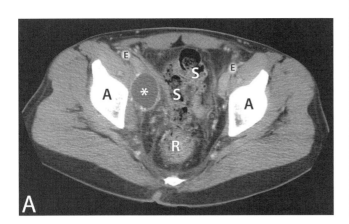

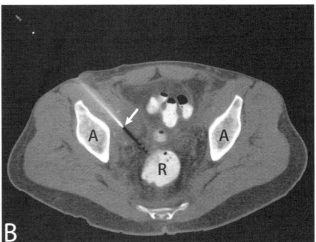

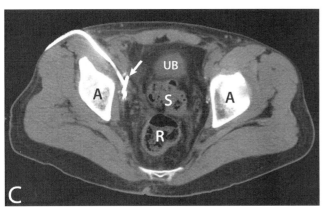

Fig. 15.8 Management process of a lymphocele. **(A)** Contrast-enhanced axial computed tomography (CT) image of the pelvis at the level of the acetabuli (A). A well-circumscribed collection with an enhancing wall is seen on the right pelvic wall medial to the right acetabulum (*). Clips/sutures are seen at its periphery. The patient is status postradical prostatectomy. Given the clinical history and the location, this is most likely a lymphocele. Laboratory samples should confirm it (S, sigmoid colon; R, rectum; E, external iliac arteries). **(B)** Oral contrast-enhanced axial CT image of the pelvis at the level of the acetabuli (A). Under CT guidance an 18-gauge needle is passed into the collection. This is followed by a drain placement over a wire (*arrow*; Seldinger technique) as described in **Figs. 15.2, 15.3, and 15.4**. Laboratory values were ordered to rule out infection and to confirm lymphatic fluid (high cell differential) (R, rectum). **(C)** Oral contrast-enhanced axial CT image of the pelvis at the level of the acetabuli (A). The study was performed after the daily drainage from the drain had dropped below 10–20 mL. The CT image demonstrates the drain to be coiled (*arrow*) in a completely obliterated lymphocele. It is time to sclerose the lymphocele (UB, urinary bladder; S, sigmoid colon; R, rectum).

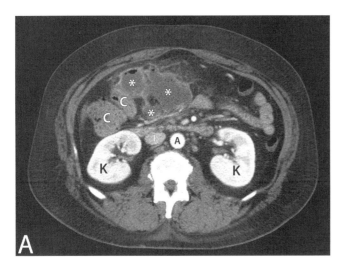

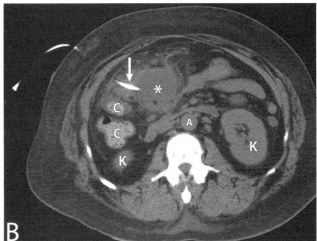

Fig. 15.9 Management process of an abdominal abscess related to bowel pathology (primary bowel disease or postoperative bowel surgery). **(A)** Contrast-enhanced axial computed tomography (CT) image of the abdomen in a patient who has had a duodenal perforation from an upper endoscopy (EGD: esophogastroduodenoscopy). The abscess is marked with asterisks (C, colon; K, kidney; A, aorta; I, inferior vena cava [IVC]). **(B)** Unenhanced axial CT image of the abdomen after drain placement in the abscess. The drain (*arrow*) is seen traversing the anterior abdominal wall heading for the collection (*) (C, colon; K, kidney; A, aorta).   *(Continued on page 208)*

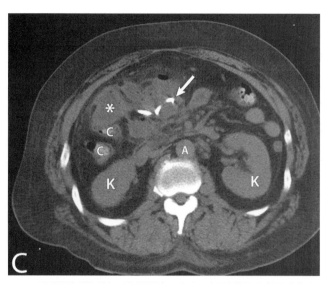

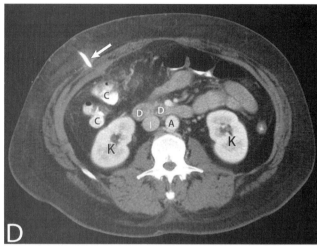

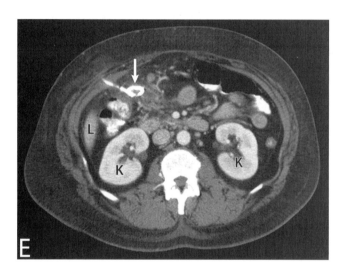

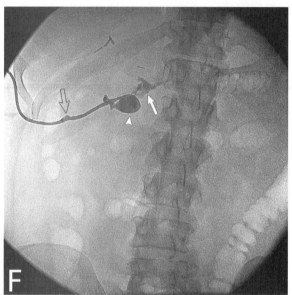

Fig. 15.9 (Continued) **(C)** Same CT exam as **Fig. 15.9B**: unenhanced axial CT image of the abdomen after drain placement in the abscess. The drain (arrow) is seen coiled in the collection. An adjacent locule is seen next to the colon and drain (C, colon; K, kidney; A, aorta). **(D)** Contrast-enhanced axial CT image of the abdomen after drain placement in the abscess. The drain is seen traversing the anterior abdominal wall (arrow). The CT exam was obtained after the drainage from the tube was less than 10 mL per day (C, colon; K, kidney; A, aorta; I, IVC; D, duodenum). **(E)** Same CT exam as **Fig. 15.9D**: Contrast-enhanced axial CT image of the abdomen after drain placement in the abscess. The drain is seen coiled in the site of the collection (arrow). There is minimal residual collection by CT (L, liver; K, kidney). **(F)** Sinogram or contrast tube-check after the CT demonstrated that the cavity has been obliterated (**Figs. 15.9D and 15.9E**). The purpose is to rule out a fistulous communication with bowel. If there is no fistulous communication, the tube can be removed. The tube is seen coiled in the cavity, which has shrunken to the size of the pigtail (arrowhead). Contrast is seen passing into a small adjacent cavity (arrow), but it does not communicate with bowel. Incidentally noted is contrast tracking back along the tract of the drain (hollow arrow) showing that this is a mature drain/tube tract (more of an issue with transvisceral tract, especially transhepatic tract, of which this is not).

- Sclerosis of fluid collections
  - Performed to sclerose and cause coaptation of the walls of the collection to prevent reaccumulation of fluid (**Figs. 15.7 and 15.8**).
  - Clinical scenarios where sclerosis can be used are
    - Lymphocele
    - Pleural effusion (pleurodesis)
    - True cysts (e.g., renal cyst)
  - Three common agents are used.
    - Doxycycline mixed with lidocaine
    - Talc powder (common for pleurodesis)
    - Absolute alcohol
- Sclerosis of the collection requires the drainage to drop significantly; the collection itself is then minimized. This maximizes the chance the walls of the collection are in close proximity of one another (chance for wall

contact/coaptation). In addition, the accumulating fluid in the potential collection can dilute the sclerosant and render it less effective.

- Absolute alcohol is injected through the drain. Approximately one-third of the estimated volume of the collection is administered; 30–60 minutes later, the residual alcohol is aspirated and the drain is removed. If the patient feels pain, sedation may be required.
- Doxycycline is used for lymphocele sclerosis when drainage is less than 30 mL per 24 hours and the size of the lymphocele has been reduced to <10% of its original size. A doxycycline mixture is injected through the percutaneous drain. This is composed of 500 mg of doxycycline hyclate powder (American Pharmaceutical Partners, Los Angeles, CA) is reconstituted in 20 mL of normal saline, and is mixed with 5 mL of 1% lidocaine. The sclerosant is left in for 60 minutes while rotating the patient every 10 minutes during the 60 minutes. The sclerosant is then aspirated in its entirety and the drain is removed.

Complications and Their Management

Please see **Table 15.1** for the list of the most common complications and their incidence following percutaneous abscess/fluid collection drainage.

Management of Pain and Pain-Related Morbidity

- Pain is usually not a problem after abscess drainage except in transgluteal drains and intercostal transhepatic drains (see below). In these cases, nonnarcotic medication usually is enough to control the pain caused by fluid collection drains.
- Narcotic medications for pain management may occasionally be required in
  ○ Intercostal transhepatic abscess drains
  ○ Transgluteal drains
    ▪ Less than 5% of cases require narcotics (my estimate).
    ▪ If pain continues despite narcotics or if narcotics are contraindicated (or complicated), remove the drain and place another one with a different traversal tract (can still be transgluteal).

Management of Bleeding Complications

- Bleeding postfluid drainage can take several forms.
  ○ Intraperitoneal hemorrhage (hemoperitoneum)
  ○ External/site bleeding (rule out a skin bleed first)
  ○ Hemothorax

  ○ Bleeding into viscera that are traversed by the drain or that are involved by the collection
- Significant bleeding affecting vital signs and patient stability should be managed by
  ○ Fluid resuscitation starting with crystalloid fluid bolus
  ○ Type and cross
  ○ Repeat hematocrit to compare with baseline
  ○ Blood transfusion to maintain hematocrit at or above 30%
  ○ Surgical/interventional radiology consult
  ○ Interventional radiology can provide visceral angiography of the vascular bed of the abscess and/or the tissues traversed by the drain with superselective embolization.

Management of Pleural/Thoracic Complications

- This is not common (1% of abdominal cases).
- If chest pain with or without reduced oxygen saturation is encountered, a chest x-ray should be obtained to rule out pneumothorax or hemothorax.
- Clinically significant hemo- and/or pneumothorax require chest tube placement, increased nasal cannula oxygenation, and fluid resuscitation/bleeding management in case of the former.

Management of Puncture of Adjacent Organs

- This is not common.
- If transgression of bowel occurs by the drain, the drain should be left in place for the tract to mature. This allows
  ○ The patient to recover from the acute situation of a procedure, renal failure, and/or sepsis.
  ○ Later management of the fistula, if it occurs, can be performed in an elective setting.

Sepsis

- Operators should not over distend the fluid collection with contrast.
- Rigors only without fever can respond to 25–50 mg of Demerol (Sanofi Aventis Pharmaceuticals, Paris, France) administered intramuscularly.
- In cases of postoperative fever, operators should continue with IV antibiotics and should check the culture and sensitivity of the fluid sample obtained from the cholecystostomy.
- Sepsis requires fluid resuscitation and even vasopressors with ICU admission (the patient may already be in the ICU).

Further Reading

Bakal CW, Sacks D, Burke DR, et al; Society of Interventional Radiology Standards of Practice Committee. Quality improvement guidelines for adult percutaneous abscess and fluid drainage. J Vasc Interv Radiol 2003;14(9 Pt 2):S223–S225

Gerzof SG, Robbins AH, Johnson WC, Birkett DH, Nabseth DC. Percutaneous catheter drainage of abdominal abscesses: a five-year experience. N Engl J Med 1981;305(12):653–657

vanSonnenberg E, Mueller PR, Ferrucci JT Jr. Percutaneous drainage of 250 abdominal abscesses and fluid collections. Parts 1 and 2. Radiology 1984;151:337–347

Lambiase RE, Deyoe L, Cronan JJ, Dorfman GS. Percutaneous drainage of 335 consecutive abscesses: results of primary drainage with 1-year follow-up. Radiology 1992;184(1):167–179

Caliendo MV, Lee DE, Queiroz R, Waldman DL. Sclerotherapy with use of doxycycline after percutaneous drainage of postoperative lymphoceles. J Vasc Interv Radiol 2001;12(1):73–77

16 Abdominal Paracentesis
Wael E.A. Saad

Indications

- Symptomatic ascites
  - Abdominal distention
  - Abdominal discomfort
  - Shortness of breath
- Question of infection (fever) – spontaneous bacterial peritonitis
- Asymptomatic ascites of unknown etiology (diagnostic)
- An abdominal paracentesis is a prerequisite for an invasive hepatic procedure, particularly a transcapsular procedure (intentional or inadvertent capsular transgression) to potentially reduce the risk of hepatic capsular bleeding (controversial, not proven to reduce bleeding, but it is a common practice). An abdominal paracentesis is done prior to the following procedures:
  - Percutaneous transhepatic procedures
    - Percutaneous liver biopsy (random versus lesion specific)
    - Percutaneous transhepatic cholangiography with or without biliary drain placement
    - Percutaneous transhepatic venography with or without venoplasty
  - Procedures that may have hepatic capsule transgression
    - Transjugular intrahepatic portosystemic shunt (TIPS) procedure
    - Transjugular liver biopsy

Contraindications

Relative Contraindication

- Uncorrected coagulopathy (relative)
- Small amount of fluid for therapeutic procedure (for therapeutic intentions)

Preprocedural Evaluation

Evaluate Prior Cross-Sectional Imaging

- Evaluate
  - The size and extent of ascites
  - If ascitic fluid is loculated or confined in a certain area. This is where to perform a limited/focused ultrasound preprocedure.
  - Whether in small to moderate amounts of ascites, fluid has accumulated in the perihepatic region only
  - If there is focal wall thickening or associated masses to help identify or confirm the suspected diagnosis. Areas of peritoneal masses/implants should be avoided because they may increase the risk of bleeding.
  - An enhancing peritoneal lining may be due to infection, tumor, or subacute/chronic hemoperitoneum
  - For the presence of high-density fluid (>30 HU), which may represent infected fluid, bile, or blood – has a high probability of septations and/or loculations
- Look for adjacent organs that can be inadvertently traversed
  - Transgression of organs is not a common problem.
  - It may be more common with small amounts of ascitic fluid.
  - Organs that may be transgressed include bowel (especially small bowel, which may float in the ascetic fluid).
  - Plan a paracentesis that is safe and away from adjacent structures and organs (**Fig. 16.1**)

Evaluate Preprocedure Laboratory Values

- Laboratory value evaluation mostly revolves around ruling out coagulopathy.
  - Suggested coagulopathy thresholds for thoracentesis are
    - International normalized ratio (INR): ≤ 2.0
    - Platelets (PLT): $\geq 50,000$
    - Activated partial thromboplastin time (aPTT): ≤ 65 seconds

Obtain Informed Consent

- Indications
  - See Indications above
  - Technical success in placing a drain in the gallbladder is high (99–100%).
- Alternatives
  - To refuse the procedure
- Procedural risks
  - Major complications occur in <1% of patients.
  - Common postprocedural complications include

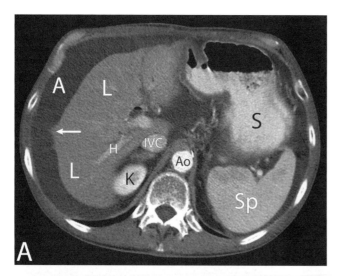

Fig. 16.1 Paracentesis performed from adjacent to the liver that has an adhesive band between the right liver lobe and the peritoneum. **(A)** Axial computed tomography (CT) image with contrast enhancement at the level of the aortic hiatus. There appears to be tenting of the hepatic parenchyma toward the peritoneum at the midaxillary line (*arrow*). Occasionally the majority, if not all, of the ascites fluid is perihepatic, which requires a right upper quadrant access paracentesis rather than the more common lower quadrant sites. It is important to avoid the liver capsule and/or mistaking a large and distended gallbladder for a loculated fluid collection (A, ascites; L, liver; IVC, inferior vena cava; H, right hepatic vein; Ao, aorta; S, stomach; Sp, spleen). **(B)** Gray-scale ultrasound image of the upper abdomen (*top*) and schematic sketch of it (*bottom*). The band is tenting toward the peritoneum (*). The operator avoided the band. In addition, the operator did not go deep with the needle avoiding transgression of the liver capsule (A, ascites; L, liver). **(C)** Gray-scale ultrasound image of the upper abdomen (*top*) and schematic sketch of it (*bottom*). The 21-gauge access needle (*arrow*) is seen traversing the peritoneum (*arrowheads*). The operator avoided the band. In addition, the operator did not go deep with the needle avoiding transgression of the liver capsule (A, ascites; L, liver).

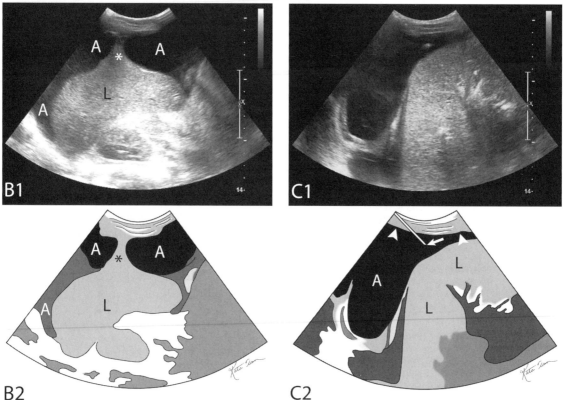

- Anterior abdominal wall/inferior epigastric artery hematoma
- Hypotension and hyponatremia
- Hemoperitoneum
- Peritonitis (theoretically)
- Bowel perforation
  - Bleeding
    - This is the most common complication (minor or major).

- Bleeding occurs in 0.2–2.0% (<1.0% if real-time ultrasound guidance is used).
- Bleeding can take several forms.
  - Skin bleeding/hematoma (0–0.5%)
  - Hemoperitoneum (rare)
  - Rectus sheath (inferior epigastric hematoma) (0–1.9%)
  - Inferior epigastric artery pseudoaneurysm (<0.5%)

- Bleeding may be transient with or without blood transfusion.
- Blood transfusion is required in 0–0.9% of cases.
- The source of bleeding is usually
  - Inferior epigastric artery
  - Anterior abdominal wall portosystemic portal hypertension collateral
  - Skin bleed

Equipment

Ultrasound Guidance

- Multiarray 3.5–5.0 MHz ultrasound transducer
- Transducer guide bracket (usually not necessary)
- Sterile transducer cover

Standard Surgical Preparation and Draping

- Chlorhexidine skin preparation/cleansing fluid
- Fenestrated drape

Local Infiltrative Analgesia Administration

- 21-gauge infiltration needle
- 10 to 20 mL 1% lidocaine syringe

Sharp Access Devices

- 11-blade incision scalpel
- 18-gauge needle that allows a 0.035-inch or 0.038-inch wire
- 21-gauge needle that allows a 0.018-inch wire
- A 15- to 20-cm-long needle (18- to 21-gauge) may be required to access the peritoneum in obese patients. The majority of patients can have their anterior abdominal wall traversed with a 7- to 8-cm-long needle.

Tubular Access Devices

- Telescoped graduate dilation system (micropuncture kit transitional dilator) to upsize 0.018-inch wire to 0.035-inch wire
- An 8-French fascial dilator that can be passed over a 0.035-inch guide wire may be used (see below).
- An 8-French self-retaining (string-locking) pigtail drainage catheter can be used.
- All-in-one sharp and tubular access – this is a tube loaded coaxially on a hypodermic needle, which leads with a spring-loaded blunt tip. Once an indicator shows that there is fluid at the needle tip, the outer plastic Teflon tubing is passed over the needle and into the

pleural space. For the purposes of this chapter, the Seldinger technique will be described.

Suction Devices

- The peritoneal tube in the peritoneal space can be drained utilizing sealed suction bottles (1-L vacuum bottles).

Technique

There are variations in the procedure part of this due to varying techniques and equipment. An all-in-one sharp and tubular access device is available. This is a tube loaded coaxially on a hypodermic needle, which leads with a spring-loaded blunt tip. Once an indicator shows that there is fluid at the needle tip, the outer plastic tubing is passed over the needle and into the peritoneal space. For the purposes of this chapter, the Seldinger technique will be described.

There are three procedure endpoints.

- Diagnostic paracentesis only
- Therapeutic paracentesis without an indwelling catheter left behind (all the fluid is removed and no catheter is left behind inside the patient)
- Therapeutic paracentesis with an indwelling catheter left behind to remove subsequent pleural fluid reaccumulation. Not commonly resorted to unless in the setting of malignant ascites with rapid reaccumulation of malignant ascitic fluid. Catheter is usually tunneled.

Intravenous Access and Medication

- Required for moderate sedation (moderate sedation is not necessary for this procedure, although some patients may require it)
- Required for albumin administration and crystalloid fluid replenishment (4–8 g per liter of ascitic fluid removed). At my institution, 12.5 g albumin bottles are given for every 3 liters of ascitic fluid removed (12.5 g/3 L = 4.2 g/L).
- Required for fluid resuscitation and rapid medication administration if there are complications

Preprocedure Ultrasound Exam

- Identify whether there is fluid in the peritoneal space
- Identify a window at which a needle can be passed into the peritoneal collection away from organs and viscera, particularly bowel
- Assess for safety – the smaller the volume of fluid the higher the risk

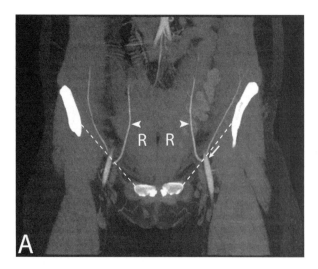 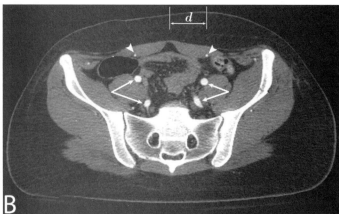

Fig. 16.2 (A) Contrast-enhanced computed tomography (CT) delineating the inferior epigastric artery anatomy. Coronal maximum intensity projection (MIP) of the pelvis of contrast-enhanced CT. As the external iliac artery passes under the inguinal ligament (*depicted by dotted line*), it gives off the inferior epigastric artery medially, which ascends the rectus abdominis sheath (*arrowheads*) along the lateral aspect of the rectus abdominis muscle (R). **(B)** Axial CT image with contrast enhancement at the level of S1. The common iliac arteries have bifurcated. The *arrows* point to the right- and left-external (*anterior*) and right- and left-interior (*posterior*) iliac arteries. The inferior epigastric arteries (*arrowheads*) are seen running posterior to the rectus muscles at this level of the pelvis. The inferior epigastric arteries run 4–8 cm from the midline (*d* = distance from midline = 4–8 cm).

- Attempt to characterize the ascitic fluid (**Fig. 16.1**)
  - Is the fluid loculated? This correlates with how difficult or how complete the drainage would be.
    - Septations, fluid complexity, and echogeneity are findings of possible infection or hemoperitoneum.
- The abdominal wall site is chosen with correlation with a safe pocket seen by ultrasound. Avoiding the course of the inferior epigastric artery is important. The course of the inferior epigastric artery passes parallel to the long axis of the abdomen (midline/linea alba) along the midclavicular line, which runs 4–8 cm from the midline (**Fig. 16.2**).
- Common sites for blinded paracentesis include
  - 2 cm below the umbilicus in the midline
  - 5 cm supramedial to the anterior superior iliac spine (ASIS)
- Common sites for ultrasound-guided paracentesis
  - First – where the greatest amount of fluid is, which is away from bowel
  - The right and left lower quadrants
  - Perihepatically where there is little fluid. Remember, one of the most dependent sites in the peritoneum when the patient is supine is the Morrison's pouch between the right hepatic lobe and the right kidney.

Standard Surgical Preparation and Draping

- Skin preparation/cleansing in the region that was chosen as an ultrasound imaging portal and a needle access needle portal

- Place a fenestrated drape at the chosen and prepared skin region

Local Infiltrative Analgesia Administration

- Utilizing a 21-gauge (by at least a 3.7-cm-long) infiltration needle, 1% lidocaine infiltration is performed (**Fig. 16.3**).
- Infiltrating down to the sensitive peritoneal lining may require needles in excess of 7 cm (up to 15- to 20-cm long may be required).

Ultrasound-Guided Sharp Access

- Use free-hand ultrasound guidance and a 21-gauge hypodermic needle to access the peritoneal cavity initially
- Free-hand ultrasound guidance allows flexibility in choosing access.
  - Once the needle traverses the skin into the subcutaneous tissue, suction is applied (operator aspirates using syringe) as the needle is advanced further.
  - Needle tip entry (seen by real-time ultrasound, **Figs. 16.1 and 16.3**) into the peritoneal space should correlate with a return of fluid into the syringe.
  - Once a peritoneal fluid sample is obtained, the syringe is removed.
- A 0.018-inch wire is passed through the 21- or 22-gauge needle, or a 0.035-inch wire is passed through a 19- or 18-gauge needle without imaging guidance (by feel).

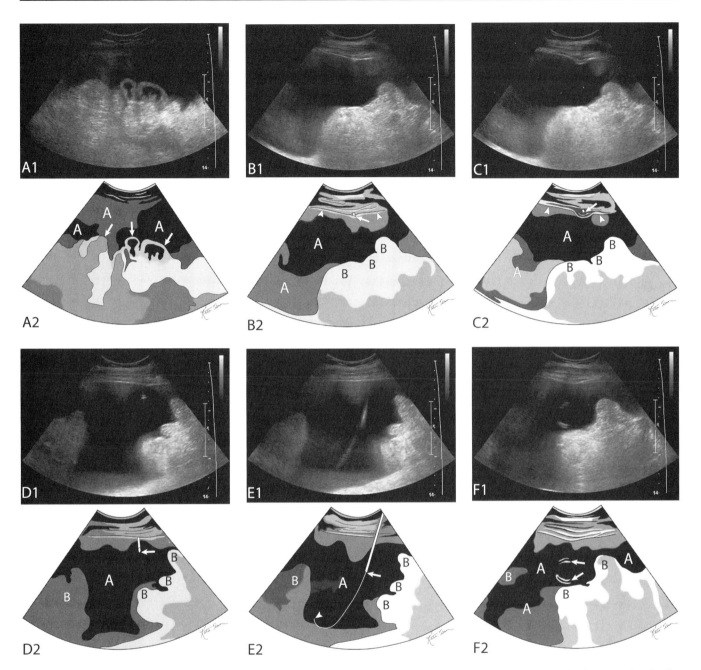

Fig. 16.3 Step-by-step real-time ultrasound-guided paracentesis.
(A) Diagnostic gray-scale ultrasound image of the right lower abdomen
(*top*) and schematic sketch of it (*bottom*). Fluid (A, ascites) is seen
between the abdominal wall and the deeper bowel loops (*arrows*).
(B) Diagnostic gray-scale ultrasound image of the right lower abdomen
(*top*) and schematic sketch of it (*bottom*). Fluid (A, ascites) is seen
between the abdominal wall and the deeper omentum and bowel
loops (B). The *arrowheads* point to the peritoneal lining. The tip of the
lidocaine needle is at the peritoneum (*arrow*). **(C)** Diagnostic gray-scale
ultrasound image of the right lower abdomen (top) and schematic
sketch of it (*bottom*). Fluid (A, ascites) is seen between the abdominal
wall and the deeper omentum and bowel loops (B). The *arrowheads*
point to the peritoneal lining. Infiltration of lidocaine forms a peritoneal
wheel at the needle tip (*arrow*). **(D)** Diagnostic gray-scale ultrasound

image of the right lower abdomen (*top*) and schematic sketch of it
(*bottom*). Fluid (A, ascites) is seen between the abdominal wall and the
deeper omentum and bowel loops (B). The tip 21-gauge definitive
access needle (*arrow*) is seen in the fluid. **(E)** Diagnostic gray-scale
ultrasound image of the right lower abdomen (*top*) and schematic
sketch of it (*bottom*). Fluid (A, ascites) is seen between the abdominal
wall and the deeper omentum and bowel loops (B). The wire (*arrowhead*) has been passed through the 21-gauge access needle (*arrow at
needle tip*). **(F)** Diagnostic gray-scale ultrasound image of the right
lower abdomen (*top*) and schematic sketch of it (*bottom*). Fluid
(A, ascites) is seen between the abdominal wall and the deeper omentum and bowel loops (B). Parts of the pigtail catheter are seen in the
peritoneal fluid (*arrows*).

- A 0.018-inch wire requires it to be upsized to a 0.035 or 0.038-inch wire utilizing a transitional micropuncture kit sheath. However, if a 15 cm needle is used, an Accu-Stick (Boston Scientific, Natick, MA) system (telescoped and stiffened dilator, see above) is used.
- Once there is a 0.035-inch wire in the peritoneal space, an 8-French fascial dilator is passed to dilate the tract.
- The dilator is removed and is quickly replaced by a self-retaining string-locking pigtail catheter (8-French). The pigtail is placed and secured ("Coped") in the peritoneal space (**Fig. 16.3**).
- The peritoneal drain is then placed to either gravity drainage (Foley collection bag) or a vacuum bottle.
- Tilting the patient toward the drain may help with drainage of ascitic fluid, especially when the paracentesis is near its end.
- Manipulating the drain including slightly pulling it out one step at a time may help maximize the amount of fluid removed.

Postparacentesis Imaging

- Once the drainage has ceased, repeat ultrasound evaluation of the abdomen can be performed to look for residual fluid. Usually this is not necessary in large volume paracentesis. The volume removed is evident clinically by inspection of the significant reduction in abdominal girth.
- Ask chronic (experienced) patients how many liters they suspect they are carrying. Experienced patients (chronic liver cirrhosis patients) usually have an accurate estimate of the amount of excess peritoneal fluid they are carrying.
- Once the endpoints (see below) of the procedure are achieved, the peritoneal drain is removed.

Endpoints

- There are three possible endpoints.
  - Diagnostic paracentesis only
  - Therapeutic paracentesis without an indwelling catheter left behind (all the fluid is removed and no catheter is left inside the patient)
  - Therapeutic paracentesis with an indwelling catheter left in (small-bore pigtail catheter placement) to remove subsequent ascitic fluid reaccumulation.
- In cases of large volume paracenteses, a limit on the maximum amount of fluid to be removed can be established.
  - A limit is set because some patients may suffer from hypotension and/or light-headedness from too much fluid extraction (intravascular hypovolemia).

- Upper level volume limits usually range between 8 and 12 L per session. However, limitations should be tailored to each patient.
- Chronic patients usually know if they have a maximum limit where they feel uncomfortable or light-headed despite albumin replenishment.
- Laboratory values that should be tested when a peritoneal fluid sample is obtained:
  - Total bilirubin
  - Amylase/lipase
  - Gram stain, culture, and sensitivity
    - Spontaneous bacterial peritonitis (SBP):
      - >90% single organism (<10% polymicrobial)
      - 50% *Escherichia coli*
      - Protein: <1 g/dL
  - Cytology evaluation to evaluate for malignant cells

Postprocedural Evaluation and Management

Postparacentesis Observation Period

- Paracenteses can be performed on both inpatients and outpatients.
- If an inpatient, the patient returns to his or her unit (regular floor or intensive care unit [ICU]).
- Check on the patient and monitor vital signs
- Outpatient paracenteses are routinely performed. Patients are usually kept for 1–2 hours.
- During this period, at least two sets of vital values are obtained and the patient should show the ability to ambulate without being light-headed.

Intravenous Fluid and Diet

- Intravenous (IV) fluid should be given until oral intake is adequate. Oral intake may not be feasible in this particular population because many can be septic and/or in the ICU. Once these patients defervesce, oral intake can be contemplated.
- IV albumin administration should be completed (4–8 g of albumin per liter of ascitic fluid removed). At my institution, 12.5 g albumin bottles are given for every 4 liters of ascitic fluid removed (12.5 g/3 L = 4.2 g/L).

Activity

- Bed rest during the period of albumin administration
- Outpatient paracentesis patients can ambulate once the IV albumin is given.
- Outpatients should show that they can ambulate without being light-headed.

Pain Management

- Usually over-the-counter analgesics will suffice for out-patients or ambulatory inpatients who have undergone a simple pleural fluid tap.

Monitoring Vital Signs

- Vital sign monitoring includes blood pressure and heart rate.
- At least two sets of vital statistics should be obtained prior to patient discharge.

Complications and Their Management

Management of Pain and Pain-Related Morbidity

- Pain is usually not encountered after completion of a paracentesis.
- Pain associated with increased abdominal girth should be suspect for intraperitoneal hemorrhage or rectus sheath hemorrhage.

Management of Bleeding Complications

- Bleeding postparacentesis can take several forms.
  - Rectus sheath hematoma/pseudoaneurysm
  - Intraperitoneal bleeding
  - Skin site bleeding

- Significant bleeding affecting vital signs and patient stability should be managed by
  - Fluid resuscitation starting with crystalloid fluid bolus
  - Type and cross
  - Repeat hematocrit to compare with baseline
  - Blood transfusion to maintain hematocrit at or above 30%
  - Surgical/interventional radiology consult
  - Interventional radiology can provide inferior epigastric angiography with super-selective embolization.
- Rectus sheath hematomas are usually self-limiting. Correction of abnormal coagulopathy parameters is recommended.

Management of Puncture of Adjacent Organs

- This is not common.
- Management of bowel injury by a needle should be by observation. If a 21-gauge needle is used, usually nothing will happen (anecdotal).
- Inadvertent drain placement in hollow viscera such as the gallbladder or colon should be managed conservatively. This includes securing the drain and waiting for tract maturity.

Further Reading

Lin CH, Shih FY, Ma MH, Chiang WC, Yang CW, Ko PC. Should bleeding tendency deter abdominal paracentesis? Dig Liver Dis 2005; 37(12):946–951

Nakamoto DA, Haaga JR. Emergent ultrasound interventions. Radiol Clin North Am 2004;42(2):457–478

Nicolaou S, Talsky A, Khashoggi K, Venu V. Ultrasound-guided interventional radiology in critical care. Crit Care Med 2007;35(5, Suppl):S186–S197

Tibbles CD, Porcaro W. Procedural applications of ultrasound. Emerg Med Clin North Am 2004;22(3):797–815

17 Thoracentesis
Wael E.A. Saad

Indications

By Presentation

- Shortness of breath
- Question of infection (fever)
- Asymptomatic effusion of unknown etiology (diagnostic)
- Recurrent effusions requiring pleurodesis (percutaneous access to pleural space)

By Etiology/Fluid Type

- Pleural effusion
  - Transudate
    - Congestive heart failure
    - Renal failure
    - Hepatic hydrothorax
    - Hypoproteinemia
    - Meig's syndrome
  - Exudate
    - Malignant effusion
    - Infections (including tuberculosis)
- Pleural space infection
  - Empyema (from pneumonia, lung abscess)
  - Postoperative infection
  - Posttranshepatic procedures (bile leak, for example)
- Hemothorax
  - Spontaneous
  - Malignant
  - Trauma
  - Postoperative
- Chylothorax
  - Posttraumatic
  - Iatrogenic

Contraindications

Relative Contraindication

- Uncorrected coagulopathy (relative)
- Small amount of fluid for therapeutic procedure (for therapeutic intentions)
- Mechanical ventilation is not a contraindication.

Preprocedural Evaluation

Evaluate Prior Cross-Sectional Imaging

- Evaluate
  - The size and extent of pleural effusion
  - If there is focal wall thickening or associated masses to help identify or confirm the suspected diagnosis
  - If enhancing pleura (collection wall) is due to infection, tumor, or subacute/chronic hemothorax
  - For hints of loculation of pleural fluid
    - Shifting of fluid from one computed tomography (CT) scan to the next, or from plain film radiographs (**Fig. 17.1**)
    - Lobulation of the pleural fluid in pockets within the thoracic cavity (**Fig. 17.1**)
    - High-density fluid (>30 HU) that may represent infected fluid, bile, or blood – has a high probability of septations and/or loculations
- Prior ultrasound images/evaluations of the pleural space may show septations within the pleural fluid (**Fig. 17.2**).
  - The septations may indicate that a simple tube/drain placement may not adequately drain all the fluid in the pleural space.
  - This is an indication that the septations may require wire break-up during the procedure (see Fluoroscopic-guided wire and tube access).
- Look for adjacent organs that can be inadvertently traversed
  - Transgression of organs is not a common problem.
  - It may be more common with small amounts of subpulmonic fluid, which raise the technical difficulty of a thoracentesis.
  - Organs that may be transgressed include the lung, spleen (left thoracentesis), and liver (right thoracentesis).
  - Plan a thoracentesis that is safe and away from adjacent structures such as the descending thoracic aorta particularly in left-sided posterior thoracentesis in the elderly with ectatic aorta

Evaluate Preprocedure Laboratory Values

- Laboratory value evaluation mostly revolves around ruling out coagulopathy.
  - Suggested coagulopathy thresholds for thoracentesis are

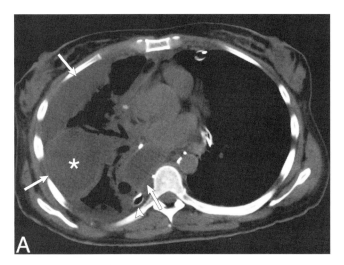

Fig. 17.1 Drainage of postoperative infected pleural space (empyema). **(A)** Unenhanced axial computed tomography (CT) image of the lower chest in a patient status postthoracic surgery demonstrated thick-walled loculated collections (*arrows*) in the pleural space. One of these locules has a thick wall (*asterisk in center of it*). A large-bore surgically placed chest tube is seen in the chest bases, posteriorly (*arrowhead*). **(B)** Gray-scale ultrasound image of the fluid collection in **Fig. 17.1A** (*top*) and schematic sketch of it (*bottom*). A 21-gauge needle has been advanced into the pleural collection (*arrow*). The underlying lung is seen (*asterisk*) (LE, loculated pleural effusion). **(C)** Gray-scale ultrasound image of the fluid collection in (*top*) and schematic sketch of it (*bottom*). A 10-French drain (*arrow*) is now seen in the target pleural collection (LE, loculated pleural effusion). The underlying lung is seen (*asterisk*).

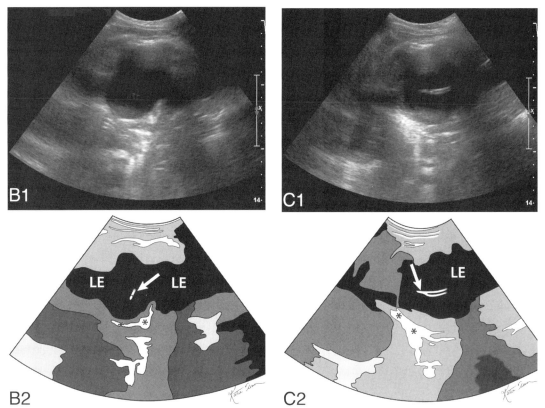

- International normalized ratio (INR): ≤1.7
- Platelets (PLT): ≥50,000–70,000
- Activated partial thromboplastin time (aPTT): ≤5 seconds

Obtain Informed Consent

- Indications
  - ○ See Indications above
  - ○ Technical success in placing a drain in the gallbladder is high (98–100%).
  - ○ Technical success of ultrasound-guided thoracentesis after failed "blind" or clinical/palpation thoracentesis is 88%.
- Alternatives
  - ○ To refuse the procedure
  - ○ Bedside, nonimage-guided thoracentesis
  - ○ Surgically placed large-bore chest tube
  - ○ Video-assisted thoracotomy drainage (VAT)
  - ○ Surgical decortication in loculated and chronically infected pleural space

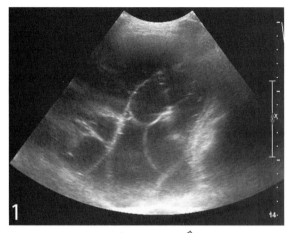

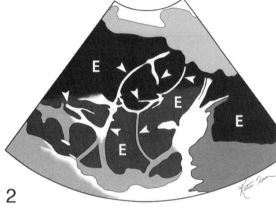

Fig. 17.2 Gray-scale ultrasound image of a septated pleural effusion (*top*) and schematic sketch of it (*bottom*). Numerous septa are seen (*arrowheads*) crisscrossing the pleural effusion (E).

- Procedural risks
  - Major complications occur in 1–5% of patients.
  - Common postprocedural morbidity symptoms (part of the spectrum of complications) are listed in **Table 17.1**.
  - Infection (**Table 17.2**)
    - This complication is not mentioned (rare) in thoracenteses studies; however, it is theoretically possible, although difficult to prove, that infection can be introduced into a sterile pleural effusion.

Table 17.1   Common Symptoms Following Percutaneous Thoracentesis

Symptoms	Incidence
Shortness of breath	1.0–2.0%
Cough	0.8%
Hemoptysis	0.1%
Pain	2.7–8.2%
Vasovagal reaction	0.6%

Table 17.2   Complications of Percutaneous Thoracentesis

Complication	Incidence
Pneumothorax	1.0–7.5%
Pneumothorax requiring chest tube	0.0–1.9%*
Hemothorax	1.6–2.0%
Hypotension†	1.1%
External bleeding (hematoma, entrance bleeding)	0.5%
Hemoptysis	0.1%
Pain	2.7–8.2%
Vasovagal reaction	0.6%
Reexpansion pulmonary edema	0.0–0.3%‡
Introduction of infection	Rare§
Infra- and supradiaphragmatic visceral or structural transgression	Rare§

*10–40% of patients with pneumothoraces require chest tube placement.

†May not necessarily be due to bleeding, but may be due to hypovolemia due to removal of large volume of pleural effusion/hydrothorax.

.‡Reexpansion pulmonary edema is associated with large volume pleural effusion tapping (>1000 mL), which is associated with a 0.5% incidence of reexpansion pulmonary edema.

§Not mentioned in large case series, but theoretically possible.

- Bleeding (**Table 17.2**)
  - Bleeding occurs in <2–3% of patients.
  - Bleeding can occur as site (peritube) bleeding/hematoma (0.5%), hemothorax (<2.0%), or hemoptysis (0.1%).
  - It may present as pain and/or hypotension and a CT scan may show
    - Enlarging hydrothorax now with high density (>45 HU) fluid (blood)
    - Active extravasation in the few cases where CT intravenous (IV) contrast is used
  - Bleeding may be transient with or without blood transfusion.
  - The source of bleeding is usually an intercostal artery; it is usually self-limiting.
  - In rare cases, bleeding may require intervention such as transcatheter intercostal arterial embolization or exploratory surgery (thoracotomy).
  - Injury to surrounding organs and/or structures (**Table 17.2**)
    - Lung
    - Spleen, liver
  - Pneumothorax (**Table 17.2**)
    - Occurs in <5% of cases

- Incidence varies depending on whether a routine chest x-ray (CXR) is performed after the thoracentesis or not. This is controversial. Some institutions perform a CXR only in symptomatic patients; other institutions perform at least one CXR after all thoracenteses.
- 33% of patients with pneumothoraces are symptomatic.
- 25% of patients with pneumothoraces have chest pain.
- 25% of patients with pneumothoraces have shortness of breath.
- 57% of patients with shortness of breath have pneumothoraces.
- 16% of patients with chest pain have pneumothoraces.
- 10–40% of patients with pneumothoraces require a chest tube to be placed.

Equipment

Ultrasound Guidance

- Multiarray 4–5 MHz ultrasound transducer
- Transducer guide bracket (usually not necessary)
- Sterile transducer cover

Standard Surgical Preparation and Draping

- Chlorhexidine skin preparation/cleansing fluid
- Fenestrated drape

Local Infiltrative Analgesia Administration

- 21-gauge infiltration needle
- 10– 20 mL 1% lidocaine syringe

Sharp Access Devices

- 11-blade incision scalpel
- 18-gauge needle that allows a 0.035-inch or 0.038-inch wire
- 21-gauge needle that allows a 0.018-inch wire

Tubular Access Devices

- Telescoped graduate dilation system (micropuncture kit transitional dilator) to upsize a 0.018-inch wire to a 0.035-inch wire
- An 8-French fascial dilator that can be passed over a 0.035-inch guidewire may be used (see Fluoroscopic-guided wire and tube access).
- An 8-French self-retaining (string-locking) pigtail drainage catheter, which is the definitive cholecystostomy tube/drain to be placed last (final product of the procedure)

- All-in-one sharp and tubular access. This is a tube loaded coaxially on a hypodermic needle, which leads with a spring-loaded blunt tip. Once an indicator shows that there is fluid at the needle tip, the outer plastic Teflon tubing is passed over the needle and into the pleural space. For the purposes of this chapter, the Seldinger technique will be described.

Suction/Water Seal Devices

- A thoracic tube in the pleural space can be drained utilizing sealed suction bottles (1 L vacuum bottles).
- The thoracic drain/chest tube can be put to water seal or be on controlled suction (common level is -20-cm water wall suction) utilizing a pleurovac system; for example, chest drain multipurpose model Oasis (Atrium Medical Corp., Hudson, NH).

Technique

There are variations in the procedure due to varying techniques and equipment and the the varying intended endpoints (aim) of the procedure. An all-in-one sharp and tubular access device is available. This is a tube loaded coaxially on a hypodermic needle, which leads with a spring-loaded blunt tip. Once an indicator shows that there is fluid at the needle tip, the outer plastic tubing is passed over the needle and into the pleural space. For the purposes of this chapter, the Seldinger technique will be described.

There are three endpoints for the procedure:

- Diagnostic thoracentesis only
- Therapeutic thoracentesis without an indwelling catheter left behind (all the fluid is removed and no catheter is left behind inside the patient)
- Therapeutic thoracentesis with an indwelling catheter left behind to remove subsequent pleural fluid reaccumulation.

Intravenous Access and Medication

- Required for moderate sedation and fluid replenishment (moderate sedation is not necessary for this procedure, although some patients may require it)
- Required for fluid resuscitation and rapid medication administration if there are complications

Preprocedure Ultrasound Exam

- Identify whether there is fluid in the pleural space
- Identify an intercostals window (an intercostals level) at which a needle can be passed into the pleural collection.

- Assess safety – the smaller the volume of fluid the higher the risk. Fluid one space above and below the intended intercostal space usually indicates an adequate amount of fluid.
- Attempt to characterize the pleural fluid
  - Is the fluid loculated? This correlates with how difficult or how complete the drainage would be.
  - Septations, fluid complexity, and echogeneity are findings of possible infection in the pleural space (empyema) (**Fig. 17.2**).
    - 73% of cases of empyema have complex stations.
    - 13% of cases of empyema are homogeneously echogenic.
- It is important to differentiate between pleural effusion and lesions that can be hypoechoic and mimic effusions. Doppler ultrasound can help differentiate between these lesions (vascular) and pleural fluid (avascular). These lesions include
  - Pleural masses/metastasis
  - Consolidated lung
- In the left hemithorax, identify the depth of vital structures such as the posterior wall of the left atrium and/or the descending thoracic aorta.

Standard Surgical Preparation and Draping

- Skin preparation/cleansing in the region that was chosen as an ultrasound imaging portal and a needle access needle portal
- Place a fenestrated drape at the chosen and prepared skin region

Local Infiltrative Analgesia Administration

- Utilizing a 21-gauge (by at least a 3.7-cm-long) infiltration needle, a 1% lidocaine infiltration is performed, infiltrating down to the sensitive hepatic capsule.

Ultrasound-Guided Sharp Access

- Use free-hand ultrasound guidance and a 21-gauge hypodermic needle to access the pleural space initially
- Free-hand ultrasound guidance allows flexibility in choosing access, particularly if there are ribs in the way. Ideally, the operator should pass the needle above the rib to avoid the intercostal neurovascular plexus, thus avoiding pain and or bleeding.
  - Once the needle traverses the skin into the subcutaneous tissue, suction is applied (operator aspirates using syringe) as the needle is advanced further.
  - Needle tip entry (seen by real-time ultrasound) into the pleural space should correlate with a return of fluid into the syringe (**Figs. 17.1, 17.3, and 17.4**).

- Once a pleural fluid sample is obtained, the syringe is removed.
  - Fluid can move in and out of the needle at its hub with respiration. This is the best proof that the needle tip is in the pleural space.
  - Pneumothorax from leaving the needle hub unsealed while the operator watches fluid leaking from it or moving in and out with respiration is not likely when a 21- to 22-gauge needle is utilized.

Fluoroscopic-Guided Wire and Tube Access

- Fluoroscopic-guided wire and tube access is used when there is loculated fluid suspected to be infected and particularly when there is a therapeutic intent to break locules/septa and leave a drain in the pleural space.
- In cases of simple thoracenteses for simple pleural fluid collections, fluoroscopy is not necessary.
- Once the needle is in place (if fluoroscopy is going to be used), radiographic contrast is injected to further confirm placement of the needle.
- A 0.018-inch wire is passed through the 21- to 22-gauge needle or a 0.035-inch wire is passed through a 19- to 18-gauge needle under fluoroscopy. The wire is coiled in the gallbladder lumen.
- A 0.018-inch wire requires it to be upsized to a 0.035 or 0.038-inch wire utilizing an AccuStick (Boston Scientific, Natick, MA) system (telescoped and stiffened dilator, see above) or a micropuncture kit transitional dilator.
- Once there is a 0.035-inch wire in the target pleural space, an 8-French fascial dilator is passed to dilate the tract.
- The dilator is removed and is quickly replaced by a self-retaining string-locking pigtail catheter (8- to 10-French for simple pleural effusion). The pigtail is placed and secured ("Coped") in the pleural space (**Figs. 17.3 and 17.4**).
- Please see Endpoints section below for appropriate chest tube/drain sizes based on the etiology/type of fluid being drained.
- The chest tube drain is then secured to the skin utilizing sutures and left to -20 cm water wall suction through a water seal system such as a pleurovac system; for example, chest drain multipurpose model Oasis (Atrium Medical Corp.).

Postthoracentesis Imaging

- Immediate postchest tube imaging is for documentation that the pigtail end of the drain is in the pleural space/fluid collection.
- Postthoracentesis imaging also includes CXRs to evaluate for pneumothoraces.

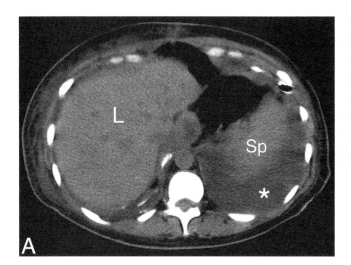

Fig. 17.3 Thoracentesis. **(A)** Unenhanced axial computed tomography (CT) image of the lower chest and upper abdomen in a patient with a left-sided pleural effusion (*) (Sp, spleen; L, liver). **(B)** Gray-scale ultrasound image of the pleural effusion (*top*) and schematic sketch of it (*bottom*). The pleural effusion (E) is again seen. The left lower lobe of the lung is collapsed (*arrows*) over the spleen (Sp). **(C)** Gray-scale ultrasound image of the patient with the pleural effusion in **Fig. 17.3A and 17.3B** (*top*) and schematic sketch of it (*bottom*). The pleural effusion (E) is again seen. The left lower lobe of the lung is collapsed (L) over the spleen (Sp). The diaphragm sits over the spleen (*between arrows*). *(Continued on page 224)*

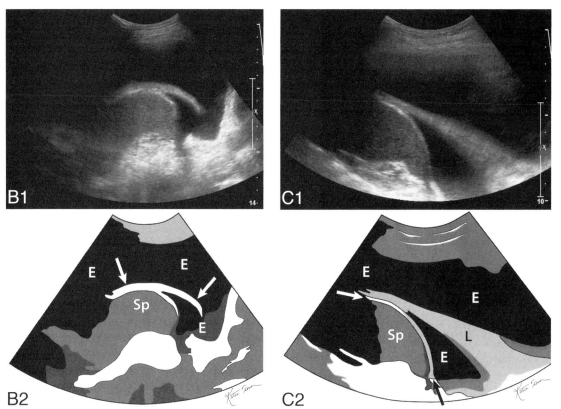

- This is controversial. Some institutions limit post-procedural CXRs to symptomatic patients. Other institutions perform two CXRs: one immediately post-thoracentesis and the other 1 hour from the start of a thoracentesis.
- Increasing size of the pneumothorax from the baseline CXR is grounds for admission with or without chest tube placement for pneumothorax (**Fig. 17.5**).

Endpoints

As mentioned above, there are three possible endpoints:

- Diagnostic thoracentesis only
- Therapeutic thoracentesis without an indwelling catheter left behind (all the fluid is removed and no catheter is left inside the patient)

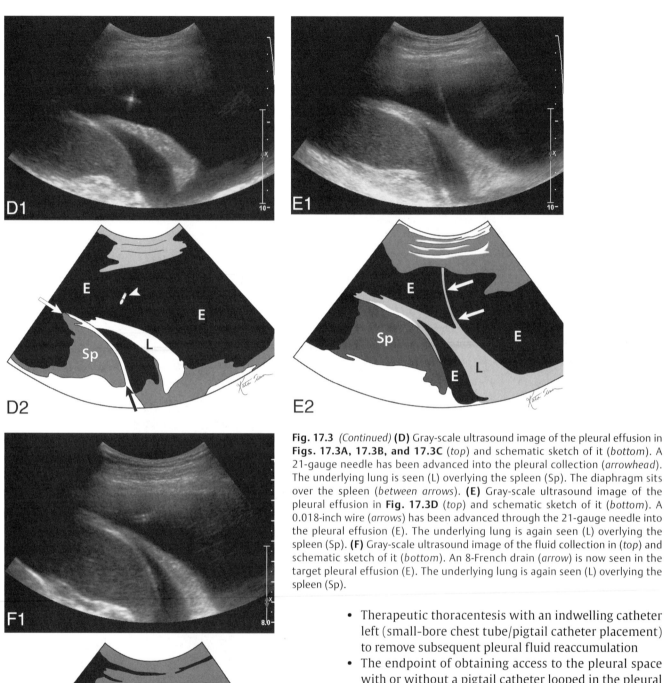

Fig. 17.3 *(Continued)* **(D)** Gray-scale ultrasound image of the pleural effusion in **Figs. 17.3A, 17.3B,** and **17.3C** (*top*) and schematic sketch of it (*bottom*). A 21-gauge needle has been advanced into the pleural collection (*arrowhead*). The underlying lung is seen (L) overlying the spleen (Sp). The diaphragm sits over the spleen (*between arrows*). **(E)** Gray-scale ultrasound image of the pleural effusion in **Fig. 17.3D** (*top*) and schematic sketch of it (*bottom*). A 0.018-inch wire (*arrows*) has been advanced through the 21-gauge needle into the pleural effusion (E). The underlying lung is again seen (L) overlying the spleen (Sp). **(F)** Gray-scale ultrasound image of the fluid collection in (*top*) and schematic sketch of it (*bottom*). An 8-French drain (*arrow*) is now seen in the target pleural effusion (E). The underlying lung is again seen (L) overlying the spleen (Sp).

- Therapeutic thoracentesis with an indwelling catheter left (small-bore chest tube/pigtail catheter placement) to remove subsequent pleural fluid reaccumulation
- The endpoint of obtaining access to the pleural space with or without a pigtail catheter looped in the pleural space has the following technical success rates:
  - Technical success occurs in 98–100% of ultrasound-guided thoracentesis.
  - Technical success of ultrasound-guided thoracentesis is 88% following failed "blind" thoracentesis.
  - Technical failures are more common when
    - Small pleural fluid is available
    - Pleural fluid is too little and very thick (viscid fluid)
- Laboratory values that should be tested when a pleural fluid sample is obtained:
  - Glucose
  - Protein
  - LDH: l-lactate dehydrogenase

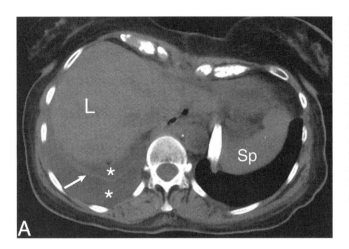

Fig. 17.4 Thoracentesis. **(A)** Unenhanced axial computed tomography (CT) image of the lower chest and upper abdomen in a patient with a right-sided pleural effusion (*) seen on both sides of a collapsed right lower lung lobe (*arrow*) (Sp, spleen; L, liver). **(B)** Gray-scale ultrasound image of the pleural effusion (*top*) and schematic sketch of it (*bottom*). The pleural effusion (E) is again seen. The right lower lobe of the lung is collapsed (Lu). The diaphragm is seen (*between the arrows*) overlying the hepatic dome (L). **(C)** Gray-scale ultrasound image of the patient with the pleural effusion in **Figs. 17.4A and 17.4B** (*top*) and schematic sketch of it (*bottom*). The pleural effusion (E) is again seen. A 21-gauge needle has been advanced into the pleural collection (*arrowhead*). The right lower lobe of the lung is collapsed (Lu). The diaphragm is seen (*between the arrows*) overlying the hepatic dome (L). *(Continued on page 226)*

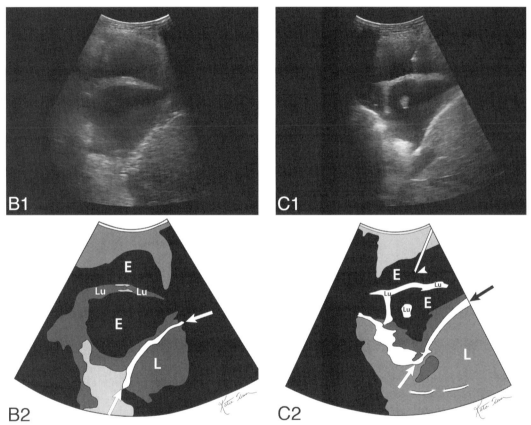

- ○ pH
- ○ Amylase/lipase
- ○ Gram stain, culture, and sensitivity
- ○ Cytology analysis to evaluate for malignant cells
- ○ Criteria for diagnosing exudative effusion (Light's criteria) – one of these three criterio is enough for a diagnosis:
  - • Pleural fluid protein: serum protein ratio >0.5
  - • Pleural fluid lactate dehydrogenase (LDH): serum LDH >0.6
  - • Pleural fluid LDH concentration >2/3 of the normal upper limit for serum LDH

- ○ Additional criteria suggestive exudative effusion
  - • Pleural fluid LDH >1000 U/L
  - • Pleural fluid pH >7.2
  - • Pleural fluid glucose <40 mg/dL
- • Tube size endpoints
  - ○ Pneumothorax: 6- to 8-French
  - ○ Simple uninfected pleural effusion: 8- to 10-French
  - ○ Hemothorax: >12-French (up to 24-French)
  - ○ Empyema: >18-French ± thrombolytics, multiple tubes
  - ○ Intent for pleurodesis: ≥16-French

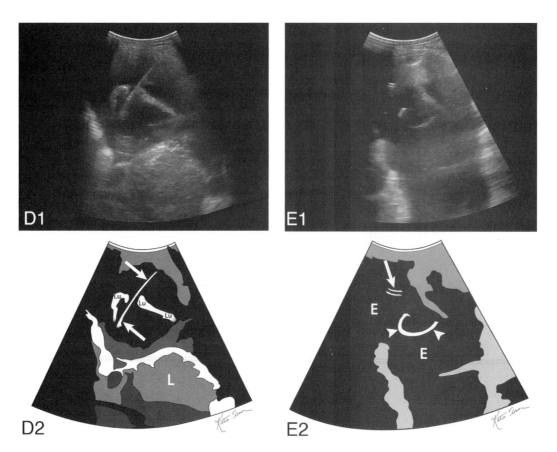

Fig. 17.4 *(Continued)* **(D)** Gray-scale ultrasound image of the patient with the pleural effusion in **Figs. 17.4A and 17.4B** (*top*) and schematic sketch of it (*bottom*). A 0.018-inch wire (*arrows*) has been advanced through the 21-gauge needle into the pleural effusion (E) and is pushing up against the right lower lobe of the lung, which is collapsed (Lu; L, liver). **(E)** Gray-scale ultrasound image of the fluid collection in (*top*) and schematic sketch of it (*bottom*). An 8-French drain (*arrow and arrowheads*) is now seen in the target pleural effusion (E). The shaft of the drain (*arrow*) can be discerned clearly from the pigtail end of the drain (*arrowheads*).

Postprocedural Evaluation and Management

Thoracentesis can be performed on both inpatients and outpatients. In cases of empyema or postoperative infection when indwelling pigtail catheters are left behind, the patients are inpatients or are admitted immediately after the thoracentesis/pigtail catheter placement.

Postthoracentesis (Chest Tube Placement) Observation Period

- If an inpatient, the patient return to his or her unit (regular floor or intensive care unit [ICU]).
- Septic patients at baseline or patients who become septic postpigtail drain placement (become worse) should be transferred to the ICU for resuscitation and even cardiopulmonary support.
- Check on the patient and monitor vital signs
- Observe the chest tube (pleural pigtail catheter) output including volume output and character

- Outpatient thoracentesis can be performed. Patients are usually kept for at least 2 hours. During this period, an immediate postprocedure CXR and a 1-hour postprocedure CXR are obtained to evaluate for postthoracentesis pneumothorax (**Fig. 17.5**).

Intravenous Fluid and Diet

- IV fluid should be given until oral intake is adequate. Oral intake may not be feasible in this particular population because many can be septic and/or in the ICU. Once these patients defervesce, oral intake can be contemplated.

Activity

- Bed rest. Many inpatients are usually not in a condition to ambulate.
- Outpatient thoracentesis patients can ambulate after an hour from the procedure.

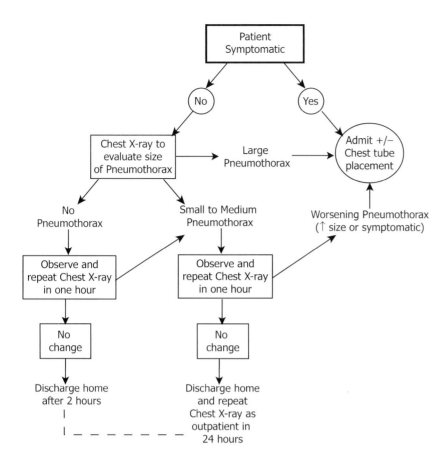

Fig. 17.5 Flow chart for the management of postprocedural pneumothorax (postlung or mediastinal biopsy or postthoracentesis).

- The indwelling chest tube/pigtail catheter should be to -20-cm water wall suction or at least water seal.
- During ambulation, the pigtail catheter should be under water seal.
- If ambulatory, patients should be instructed on how to maneuver with the small-bore chest tubes/pigtail catheters and to be reminded that they are tethered to a water seal/suction device (a pleurovac system; for example, chest drain multipurpose model Oasis [Arium Medical Corp.]).

Pain Management

- Usually over-the-counter analgesics will suffice for outpatients or ambulatory inpatients who have undergone a simple pleural fluid tap.
- Narcotics may be required in patients with indwelling chest tubes, particularly when they rub against the intercostal neurovascular bundle.

Monitoring Vital Signs

- Vital sign monitoring includes blood pressure and heart rate. Occasionally, oxygen saturation monitoring is required in cases of shortness of breath and/or chest pain.
- In cases of shortness of breath, one must be able to differentiate between splinting due to pain and pleural compli-

cations (pneumothorax or hemothorax). Clinical exam and a CXR would help differentiate between the two.
- Hypotension may be a result of sepsis. Careful postprocedural clinical evaluation to differentiate sepsis versus hypovolemia is required.

Complications and Their Management

Please see **Table 17.2** for a list of the most common complications and their incidence following thoracentesis.

Management of Pain and Pain-Related Morbidity

- See *Pain Management* in the Postprocedural Evaluation and Management section above
- If pain from an indwelling chest tube is refractory to narcotics or requires unreasonably large amounts of narcotics, then there are two main options:
  ○ Remove chest tube ± place it at a different site
  ○ Pain management consult ± nerve block therapy

Management of Bleeding Complications

- Bleeding postchest tube placement can take several forms:
  ○ Hemothorax
  ○ Site bleeding around chest tube or site hematoma
  ○ Hemoptysis

- Significant bleeding affecting vital signs and patient stability should be managed by
  - Fluid resuscitation starting with crystalloid fluid bolus
  - Type and cross
  - Repeat hematocrit to compare with baseline
  - Blood transfusion to maintain hematocrit at or above 30%
  - Surgical/interventional radiology consult
  - Interventional radiology can provide intercostal angiography with super-selective embolization.
- The source of new onset postprocedural hemothorax and/or site bleeding is usually an intercostal artery.
- Intercostal artery bleeding after chest tube placement is usually self-limiting as long as there is no coagulopathy.
- However, there are criteria that form a threshold where surgical consultation/interventional angiography and embolization should be entertained. These criteria include
  - Chest tube output is >1000 mL of fresh blood at placement.
  - Chest tube output is >200 mL of fresh blood per hour for several hours.
  - Chest tube output is >1500 mL of fresh blood in 24 hours.
  - Unstable patient

Management of Pleural/Thoracic Complications

- This is the most common major complication occurring 2–7% of thoracentesis cases.
- If chest pain with or without reduced oxygen saturation is encountered, a CXR should be obtained to rule out pneumothorax or hemothorax (see above Management of Bleeding Complications section) (**Fig. 17.5**).
- Clinically significant hemo- and/or pneumothorax require chest tube placement (see above), increased nasal cannula oxygenation, and fluid resuscitation/bleeding management in case of the former (see above Management of Bleeding Complications section) (**Fig. 17.5**).

Management of Puncture of Adjacent Organs

- This is not common.
- If transgression of liver occurs by the drain:
  - The patient should be admitted for at least 24 hours.
  - The drain should be left in place for the tract to mature; this allows the drain to be removed usually without additional invasive procedures.
- If transgression of spleen occurs by the drain:
  - The patient should be admitted for at least 24 hours.
  - Surgical consult should be obtained. The patient is to be treated as for a posttraumatic splenic fracture/laceration.
  - If the patient is stable (stable patient with splenic laceration), continued observation should be made. The drain should be left in place for the tract to mature; this allows the drain to be removed usually without additional invasive procedures.
  - If the patient is unstable (unstable patient with splenic laceration/fracture), resuscitation should be made with or without splenic artery embolization/exploratory laparotomy with splenectomy.

Further Reading

Beaulieu Y, Marik PE. Bedside ultrasonography in the ICU: part 1. Chest 2005;128(2):881–895

Capizzi SA, Prakash UBS. Chest roentgenography after outpatient thoracentesis. Mayo Clin Proc 1998;73(10):948–950

Feller-Kopman D. Ultrasound-guided thoracentesis. Chest 2006;129(6):1709–1714

Heidecker J, Huggins JT, Sahn SA, Doelken P. Pathophysiology of pneumothorax following ultrasound-guided thoracentesis. Chest 2006;130(4):1173–1184

Jones PW, Moyers JP, Rogers JT, Rodriguez RM, Lee YCG, Light RW. Ultrasound-guided thoracentesis: is it a safer method? Chest 2003;123(2):418–423

Mynarek G, Brabrand K, Jakobsen JA, Kolbenstvedt A. Complications following ultrasound-guided thoracocentesis. Acta Radiol 2004;45(5):519–522

Nakamoto DA, Haaga JR. Emergent ultrasound interventions. Radiol Clin North Am 2004;42(2):457–478

Nicolaou S, Talsky A, Khashoggi K, Venu V. Ultrasound-guided interventional radiology in critical care. Crit Care Med 2007;35(5, Suppl): S186–S197

Shoseyov D, Bibi H, Shatzberg G, et al. Short-term course and outcome of treatments of pleural empyema in pediatric patients: repeated ultrasound-guided needle thoracocentesis vs chest tube drainage. Chest 2002;121(3):836–840

Tibbles CD, Porcaro W. Procedural applications of ultrasound. Emerg Med Clin North Am 2004;22(3):797–815

Tu CY, Hsu WH, Hsia TC, et al. Pleural effusions in febrile medical ICU patients: chest ultrasound study. Chest 2004;126(4):1274–1280

18 Musculoskeletal Joint Interventions
Ralf Thiele

Ultrasonography has been used to guide interventions for several decades. Interventional ultrasonography can be an office-based or bedside technique, or performed in a dedicated suite. Interventional ultrasonography in musculoskeletal medicine is used for diagnostic and therapeutic purposes.

Indications

- Fluid aspiration
- Biopsy guidance
- Targeted injection of therapeutics

Fluid obtained is examined for

- Presence of crystals
- Cell count
- Cell culture
- Gram stain

Possible Diagnoses

- Crystal-induced arthropathy
- Inflammatory arthritis
- Noninflammatory arthropathy
- Septic arthritis
- Tendinitis

In comparison with blind aspiration, the yield of sonographically guided aspirations is significantly higher, particularly in the small joints of the hands and feet. Guided-diagnostic aspirations are therefore more accurate, there is less delay in diagnosis and treatment, and referrals can frequently be avoided.

Analysis of synovial tissue following biopsy can provide valuable insights into

- Pathophysiology
- Disease status
- Treatment effect and prognosis of inflammatory joint diseases

Ultrasound guidance can improve the yield of such biopsies because hypertrophied and hypervascularized synovial tissue can be accurately located. If ultrasound guidance is employed, even small joints will be accessible to biopsy.

Intralesional, Intraarticular, and Tendon Sheath Injections of Steroids and Other Therapeutic Agents

- Daily practice in emergency medicine, primary care, orthopedics, physiatry, rheumatology, and interventional radiology
- Ultrasound guidance has been reported to improve accuracy of injections as well as clinical outcomes.

Adverse Effects

They include

- Tissue necrosis
- Tendon rupture

Adverse effects can be avoided if

- Steroids are placed correctly within joint cavities, bursae, and tendon sheaths.

Contraindications

- Patient with bleeding disorders
- Patient on anticoagulants therapy

Preprocedural Evaluation

Typical indications for diagnostic joint aspirations are

- Redness
- Joint swelling and pain
- Remember, joint swelling can be mimicked by swelling of structures outside of the joint such as subcutaneous edema due to heart failure venostasis, lymph edema, and cellulitis.

These etiologies can be readily determined sonographically and an unnecessary joint aspiration can be avoided. Preprocedure sonographic examination can also determine

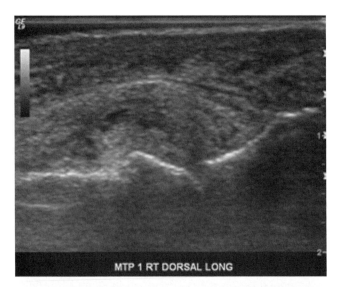

Fig. 18.1 Dorsal, long axis views centered over joint line of first metatarsophalangeal (MTP) joint in three different patients. All patients present similarly with pain and swelling of the first toe. **(A)** Shows distension of joint capsule by hyperechoic, crystalline material in a patient with chronic tophaceous gout. No significant amounts of anechoic fluid are seen. This preaspiration image indicates that a "dry tap" can be expected. **(B)** Shows distension of the joint capsule by synovial tissue in a patient with rheumatoid arthritis. No anechoic free fluid is seen, again indicating a "dry tap." In **(C)**, hypoechoic synovial proliferation is seen lining the more hyperechoic joint capsule in a patient with inflammatory arthritis. Anechoic free fluid is seen that can be aspirated.

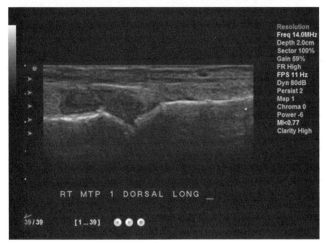

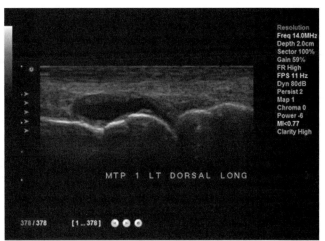

- The joint capsule is distended by material other than synovial fluid.
- Proliferative synovial tissue or tophaceous material can distend the joint capsule even if no or very little free synovial fluid is present.
- In these scenarios, a "dry tap" would ensue unless saline is injected first (**Fig. 18.1**).
- If fluid is detected, the viscosity of this fluid can be estimated sonographically.
- Thin, anechoic synovial fluid is readily displaceable with pressure of the probe. Particles of increased echogenicity float around freely in such fluid.
- In contrast, fluid that is entrapped chronically in ganglia or bursae becomes gelatinous and is less readily displaceable. Contained particles of increased echogenicity or bubbles do not float freely.
- Intraarticular or intrabursal material of higher viscosity is more difficult to aspirate and requires a larger bore needle.

Synovial tissue can be distinguished from synovial fluid by its often higher echogenicity and decreased compressibility. In inflammatory arthritis, Doppler signals may be detected in synovial tissue, but not in synovial fluid if the probe is kept steady.

Room Setup, Patient Positioning, and Equipment

Setup and Positioning

- The patient's joint is positioned between the operator and ultrasound machine's screen. This allows syringe, joint, and screen to keep in one line of sight (**Fig. 18.2**).
- Handling of syringe and following the path of the needle on the screen can be performed without the need for the operator to turn his or her head to the screen and look away from the injection site.

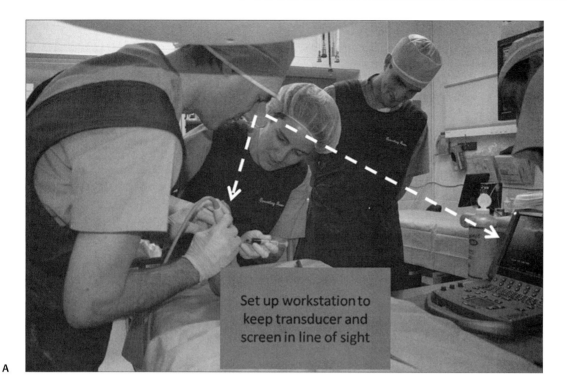

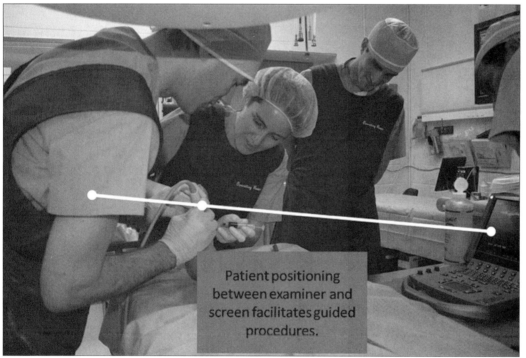

Fig. 18.2 When arranging a patient and equipment for a guided injection, it is helpful to place the patient and ultrasound screen so that the examiner can see the injection site and ultrasound image without the need to turn the head. This way the injection site can be observed throughout the procedure.

- Injections of the hip, knee, ankle, and foot joints can be performed with the patient lying on the examination table.
- Injections of the shoulder can be performed with the patient sitting. Rotating stools for both the patient and operator allow for easy positioning during sonographic shoulder evaluation and injection.
- For injections of the elbow, wrist, and hand, the extremity can be placed on a table with the patient sitting on a chair.

Equipment

- Use linear array transducers for joint injections
- A linear high-frequency transducer (between 10 and 18 MHz) is useful to visualize the soft tissues between skin and joint capsule. The same transducer can be used for joint injections.
- Particularly in obese patients, lower frequencies and curved array transducers may be required to visualize the deep-seated hip joint.
- All necessary equipment must be prepared and positioned within easy reach if the procedure is performed without an assistant.
- For a single-operator ultrasound-guided aspiration or injection, a foot switch for the ultrasound machine is helpful to freeze and save images and record video clips during the procedure.
- If an assistant is present, he or she can operate the machine and provide the equipment during the procedure.

Preparation of Injection Equipment for Aspirations and Injections

- Needles between 18- and 25-gauge are used for both aspirations and injections.
- The required length of the needle needs to be determined by measuring the distance from skin to joint capsule during an ultrasonographic examination prior to the procedure.
- For injections of shoulders, elbows, wrists, finger joints, knees, ankles and feet, standard needles up to 1.5-inch length are often appropriate.
- Injections of hip joints usually require longer needles: spinal needles can be used.
  ○ For hip aspirations, 20-gauge needles can be used.
  ○ For hip injections without aspiration, a 22-gauge needle is sufficient.

- In obese patients, spinal needles may also be required for guided injections of trochanteric bursa and shoulder joints.
- 27-gauge and 30-gauge needles can be used for injection of local anesthetic agents prior to the actual aspiration or injection.
- If larger volumes of joint fluid are aspirated or if a medication is injected after an aspiration, the needle should stay in place in the joint and syringes should be changed using a straight or curved-end hemostat to hold the needle steady and twist off the syringe.
- Parker-Pearson needles, grasping forceps, or fine-needle aspiration equipment can be used to obtain tissue samples (**Fig. 18.3**).

Preparation of Skin

- Aseptic techniques are used as they are for blind injections.
- Iodine and alcohol-based disinfectants are often used.
- Ethyl chloride spray can decrease injection site discomfort.

Technique

- Perform an ultrasound of the joint and assess for joint effusion and soft tissue thickness between skin and joint capsule.
- Once the joint is visualized sonographically, the probe is kept over the joint and the needle is inserted at an angle of 45 degrees or less. The steeper the angle, the less the needle is visible sonographically. This is done in real-time.
- The joint capsule is identified as a hyperechoic, fibrous structure and joint fluid appears anechoic to hypoechoic under ultrasound examination. The needle can be advanced into the joint from any approach and fluid

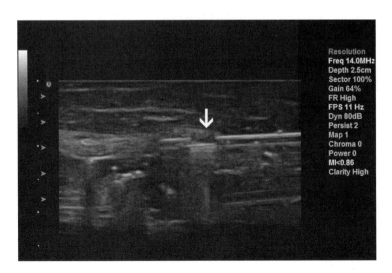

Fig. 18.3 Parker-Pearson needle inserted in target tissue. The opening is marked by an *open arrow*. Suction of an attached syringe draws tissue into the needle.

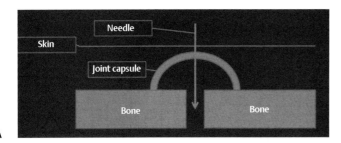

A

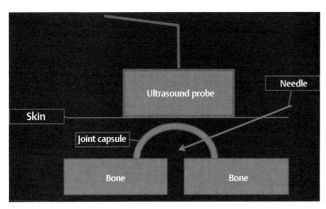

B

Fig. 18.4 The difference between palpation guidance and ultrasound guidance of arthrocenteses is illustrated. **(A)** With palpation guidance, the shortest route between skin and joint space is usually taken for the pass of the needle. **(B)** Ultrasound guidance using free-hand technique. The joint space is identified sonographically, and the needle is inserted at an angle so that it can be visualized deep to the probe.

can be successfully aspirated, or medication can be injected. The needle does not need to be buried in the joint space (**Fig. 18.4**).

- The approach can be individualized. An approach that allows passage of the needle from skin to joint with visualization of the length of the needle is typically used.

Shoulder

Positioning

- The patient sits on a stool between the operator and screen.
- Fluid in the glenohumeral joint is best visualized from a posterior horizontal or transverse view that visualizes the humeral head and glenoid as bony landmarks and the glenoid labrum and fibrous capsule with overlying infraspinatus tendon and fibrous landmarks.
  - Fluid can be seen surrounding the fibrous glenoid labrum and distending the capsule.

Procedure

- Once this area is visualized, a needle can be inserted under the probe from a medial or lateral approach, pointing toward the fluid near the glenoid labrum.

- A lateral approach provides more room for handling the probe and syringe.
- Alternate approach: Use an anterior approach with insertion of the needle into the intertubercular sheath of the proximal biceps tendon, particularly if fluid is visualized surrounding the proximal biceps tendon.
- The proximal biceps tendon runs in the intertubercular groove of the humerus, surrounded not by a true tendon sheath, but by a duplication of the joint capsule of the shoulder joint.
- This space is therefore continuous and can therefore be used as a safe and convenient entry.
- Proximal biceps tendon and surrounding fluid are visualized with an anterior, long axis view with the arm in neutral position.
- The hand of the patient rests palm up on the ipsilateral knee.
- The needle enters cranially proximal to the probe and is advanced toward fluid collections in the intertubercular sheath (**Fig. 18.5**).

For examination of the subacromial/subdeltoid bursa:

- The patient will internally rotate and adduct the arm to expose the bursa from under the acromion.
- The bursa can then be visualized from an anterior long or short axis view overlying the supraspinatus tendon.
- With the probe placed horizontally over the anterior shoulder, the needle can be inserted laterally and advanced under the probe toward the bursa.

Elbow

Procedure

- Fluid collections in the elbow or synovial proliferation will displace the posterior fat pad in the olecranon fossa.
- Aspiration and injection in this posterior recess provides a safe and convenient approach because no neurovascular bundles are present.
- The patient positions the elbow on a cushion in 90-degree flexion, or places the hand flat on the table with the elbow in 90-degree flexion.
- The probe is placed over the posterior elbow in long axis. The triceps muscle and triceps tendon are muscular and fibrous landmarks, and the olecranon will be the distal, bony landmark. The bony outline of the olecranon fossa is identified in the depth. Filling the olecranon fossa is the hyperechoic posterior fat pad. This may be displaced superficially by hypoechoic synovial tissue or anechoic synovial fluid.
- The needle can be advanced from proximal or distal to the probe at a steep angle to the "bottom" of the olecranon fossa. Contact with bone may be felt at the needle

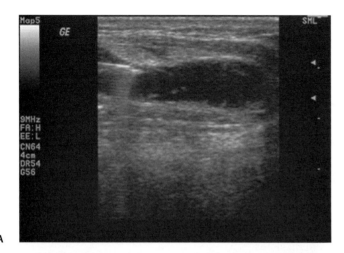

A

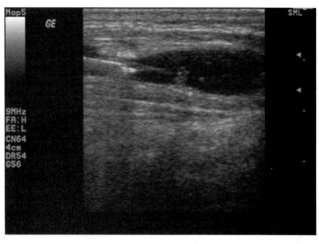

B

C

Fig. 18.5 Aspiration of a fluid collection in the intertubercular sheath that surrounds the proximal portion of the tendon of the long head of the biceps muscle. This space is continuous with the glenohumeral joint. If a full-thickness supraspinatus tendon tear is present, it is also continuous with the subdeltoid/subacromial bursa space. **(A)** The needle enters the distended sheath from cranial. **(B)** Fluid is aspirated. **(C)** A therapeutic agent is injected. The jet of the injection is seen at the needle tip.

tip. Fluid can be aspirated; synovial tissue can be injected here.

Alternatively, fluid or synovial tissue can be visualized in the lateral recess of the elbow.

- The shallowest point of entry can be identified and marked; the needle can be inserted without direct visualization.
- If direct visualization is required here, the forearm can be placed on the table with the elbow in 90-degree flexion.
- The probe is then kept over the fluid collection in long axis, the needle enters posteriorly under the probe.

Wrist

Procedure

- The radiocarpal and midcarpal joint can be examined for synovial proliferation or fluid collections.
- A dorsal, long axis, midline view can be used.
- Anechoic synovial fluid or hypoechoic synovial tissue can be found distal to the radius in the radiocarpal joint, and distending the recess between the hyperechoic capitate and hamate bones and hyperechoic joint capsule in the midcarpal joint.
- With the probe placed in long axis, the needle can be inserted distally to proximally under direct visualization (**Fig. 18.6**).

Hip

Technique

- A curvilinear probe with a frequency between 5 and 10 MHz may be needed to assess the hip joint in patients of heavier build.
- The patient is placed supine on the exam table with the leg in mild external rotation. (Internal rotation will distend the joint capsule and can lead to a false-positive assessment of a hip effusion).
- The probe is placed over the anterior proximal thigh along the femoral neck axis.
- The anatomic neck of the femur forms an angle of ~126 degrees with the anatomic axis of the femur, which is therefore also the angle the probe assumes relative to the shaft of the femur.

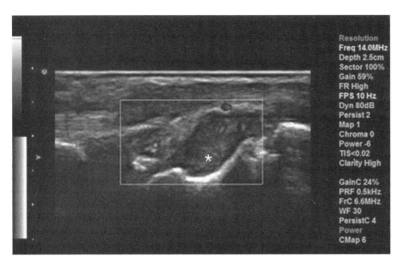

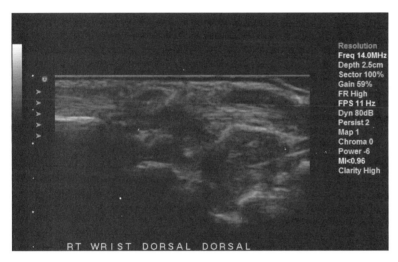

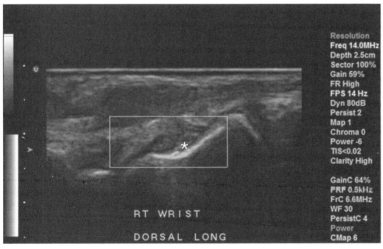

Fig. 18.6 Wrist injection and follow-up study in a patient with rheumatoid arthritis. **(A)** Shows distension of dorsal portion of midcarpal joint by synovial proliferation. A power Doppler study shows physiologic flow in the overlying dorsal carpal branch of the radial artery and hyperemia of the hypoechoic synovial tissue (*). **(B)** Shows insertion of the needle into the midcarpal joint; **(C)** was taken 4 weeks after the injection and shows involution of the previously hypertrophic synovial tissue (*). The distance between hyperechoic joint capsule and hyperechoic bone is now decreased.

- The bony-acoustic landmarks include the acetabular rim and femoral head proximally, and the concavity of the femoral neck in depth.
- The hyperechoic fibrous capsule that inserts into the distal portion of the anatomic neck is then sought.
- The distance between the concavity of femoral neck and fibrous capsule is measured.
- In a normal control, the distance should not exceed 7–9 mm. An effusion is present if the measurement exceeds this number, or if the difference of the measurement to the contralateral hip exceeds 2 mm if the same anatomic location is found. The probe is kept anteriorly over the anatomic neck of the femur.
- The point of needle entry is distal to the probe, with the needle tip aiming proximally and deep toward the concavity of the femoral neck.
- Prior to the procedure, the distance from point of entry to joint capsule can be measured sonographically, and the required length of the needle can be determined.
- If the position of the needle is lost during the insertion, a forward and backward rocking of the needle can help with identification of the position. This movement should be performed only in the axis and the canal of the needle.
- Lateral or shearing excursions of the needle increase the trauma of the procedure.
- Contact of the needle tip with the bony surface of the femoral neck and visualization of a small amount of steroid or anesthetic that is injected can also help verify a correct position of the needle tip.
- If the needle tip cannot be correctly identified within the capsule, or if the needle is inserted more than the previously determined distance, it may need to be withdrawn and reinserted.

Advantages

- Fluid collections, joint capsule, and needle can be visualized in one view in this anterolateral approach.
- The anteromedial neurovascular bundle is avoided.

Disadvantages

- The needle has to travel a longer distance through muscle tissue compared to other approaches that are used with examination- or fluoroscopy-guided needle insertions.

Knee

Assessment of Knee Effusion

- Frequent indication for knee aspirations
- The injection of corticosteroids or viscosupplements is frequently performed in musculoskeletal medicine.

- In knee effusions, a large part of synovial fluid collects in the suprapatellar recess of the knee joint.
- The area can be readily assessed sonographically.

Assessment

- The probe is placed suprapatellar in long axis, with the patient placed supine.
- The proximal pole of the patella serves as the distal landmark.
- The shaft of the femur is the bony landmark in the depth.
- The strong distal quadriceps tendon is the fibrous landmark.
- The suprapatellar recess is a Z-shaped structure lined superficially by the suprapatellar fat pad and deep by the prefemoral fat pad, frequently collapsed in normal individuals in a neutral position.
- With the probe kept steady over the distal quadriceps tendon, slow flexion of the knee allows appreciation of movement of the fat pads against each other, with the suprapatellar recess in between.
- Small fluid collections can be identified with this maneuver. Lateral and medial portions of the suprapatellar recess are examined for fluid collections as well.
- Aspiration and injection of the suprapatellar pouch can be performed under direct ultrasound visualization.
- The probe can be placed in transverse, short axis over the medial or lateral aspect of the suprapatellar pouch, and fluid collections are identified.
- The needle can then be inserted from a medial or lateral approach and directed toward the fluid collection. With this technique, the needle can be visualized in its length.
- Alternatively, the probe can be kept in the long axis view.

- If the needle is inserted from a medial or lateral approach to the suprapatellar pouch, it will be seen as a bright, hyperechoic point (**Fig. 18.7**).
- If it is located too superficial in the suprapatellar fat pad, tendon, or muscle, or too deep in the prefemoral fat pad, it may be withdrawn and redirected.
- The most superficial area of the knee effusion can be identified and marked in the suprapatellar area or adjacent to medial or lateral femoral condyles.

- The needle can be inserted perpendicular to the skin without direct visualization.

Baker Cysts

- Can be identified sonographically as fluid collections surrounding the medial edge of the medial head of the

——— Cephalad

Patellar Reflex

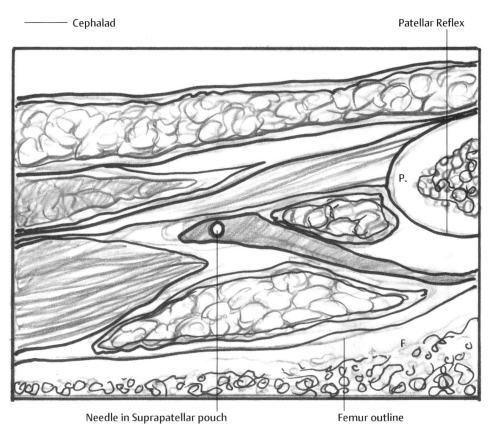

Needle in Suprapatellar pouch

Femur outline

A

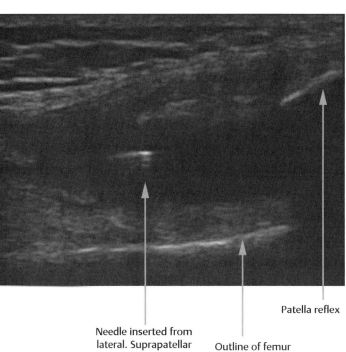

Needle inserted from lateral. Suprapatellar long axis view shows needle on end as bright dot.

Outline of femur

Patella reflex

B

Fig. 18.7 Injection of suprapatellar pouch. The needle is inserted from lateral. **(A,B)** Long axis view shows the needle on end as a hyperechoic dot with metallic artifacts. This view documents that the needle is positioned in the center of the surrounding anechoic fluid collection. **(C,D)** Short axis view demonstrates the length of the needle. Position of the needle tip can be visualized with this view. *(Continued on page 238)*

Suprapatellar pouch   Prefemoral fat pad   **Fig. 18.7** *(Continued)*

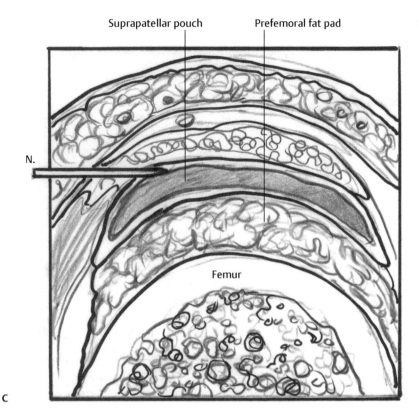

N.

Femur

C

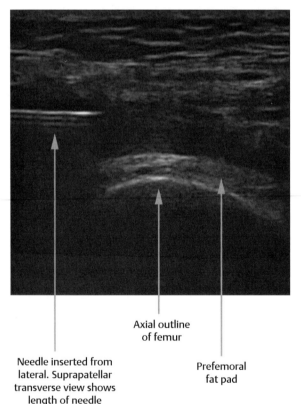

Axial outline
of femur

Needle inserted from
lateral. Suprapatellar   Prefemoral
transverse view shows   fat pad
length of needle

D

gastrocnemius muscle in the posterior knee, seen on transverse and long axis views

- If a decision is made to aspirate this fluid, the most superficial area of this fluid collection can be identified and marked in short axis views.
- It is often practical to insert the needle perpendicularly at this shallow location without direct needle visualization.
- Evacuation of the cyst can be verified sonographically after the procedure (**Fig. 18.8**).
- If direct needle visualization is required, the needle can be inserted at an angle to the probe with the probe placed over the fluid collection.

Ankle

Effusions and Synovial Proliferation in Tibiotalar and Subtalar Joints

- For an examination of the tibiotalar joint, the probe is placed in the midline over the anterior ankle.
- Bony-acoustic landmarks are the sloping tibia proximally and the curve of the dome of the talus distally.
- A hyperechoic fat pad, which normally fills out the joint space, is sought in between the bones.
- Slow excursions of dorsiflexion and plantarflexion of the ankle with the probe kept steady can help identify the relation of the anatomic structures to each other.

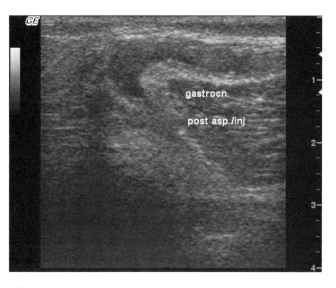

Fig. 18.8 Short axis view of posterior knee. **(A)** The almost triangular medial edge of the medial head of the gastrocnemius muscle is surrounded by anechoic fluid. Multiple hyperechoic echoes that are not floating readily indicate a gelatinous consistency. Centimeter scale on right of images documents the shallow depth of this popliteal cyst. Postprocedure image **(B)** documents evacuation of fluid.

- The fat pad should be identifiable extending into the depth of the joint. Increased fluid collections or tissue proliferation will displace this fat pad anteriorly.
- Pathologic findings can be confirmed in a short, transverse axis.
- Aspirations and injections under guidance can be performed in long and short axis.

In the long axis, the probe is kept in a position that allows visualization of the fluid collection or tissue proliferation.

- The needle is inserted proximal to the probe, pointing toward the joint space.

Using the short axis, transverse approach, the probe is

- Placed over the anterior ankle, with the hyperechoic bony contour of the talus demonstrated horizontally across the screen
- The needle is then inserted from medial or lateral, anterior to the malleoli and deep to the anterior tendons.
- When the needle is advanced toward the talus, the dorsalis pedis artery must be avoided and tendons should be avoided.
- To find the subtalar joint, the probe is placed over the lateral ankle just distal to the fibula.
- The long axis of the probe follows the superficially appearing peroneus longus and peroneus brevis tendons as fibrous landmarks.

- With supination of the ankle, fluid collections can be found deep to the tendons overlying the convexity of the calcaneus.
- The bony landmark of the tip of the fibula and the talus in between fibula and calcaneus can be identified for orientation.
- The shallowest area of the subtalar joint can be marked and the needle can be inserted perpendicularly, without direct visualization just posterior to the peroneal tendons and distal to the tip of the fibula.

Small Joints

- Metacarpophalangeal and metatarsophalangeal joints can be aspirated for diagnostic purposes and injected for therapeutic purposes under ultrasound guidance
- Joints are examined sonographically prior to the procedure.
- The probe is placed dorsally in the long axis over the joint line.
- Metacarpal head or metatarsal head, respectively, are identified proximally and the proximal phalanx is identified distally.
- For the initial orientation, the joint line is demonstrated in the center of the screen.
- A hyperechoic joint capsule is sought. Fluid, synovial tissue, or crystalline material may distend the joint capsule.
- The distance from hyperechoic, bony anatomic neck to hyperechoic joint capsule can be measured. A distension

of up to 3 mm is physiologic in first metatarsophalangeal (MTP) joints and up to 2 mm in second MTP joints dorsally.

For a guided injection, the probe can be

- Placed more proximally to allow for shorter travel of the needle under the probe
- The needle is inserted distal to the probe and directed proximally until the joint capsule is perforated. It does not need to be buried in the joint space between bones.
- For injections of proximal interphalangeal, distal interphalangeal, and tarso-metatarsal joints, an analogous technique can be used.

Tendon Sheath Injections

The tendon sheath shares anatomic and physiologic characteristics with the joint capsule.

- A fibrous outer sheath is lined with synovial tissue.
- The tendon itself is covered by an inner synovial lining that is firmly attached to the tendon.
- The tendon is tethered to the outer sheath by the mesotendineum that also supplies the inner synovial sheath and tendon with blood vessels.
- Synovial tissue can proliferate toward the interspace from the outer and inner synovial lining.
- Synovial fluid is secreted into the interspace, leading to a distension of the tendon sheath (**Fig. 18.9**).
- Compressibility confirms presence of fluid (**Fig. 18.10**).

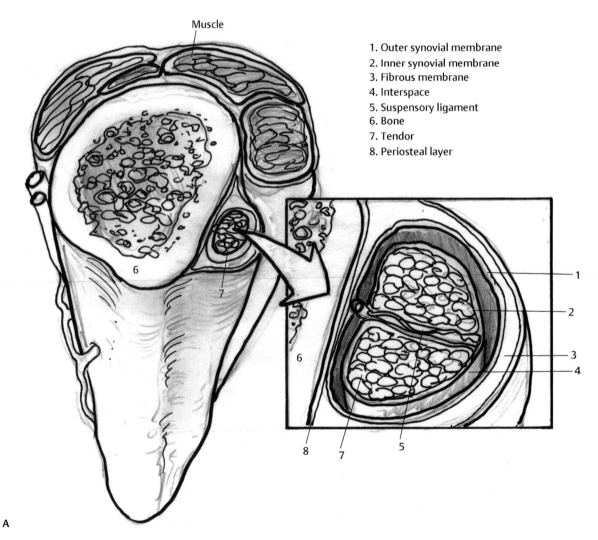

1. Outer synovial membrane
2. Inner synovial membrane
3. Fibrous membrane
4. Interspace
5. Suspensory ligament
6. Bone
7. Tendor
8. Periosteal layer

A

Fig. 18.9 Tendon, surrounding fluid, and synovial sheath need to be identified for ultrasound-guided aspirations and injections.

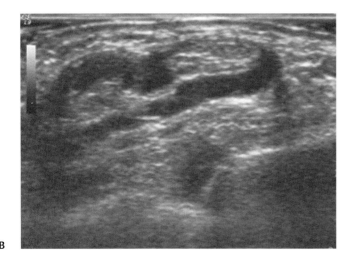

Fig. 18.9 *(Continued)*

For tendon sheath aspirations or injections to be successful:

- The needle needs to be placed into the interspace.
- Steroid injections into the tendon body may increase tendon fragility, and injections outside the interspace may be ineffective in reducing tenosynovitis.
- Distension of the tendon sheath by hypoechoic synovial tissue or anechoic synovial fluid can readily be visualized sonographically, which facilitates needle insertion (**Fig. 18.11**).

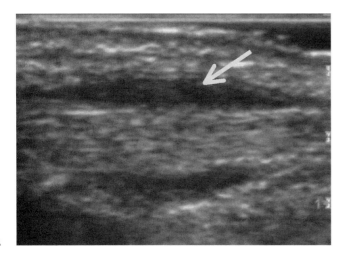

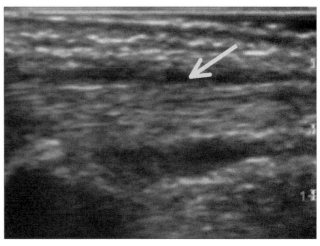

Fig. 18.10 wrist swelling. Fluid is seen surrounding the extensor carpi ulnaris tendon (*arrow*). **(A)** No pressure exerted; **(B)** pressure exerted. Displaceability confirms presence of synovial fluid.

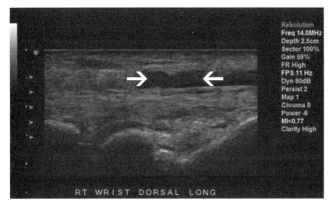

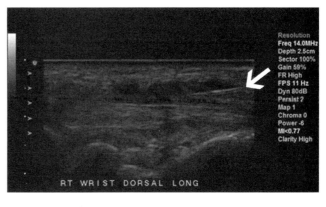

Fig. 18.11 Dorsal long axis view over wrist. **(A)** Anechoic fluid is seen overlying the hyperechoic extensor tendons (*between arrows*). **(B)** A needle is inserted into the interspace between hyperechoic tendon and hyperechoic sheath (*arrow*). Direct visualization of needle tip allows avoidance of tendon. **(C)** Steroids appear hyperechoic after injection (*arrow*). **(D)** A follow up study 3 weeks later confirms absence of tenosynovitis. *(Continued on page 242)*

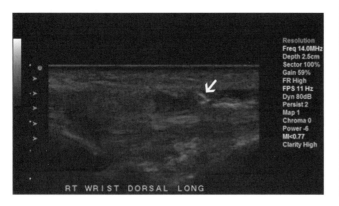

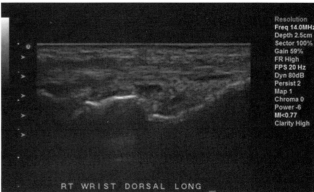

C   D

Fig. 18.11 *(Continued)*

Postprocedure Evaluation

Evacuation of fluid collections can be visualized sonographically directly after the procedure (**Fig. 18.8**).

- The placement of intraarticular medication can be verified during and after the procedure.
- Steroid crystals will appear as small, hyperechoic free-floating reflexes (**Fig. 18.10**).
- Viscosupplements will not disperse as quickly after injection and have a more hypoechoic to anechoic appearance, similar to surrounding synovial fluid.
- Can be distinguished within a joint by interface reflections between viscosupplement and synovial fluid.
- If steroids are injected into proliferative, inflamed synovial tissue, a follow-up ultrasound study can document the decrease of synovial thickness and hyperemia (**Figs. 18.6 and 18.10**).

Complications

- Bleeding into soft tissues or the joint can occur even with correct technique.
- The use of ice packs or spray before and after the procedure can help decrease swelling and limit hematoma formation.
- If intraarticular bleeding occurs, this can be visualized as hypo- to hyperechoic free blood or incompletely compressible hematoma.

Further Reading

Backhaus M, Burmester GR, Gerber T, et al; Working Group for Musculoskeletal Ultrasound in the EULAR Standing Committee on International Clinical Studies including Therapeutic Trials. Guidelines for musculoskeletal ultrasound in rheumatology. Ann Rheum Dis 2001;60(7):641–649

Balint PV, Kane D, Hunter J, McInnes IB, Field M, Sturrock RD. Ultrasound guided versus conventional joint and soft tissue fluid aspiration in rheumatology practice: a pilot study. J Rheumatol 2002;29(10):2209–2213

Bianchi S, Martinoli C. Ultrasound of the musculoskeletal system. Berlin/New York: Springer; 2007

Bradley M, O'Donnell P. Atlas of musculoskeletal ultrasound anatomy. London/San Francisco: Greenwich Medical Media; 2002

Chhem R, Cardinal E. Guidelines and gamuts in musculoskeletal ultrasound. New York: Wiley-Liss; 1999

del Cura JL. Ultrasound-guided therapeutic procedures in the musculoskeletal system. Curr Probl Diagn Radiol 2008;37(5):203–218

Epis O, Iagnocco A, Meenagh G, et al. Ultrasound imaging for the rheumatologist. XVI. Ultrasound-guided procedures. Clin Exp Rheumatol 2008;26(4):515–518

Eustace JA, Brophy DP, Gibney RP, Bresnihan B, FitzGerald O. Comparison of the accuracy of steroid placement with clinical outcome in patients with shoulder symptoms. Ann Rheum Dis 1997;56(1):59–63

Fam AG, Lawry GV, Kreder HJ. Musculoskeletal examination and joint injections techniques. Philadelphia, PA: Mosby Elsevier; 2006

Harmon D, O'Sullivan M. Ultrasound-guided sacroiliac joint injection technique. Pain Physician 2008;11(4):543–547

Holm HH, Kristensen JK, Rasmussen SN, Northeved A, Barlebo H. Ultrasound as a guide in percutaneous puncture technique. Ultrasonics 1972;10(2):83–86

Jacobson JA. Fundamentals of musculoskeletal ultrasound. Philadelphia, PA: Saunders/Elsevier; 2007

Joines MM, Motamedi K, Seeger LL, DiFiori JP. Musculoskeletal interventional ultrasound. Semin Musculoskelet Radiol 2007;11(2):192–198

Khosla S, Thiele RG, Baumhauer JF. Injection of foot and ankle joints: comparison of guidance by palpation, ultrasonography and fluoroscopy with anatomic dissection as gold standard. Arthritis Rheum 2008;58(Suppl 9):S408

Koski JM, Anttila P, Hämäläinen M, Isomäki H. Hip joint ultrasonography: correlation with intra-articular effusion and synovitis. Br J Rheumatol 1990;29(3):189–192

Koski JM, Anttila PJ, Isomäki HA. Ultrasonography of the adult hip joint. Scand J Rheumatol 1989;18(2):113–117

Koski JM, Helle M. Ultrasound guided synovial biopsy using portal and forceps. Ann Rheum Dis 2005;64(6):926–929

Koski JM, Hermunen HS, Kilponen VM, Saarakkala SJ, Hakulinen UK, Heikkinen JO. Verification of palpation-guided intra-articular injections using glucocorticoid-air-saline mixture and ultrasound imaging (GAS-graphy). Clin Exp Rheumatol 2006;24(3):247–252

Koski JM, Isomäki H. Ultrasonography may reveal synovitis in a clinically silent hip joint. Clin Rheumatol 1990;9(4):539–541

Koski JM. Ultrasonographic evidence of hip synovitis in patients with rheumatoid arthritis. Scand J Rheumatol 1989;18(3):127–131

Koski JM. Ultrasonography of the metatarsophalangeal and talocrural joints. Clin Exp Rheumatol 1990;8(4):347–351

Koski JM. Ultrasound guided injections in rheumatology. J Rheumatol 2000;27(9):2131–2138

McNally EG. Practical musculoskeletal ultrasound. Philadelphia: Elsevier; 2005

Naredo E, Cabero F, Beneyto P, et al. A randomized comparative study of short term response to blind injection versus sonographic-guided injection of local corticosteroids in patients with painful shoulder. J Rheumatol 2004;31(2):308–314

Raza K, Lee CY, Pilling D, et al. Ultrasound guidance allows accurate needle placement and aspiration from small joints in patients with early inflammatory arthritis. Rheumatology (Oxford) 2003; 42(8):976–979

Schmidt WA, Schicke B, Krause A. [Which ultrasound scan is the best to detect glenohumeral joint effusions?]. Ultraschall Med 2008;29(Suppl 5):250–255

Schmidt WA, Schmidt H, Schicke B, Gromnica-Ihle E. Standard reference values for musculoskeletal ultrasonography. Ann Rheum Dis 2004;63(8):988–994

Sofka CM, Saboeiro G, Adler RS. Ultrasound-guided adult hip injections. J Vasc Interv Radiol 2005;16(8):1121–1123

Thiele R. Doppler ultrasonography in rheumatology: adding color to the picture. J Rheumatol 2008;35(1):8–10

Thiele RG, Anandarajah AP, Tabechian D, Schlesinger N. Comparing ultrasonography, MRI, high-resolution CT and 3D rendering in patients with crystal proven gout. Ann Rheum Dis 2008;67 (Suppl II):248

Thiele RG, Schlesinger N. Diagnosis of gout by ultrasound. Rheumatology (Oxford) 2007;46(7):1116–1121

Thiele RG, Tabechian D, Anandarajah AP. Ultrasonographic demonstration of tenosynovitis preceding joint involvement in early seropositive rheumatoid arthritis. Arthritis Rheum 2008;58(Suppl 9):S407

Umphrey GL, Brault JS, Hurdle MF, Smith J. Ultrasound-guided intra-articular injection of the trapeziometacarpal joint: description of technique. Arch Phys Med Rehabil 2008;89 (1):153–156

Van Holsbeeck M, Introcaso JH. Musculoskeletal ultrasound (2nd ed.). St. Louis: Mosby; 2001

III Ultrasound-Guided Percutaneous Therapy

19 Thermal Ablation of Liver Lesion

Wael E.A. Saad and Daniel B. Brown

Classification and Indications

Liver lesions that can be thermally ablated are classified into primary liver lesions (hepatocellular carcinoma [HCC]) and secondary liver lesions (metastases).

Primary Liver Malignancy: Hepatocellular Carcinoma

This is the main indication (utilization) of hepatic radiofrequency ablation in the United States and worldwide.

- Liver cirrhosis with super-added HCC
- Nonsurgical patients
- Lesions confined to liver (no extrahepatic dissemination)
- No evidence of intrahepatic vascular invasion

Secondary Liver Malignancy: Metastasis

This is the less common utilization of hepatic thermal ablation.

- Nonsurgical candidates
- Postoperative candidates (non-reoperative candidates)
  - Percutaneous thermal ablation increases the possibility of curative treatment in patients with liver recurrence after hepatectomy from 17 to 26% and is preferred over repeat surgery because it is less invasive (lower procedural morbidity).
- Less than five lesions, with each lesion having a maximum diameter of ≤3 cm (preferable)
- Metastasis reported to be ablated:
  - Colorectal metastasis (most common metastasis)
    - 20–25% of colon cancer patients have resectable disease in the liver; surgical resection is the curative modality and not percutaneous thermal ablation.
    - Percutaneous thermal ablation increases the possibility of curative treatment in patients with liver recurrence after hepatectomy from 17 to 26% and is preferred over repeat surgery because of its less invasiveness (lower procedural morbidity).
  - Neuroendocrine metastasis
  - Gastric metastasis
  - Renal metastasis
  - Melanoma metastasis
  - Pulmonary (bronchogenic) metastasis
  - Uterine metastasis
  - Ovarian metastasis
  - Breast metastasis

Contraindications

Absolute Contraindications

- Uncorrected coagulopathy (see **Table 19.1** for suggested thresholds)
- Suggested coagulopathy
  - International normalized ratio (INR): ≤1.4
  - Platelets (PLT): ≥50,000
  - Activated partial thromboplastin time (aPTT): ≤65 seconds

Relative Contraindications

- Ascites (can be drained just prior to biopsy procedure)
- Hepatorenal failure
- Obstructive jaundice (bilirubin level >3 mg/dL)
- Vascular invasion (portal venous tumor thrombus)

Noncandidates for Treatment

- Disease not confined to liver (extrahepatic dissemination)
- Hepatorenal failure including high bilirubin (bilirubin level >3 mg/dL)
- Vascular invasion (portal venous tumor thrombus)
- Diffuse/infiltrative (nonnodular HCC)
- Numerous lesions (primary or metastatic) – defined as more than five lesions
- Location related (unfavorable lesions/technically more difficult lesions):
  - Lesions close to hilum
    - Increased risk of iatrogenic biliary injury
    - Higher probability to be close to vessels
  - Lesion adjacent to vessels
    - Usually no injury to the vessels themselves because the flowing blood "refrigerates" the vessel wall and thus protects against thermal injury
    - However, there is a higher risk of direct (old fashioned) needle injury of the vessels and resultant bleeding.
    - Vessels act as heat sumps and increase the risk of incomplete ablation of the neoplastic tissue adjacent to the vessel.

Table 19.1 Complications of Ultrasound-Guided Liver Radiofrequency Ablation (RFA)

Complication	Incidence
Abdominal and/or shoulder pain	Not uncommon
Fevers	Common
Peritoneal bleeding	0.3–0.5%*
Abscess formation	0.3–2.0%†
Pericapsular hematoma	0.3–0.5%‡
Portal vein thrombosis	<0.1%
Hemo- and/or pneumothorax	0.17–2.2%§
Hepatic decompensation/liver failure	0.04–0.3%
Cholecystitis	0.0–0.04%
Sepsis	0.0–0.04%
Bowel perforation	0.22%
Mortality	0.1–0.5%
Grounding pad burns	0.04–1.4%
Tumor seeding of RFA needle tract	0.3–0.5%

Source: Data from Crum CD, vanSonnenberg E, Silverman SG, Morrison PR, Tuncali K. Cryotherapy of liver tumors. In: Mauro M, Murphy K, Thomson K, Venbrux A, Zollikofer C, eds. Image Guided Interventions. Philadelphia: Saunders; 2008: 1516–1522; de Baère T, Risse O, Kuoch V, et al. Adverse events during radiofrequency treatment of 582 hepatic tumors. AJR Am J Roentgenol 2003;181(3):695–700; Lencioni R, Crocetti L, Bozzi E, Bartolozzi C. Thermal (heat) ablation of hepatocellular cancer. In: Mauro M, Murphy K, Thomson K, Venbrux A, Zollikofer C, eds. Image Guided Interventions. Philadelphia: Saunders; 2008: 1491–1504; Livraghi T, Solbiati L, Meloni MF, Gazelle GS, Halpern EF, Goldberg SN. Treatment of focal liver tumors with percutaneous radiofrequency ablation: complications encountered in a multicenter study. Radiology 2003;226(2):441–451; Solbiati L, Lerace T, Cova L, Zaid S. Thermal (heat) ablation of other liver lesions. In: Mauro M, Murphy K, Thomson K, Venbrux A, Zollikofer C, eds. Image Guided Interventions. Philadelphia: Saunders; 2008: 1505–1515.

*75% require blood transfusion, 25% require surgery or embolization.

†67% require surgical management or percutaneous drainage (more common).

‡Incidence is most likely higher than this.

§Pneumothorax: 0.04%, hemothorax: 0.13%, pleural effusion: up to 2.0%.

- Lesion next to gallbladder
  - Increased risk of iatrogenic cholecystitis
  - Iatrogenic cholecystitis is usually transient.
- Lesions at surface of the liver
  - Increased risk of iatrogenic injury to the gastrointestinal tract
  - The large bowel is more vulnerable to iatrogenic thermal injury compared with the small bowel and stomach.
  - Percutaneous techniques can be utilized to displace bowel from superficial hepatic lesions

during the ablation procedure. This includes displacing colon by saline injection between the lesion and the colon.

- Tumor seeding (HCC)

Preprocedural Evaluation

Evaluate Prior Cross-Sectional Imaging

- Look for ascites
  - When there is no ascites, bleeding can stop due to the tamponade effect of adjacent organs and particularly the chest wall (rib cage).
  - Some operators consider ascites an increased risk for bleeding (controversial).
  - Many operators would drain ascites prior to the percutaneous thermal ablation of liver lesions.
  - Ascites may act as a heat sump for hepatic lesions at the surface of the liver adjacent to the ascites.
- Look for adjacent organs that can be inadvertently traversed
  - This helps plan the needle trajectory (ablative approach).
  - This can help reduce transgression of adjacent organs with subsequent potential major complications.
  - Particular organs that may be traversed include the colon, gallbladder, lung (pleura), stomach, and less likely the small bowel.
- Look for normal hepatic parenchymal segments for peripherally located subcapsular lesions
  - This helps plan the biopsy needle trajectory so normal hepatic parenchyma is traversed by the needle prior to entering the target lesion.
  - Traversing normal hepatic parenchyma may reduce the risk of bleeding.
  - Traversing normal hepatic parenchyma may reduce the risk of tumor seeding.
- Avoid intrahepatic structures: they include
  - Portal triads to avoid injury to their contents (portal veins and main bile ducts) in the hilum
  - Nontarget vascular lesions (for example, a large hemangioma), which cause bleeding complications
  - Transjugular intrahepatic portosystemic shunts (TIPS)
  - Transhepatic biliary drains

Evaluate Preablative Laboratory Values

- Laboratory value evaluation to rule out coagulopathy. Suggested coagulopathy thresholds are
  - INR: ≤1.4
  - PLT: ≥50,000
  - aPTT: ≤65 seconds

- Laboratory value evaluation to rule out hepatic failure or obstructive jaundice
  - Bilirubin: >3 mg/dL

Obtain Informed Consent

- Indications
  - To locally control malignant liver disease
    - Primary liver disease (HCC)
    - Metastatic liver disease
  - Local control of malignant liver disease can be intended to
    - Cure
    - Temporize and for local control while awaiting liver transplantation (for HCC only and not for liver metastasis)
    - Be palliative (painful metastasis stretching Glisson, capsule)
  - Result summary for percutaneous thermal ablation of HCC
    - Local tumor control (technical success): 95–100%
    - Progression of disease after treatment over 2 years: 2–18%
    - Overall 3-year survival rate is 74–80%, but depends on the underlying liver disease as well.
  - Result summary for percutaneous thermal ablation of colorectal metastasis
    - Local tumor control (technical success): 83–90%
    - Progression of disease after treatment: 17% (especially with tumor metastasis >3 cm in diameter)
    - Overall 3-year survival rate: 28–68%
    - Overall 5-year survival rate: 24–44%
    - Distant metachronous metastases occur in 35% of patients.
    - However, survival rates of patients undergoing percutaneous thermal ablation are similar to those of patients who undergo surgical resection with the same level of local control of metastases and probably less morbidity and mortality.
  - Result summary for percutaneous thermal ablation of breast metastasis
    - Local tumor control (technical success): >95%
    - Progression of disease with development of new metastasis occurs in up to 58% of patients.
- Alternatives
  - There is no firm evidence to establish the optimal first-line treatment of early stage HCC because of lack of randomized controlled trials.
  - To refuse the percutaneous ablation or any other therapy
  - Surgery (hepatic resection)
    - Treatment of choice for noncirrhotic patients with HCC (5% of HCC patients)
    - Procedure-related mortality: <1–3%

- Overall 5-year survival rate (with good quality care): >70%
- 5-year survival rate in patients with portal hypertension: 50%
- 5-year survival rate in patients with portal hypertension and high bilirubin: 30%
  - Liver transplantation
    - Best treatment for patients with solitary lesion <5 cm or early multifocal lesions, providing that there are ≤three lesions and all <3 cm in diameter
    - Only option that provides potential cure for both HCC and the underlying liver disease
    - Local control of tumor while awaiting liver transplantation can be achieved utilizing percutaneous thermal ablation techniques.
  - Laparoscopic-guided thermal ablation
    - Applicable to superficial lesions that can be identified and are accessible laparoscopically
    - Ability to displace/remove bowel away from the target lesion
- Advantages of percutaneous thermal ablation
  - Can be performed on nonsurgical candidates
  - Can be performed on postoperative patients
  - Repeatability of treatment if initial treatments are incomplete
  - Can be used with regional and systemic chemotherapy
  - Minimally invasive
    - Limited complications
    - Usually preserves hepatic function
    - Limited hospital stay/outpatient
    - Limited procedural cost
    - Can be performed on nonsurgical candidates or postoperative cases
- Procedural risks
  - Mortality (**Table 19.1**)
    - This is rare (0.1–0.5%).
    - Usually due to
      - Colon perforation/peritonitis (0.09%)
      - Sepsis (0.04%)
      - Hepatic failure (0.04%)
      - Tumor rupture and bleeding (0.04%)
      - Portal vein thrombosis (PVT) (0.04%)
  - Major complications (**Table 19.1**)
    - Occur in 0.7–3.1% of cases
    - Usually include
      - Intraperitoneal bleeding (25% require surgery or embolization)
      - Hepatic abscess (two-thirds require surgical evacuation or percutaneous drainage)
      - Pneumothorax, hemothorax requiring chest tube
      - Hepatic decompensation/liver failure
      - Tumor lysis syndrome

- ○ Grounding pad burns (second or third degree burns)
- ○ Central biliary duct injury
- ○ Minor complications
  - Occur 5.0–8.9% of cases
  - Usually include
    - ○ Peripheral biliary duct injury
    - ○ Cholecystitis (usually transient)
    - ○ Pneumothorax not requiring chest tube
    - ○ Subcapsular hematoma
- ○ Tumor seeding
  - Occurs in 0.3–0.5% of cases
  - Increases in incidence with
    - ○ Superficial lesions
    - ○ Poorly differentiated HCC/metastasis

Equipment

Ultrasound Guidance

- Ultrasound machine with Doppler capability
- Multiarray 4–5 MHz ultrasound transducer
- Transducer guide bracket
- Sterile transducer cover

Standard Surgical Preparation and Draping

- Chlorhexidine skin preparation/cleansing fluid
- Fenestrated drape

Local Infiltrative Analgesia Administration

- 21-gauge infiltration needle
- 10–20 mL 1% lidocaine syringe

Sharp Access

- 11-blade incision scalpel
- Coaxial access needle
  - ○ Some thermal probes are introduced through coaxial needles.
  - ○ Coaxial needles allow a coaxial biopsy needle placement followed by ablative probe placement without losing access.
  - ○ Coaxial needle may reduce the risk of tract seeding (anecdotal).
- Thermal ablative probes

Thermal Ablation Probes

The following are summaries of types of probes. Details of the probes' biomedical engineering are beyond the scope of this book.

- Radiofrequency ablation (RFA) systems
  - ○ The radiofrequency generator and the patient are the main components of an electric circuit.
  - ○ The generator is the source of the alternating current and the patient's body is the resistor.
  - ○ The resistance in the tissue (impedance) to the radiofrequency current is what generates heat and creates a thermal ablation effect.
  - ○ The thermal ablative (radiofrequency) electrode enters the body and alternating electric current passes directly into the body. However, a return connection to the generator is required. This return is established by grounding pads usually placed on the patient's thighs.
  - ○ RFA systems include
    - Radionics RFA Probe (Cool-Tip Radionics, Burlington, MA)
      - ○ This is a monopolar RFA electrode needle.
      - ○ Single 17-gauge needle
      - ○ Cluster design of three 17-gauge needles
      - ○ Cooled by continued flow of cold water that is not deposited in the body
    - LeVeen Needle Electrode (Boston Scientific Corp., Natick, MA) (**Figs. 19.1, 19.2, 19.3, and 19.4**)
      - ○ This is an array monopolar RFA electrode.
      - ○ It is a single needle with 10 tines, which splay radially and arch back in a "palm tree" appearance.
      - ○ The array diameters (2.0, 3.0, 3.5, 4.0, and 5.0 cm) can be selected to match the tumor size.
      - ○ The unique feature of this system is its impedance feedback mechanism. No measure of temperature is made by this device.
    - RITA StarBurst RFA Probe (RITA Medical, Mountain View, CA)
      - ○ This is an array monopolar RFA electrode.
      - ○ It is a single needle with 7–9 tines, which splay forward and radially in a "starburst" appearance.
      - ○ The array diameters (2–5 cm) can be selected to match the tumor size (7-tine array for diameters 2–3 cm and 9-tine array for 3–5 cm).
      - ○ The unique features of this system are its measure of temperature and its infusion of saline through select elements of the array.
      - ○ The StarBurst array probe is composed of a 14-gauge trocar.
    - Other RFA systems include
      - ○ Celon ProSurge applicators (Celon AG Medical Instruments, Berlin, Germany)
      - ○ Berchtold HiTT electrode (Berchtold, GmbH, Tuttlingen, Germany)
- Cryoablation systems include
  - ○ Galil-CryoHit Ablation System (Galil Medical, Westbury, NY)

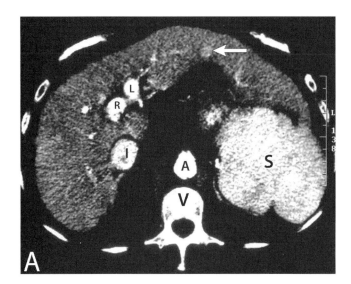

Fig. 19.1 Left lateral segment ultrasound-guided radiofrequency ablation. **(A)** Contrast-enhanced axial computed tomography (CT) image at the level of the aortic hiatus. An enhancing lesion is seen in the left lateral segment (*arrow*) (R, right portal vein; L, Left portal vein; I, Inferior vena cava [IVC]; A, aorta; V, vertebra; S, spleen). **(B)** Gray-scale ultrasound image (*top*) and schematic sketch (*bottom*) of the left hepatic lobe after the operator has advanced the radiofrequency probe (*arrow*) and after deploying the tines (*arrowheads*). **(C)** Gray-scale ultrasound image (*top*) and schematic sketch (*bottom*) of the left hepatic lobe during radiofrequency ablation. Due to cavitation, there is increased echogenicity around the probe/tines (*arrowheads*). The *arrow* points to air in an adjacent vessel (bile duct/portal vein). *(Continued on page 252)*

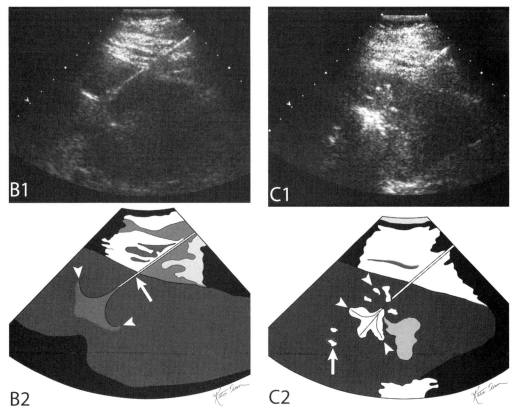

- Gas-based probe that uses argon and helium
- Up to seven probes can be used at once by the machine
- Temperatures include a freeze temperature of −180°C and a thaw temperature of +35°C.
- A "stick mode" temperature is usually set at −20°C. This provides a limited freeze to the probe, so that the probe adheres (anchors) to the immediate

tissue and prevents migration of the probe while other probes are placed.
- The operator has to add a separate thermistor needle to get real-time temperature measurements during ablation.
- Cryoablation treatments are composed of a timed freeze (usually 15 minutes) with a thaw, with or without an additional freeze.

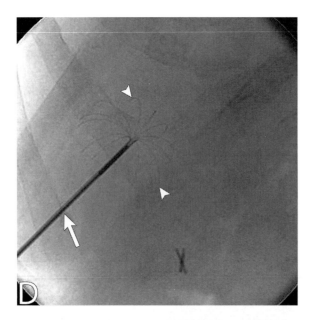

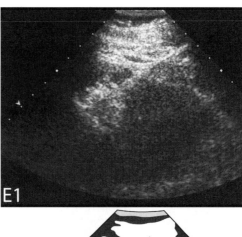

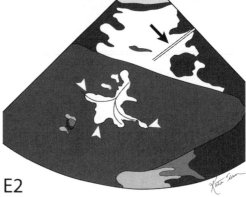

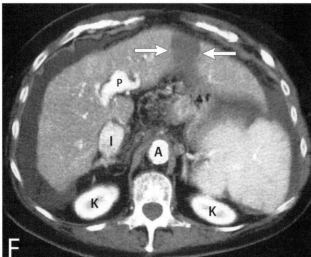

Fig. 19.1 *(Continued)* **(D)** Fluoroscopic image during the radiofrequency ablation of the lesion in **Fig. 19.1A**. The tines are seen deployed (*arrowheads*) through the probe shaft (*arrow*). Fluoroscopy is used to redeploy the LeVeen probe when performing radiofrequency ablation at multiple stations. **(E)** Gray-scale ultrasound image (*top*) and schematic sketch (*bottom*) of the left hepatic lobe after radiofrequency ablation. Due to cavitation there is increased echogenicity around the probe/tines (*arrowheads*). Still noted is the probe shaft (*arrow*). To remove the probe, the tines are retracted and the probe is removed. **(F)** Contrast-enhanced axial CT image at the level of the aortic hiatus months after the radiofrequency ablation. An unenhanced area where the enhancing lesion lay (**Fig. 19.1A**) is now seen in the left lateral segment (*between arrows*) (P, portal vein; I, IVC; A, aorta; K, kidney).

- CRYOcare System (Endocare, Inc. Irvine, CA)
  - Gas-based probe that uses argon and helium
  - Up to 8 probes can be used at once by the machine.
  - Temperatures include a variable freeze temperature ranging from −130 to −150°C and a thaw temperature of +40°C.
  - A "stick mode" temperature is usually set at −10°C. This provides a limited freeze to the probe, so that the probe adheres (anchors) to the immediate tissue and prevents migration of the probe while other probes are placed.

- Cryoablation treatments are composed of a timed freeze with a thaw, with or without an additional freeze.

Technique

Intravenous Access

- Required for moderate sedation administration or for administration of muscle relaxants and general anesthetic administration

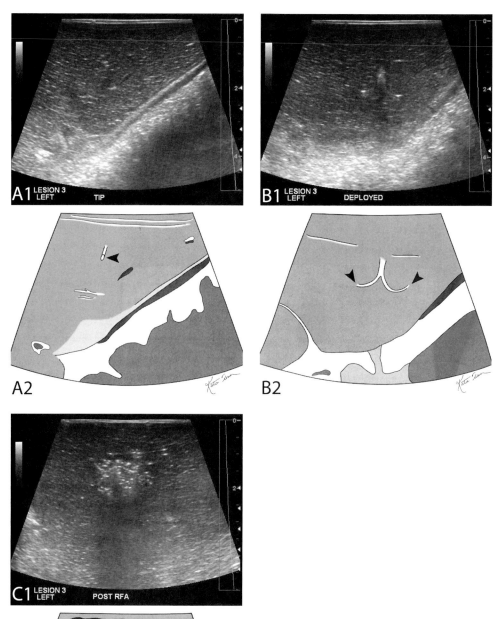

Fig. 19.2 Ultrasound-guided radiofrequency ablation of a normal swine liver using a high-frequency ultrasound probe. **(A)** Gray-scale ultrasound image (*top*) and schematic sketch (*bottom*) of the right hepatic lobe after the operator has advanced the 2-cm radiofrequency probe (*arrowhead at probe tip*). **(B)** Gray-scale ultrasound images (*top*) and schematic sketch (*bottom*) of the right hepatic lobe after the operator has deployed the tines of the 2-cm radiofrequency probe (*arrowheads at probe tip*). **(C)** Gray-scale ultrasound image (*top*) and schematic sketch (*bottom*) of the right hepatic lobe after radiofrequency ablation. Due to cavitation, there is increased echogenicity in the ablated area (*arrowheads*) with shadowing.

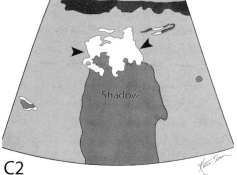

- Moderate sedation versus general anesthesia is operator/institution dependent.
- When tailoring general anesthesia versus moderate sedation

- General anesthesia may be more commonly used in
  - Uncooperative, nervous patients
  - Superficial lesions near liver capsule (painful)
  - Large lesions (longer procedure)

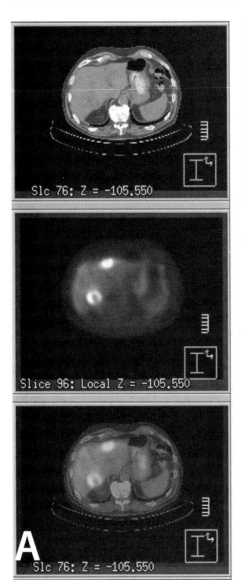

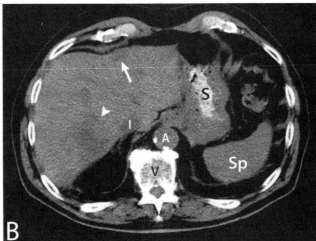

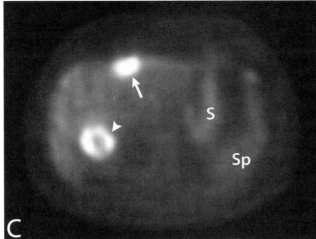

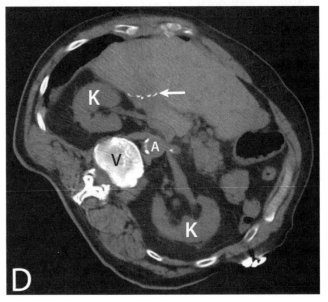

Fig. 19.3 (A,B,C) CT-guided radiofrequency ablation of a liver lesion. Positron emission tomography–computer tomography (PET-CT) exam of the liver demonstrating two lesions (*arrow: left lobe lesion and arrowhead: right lobe lesion*). **Figure 19.3A** are three images: Top = noncontrast CT (magnified image is **Fig. 19.3B**); Middle = PET image (magnified image is **Fig. 19.3C**); Bottom = fused PET and CT (S, stomach; Sp, spleen).

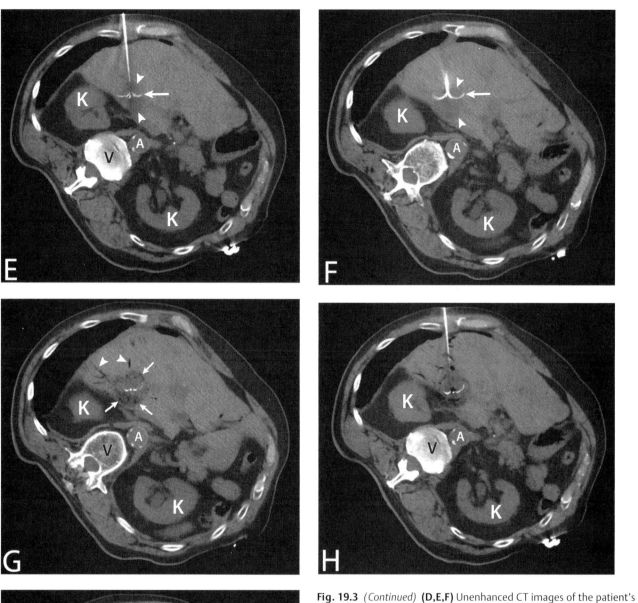

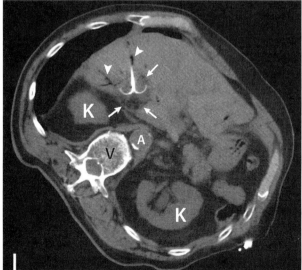

Fig. 19.3 *(Continued)* **(D,E,F)** Unenhanced CT images of the patient's images in **Figs. 19.3A–19.3C** just after a radiofrequency ablation probe has been deployed in the right hepatic lobe lesion (*arrowheads*). The tines (*arrows*) have been deployed. Ablation has not yet commenced (A, aorta; V, vertebra; K, kidney). **(G,H,I)** Unenhanced CT images of the patient's images in **Figs. 19.3A-19.3F** just after the radiofrequency ablation has been performed on the right hepatic lobe lesion. A low attenuation sphere (*arrows*). The tines are still deployed. Air is seen in adjacent vessels (portal vein/biliary ducts) (*arrowheads*) (A, aorta; V, vertebra; K, kidney).   *(Continued on page 256)*

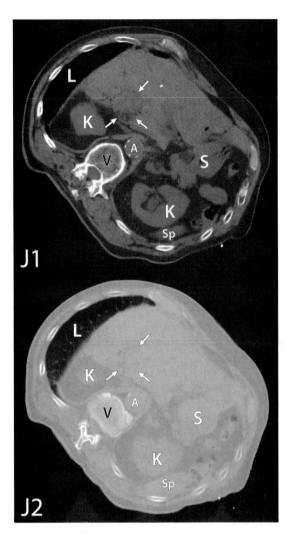

Fig. 19.3 *(Continued)* **(J)** Unenhanced CT images of the patient's images in **Figs. 19.3A–19.3I** *(above in soft tissue windows, and below in lung window)* just after the radiofrequency probe has been removed. Again, seen is the low attenuation sphere *(arrows)* (A, aorta; V, vertebra; K, kidney; S, stomach; Sp, spleen; L, lung [right lung]).

- ○ Multiple tumors (longer procedure)
- Moderate sedation
  - ○ May be more commonly used in small (<2 cm) lesions
  - ○ May be more commonly used in deep but easily accessible lesions
  - ○ Has increased comorbidity, high risk for general anesthesia
- Intravenous (IV) access is required in case of any complication (including pain-related complications), or if the need arises to administer sedation.

Preablative Ultrasound Exam

- Assess whether imaging/disease progression has changed from prior imaging that prompted the percutaneous ablation procedure. The patient may no longer be a percutaneous ablation candidate with progression of disease (tumor size and number).
- Determine easiest visibility of lesion in cases of target lesion biopsy

- Determine access (intercostal, subcostal, subxyphoid)
- Look for ascites
- Look for adjacent organs that can be traversed
- Look for normal hepatic parenchymal segments that are peripherally located (subcapsular lesions) to traverse this segment to reduce bleeding and tumor seeding complications

Standard Surgical Preparation and Draping

- Skin preparation/cleansing in the region that was chosen as an ultrasound imaging portal and a needle access needle portal
- Place a fenestrated drape at the chosen and prepared skin region

Local Infiltrative Analgesia Administration

- Utilizing a 21-gauge (by at least a 3.7-cm-long) infiltration needle, 1% lidocaine infiltration is performed. The infiltration should not be limited to the skin

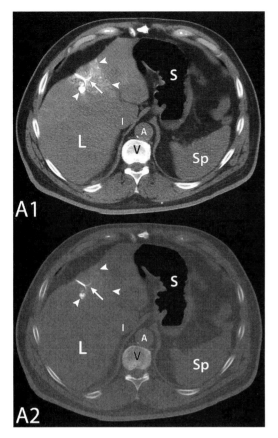

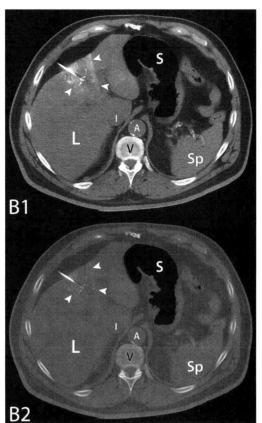

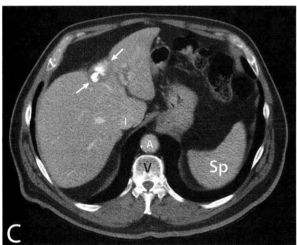

Fig. 19.4 CT-guided radiofrequency ablation of a liver lesion after selective chemoembolization. **(A)** Unenhanced CT images of a patient with a liver lesion (*above in soft tissue windows*, and *below in lung window*) just after the radiofrequency probe has been deployed (*arrow*). The high-density area is from Lipiodol from the selective chemoembolization (*arrowheads*) (S, stomach; Sp, spleen; I, IVC; A, aorta; V, vertebra; L, liver). **(B)** Unenhanced CT images of a patient with a liver lesion (*above in soft tissue windows, and below in lung window)* just after radiofrequency ablation. The radiofrequency probe is still in place within the high attenuation lesion (*arrowheads*) (S, stomach; Sp, spleen; I, IVC; A, aorta; V, vertebra; L, liver). **(C)** Contrast-enhanced axial CT image follow-up exam obtained months after the combined chemoembolization and radiofrequency ablation. An unenhanced area where the lesion lay (*between arrows*) is now seen. The lesion has shrunk. The enhancing center is due to the now aggregated Lipiodol that has aggregated over time due to tumor shrinkage (I, IVC; A, aorta; Sp, spleen).

and subcutaneous tissue, but should include infiltration of the very sensitive hepatic capsule (Glisson's capsule).

Sharp Access

- An incision is made utilizing an 11-blade scalpel usually by a 3-mm-depth stab of the 11-blade.
- A coaxial access needle can be passed under real-time ultrasound guidance.

- When utilizing a midaxillary intercostal approach, the coaxial needle (or ablative needle itself) should be passed over (cephalad) the ribs to avoid injury to the intercostal neurovascular bundle (intercostal vessels and nerve).
- The coaxial access needle
  - Allows biopsy acquisition/sampling, followed by ablation without reaccessing
  - May reduce tumor seeding of the tract
  - Used in embolization of the tract in patients with coagulopathy

Pathology Sample Acquisition (Preablation Biopsy)

- An automated spring-loaded core biopsy needle is passed to the end of a coaxial needle and "fired" (automatically deployed) and withdrawn.
- Usually one to five core (18-gauge or larger) biopsy needle passes/deployments are made.

Thermal Ablation

- The thermal ablation probe is connected to its thermal generator (see the above *Thermal Ablation Probes* subsection under Equipment).
- The thermal ablation probe is advanced under real-time ultrasound. The probe's positioning depends on
  - The type of probe
    - A cryo-probe requires its probe tip to be placed past the center of the target lesion (on the deep-end of the lesion) because the ice-ball forms at the tip and is usually longitudinal along the axis/shaft of the probe.
    - A RFA LeVeen probe requires its probe tip to be placed at, or just short-of, the center of the target lesion because the secondary probes (tines) open at the level of the probe tip or slightly forward.
    - A RFA RITA probe requires its probe tip to be placed at the superficial aspect of the target lesion because the secondary probes (tines) open forward (deeper to the probe/needle tip).
  - The number of probes (if manufactured in clusters)
  - The size of the ablation area
  - The shape of the ablation area
  - The shape and size of the lesion and how to tailor the size and shape of the proposed ablation area of the probe
  - The details are so varied, especially probe type, that it is beyond the scope of this book.

As an example, details of the RFA system that utilizes the LeVeen needle electrode are given in the section below.

- The RFA LeVeen probe is advanced into the target lesion. The probe placement is
  - At the center of small lesions using smaller probes (≤3 cm)
  - Just short of the center of the target lesion (probe size >3 cm)
- If the lesion is egg-shaped and the operator is passing the RFA probe along the long axis of a lesion (diameter of ablation more than short axis diameter of lesion, but less than the long access of the lesion):
  - A multiple station ablation is required.
  - The probe is deployed on the deep-end of the lesion and is then pulled back with a lesion overlap.
    - Pulling back the probe requires retraction of tines, withdrawal of the probe with a lesion overlap, and redeployment of the tines.
    - Pulling back for a more superficial overlapping station in the same lesion can be performed (including tine retraction and redeployment) under real-time fluoroscopy complimenting the initial real-time ultrasound probe deployment. Ultrasound is difficult to use to visualize RFA probe redeployment after ablation because of post-RFA shadowing.
    - Using computed tomography (CT) from the beginning does not require a change in modality.
- The RFA protocol utilizing the LeVeen probe is depicted in **Figs. 19.5 and 19.6**.

Transhepatic Tract Embolization

- This is not routinely performed.
- It may be performed in significantly coagulopathic patients and/or if there is inadvertent active bleeding.
- Transhepatic needle tract embolization requires a coaxial access needle (see Chapter 1, Liver Biopsy).
- Gelfoam (Pfizer Pharmaceuticals, New York, NY) pledgets, Gelfoam slurry, or metal coils can be blindly deployed through the coaxial needle as it is slowly withdrawn along the transhepatic tract.
- If fluoroscopy is available, the coils can be deployed under fluoroscopy. Deploying Gelfoam pledgets under fluoroscopy guidance requires the Gelfoam pledgets to be soaked in contrast for them to be visualized.

Immediate Postablation Ultrasound Imaging

- Immediate postablation ultrasound imaging is usually nondiagnostic as far as the lesion is concerned due to shadowing artifact (unless the lesion was missed) (**Figs. 19.1 and 19.2**).
- However, it can be used for documentation and obtaining a baseline image of a capsular or subcapsular hematoma.
- Visualizing a hepatic capsular hematoma does not alter postprocedural care or management.

Endpoints

Endpoint of Target Liver Biopsy

- A liver biopsy immediately prior to a liver RFA is not commonly performed.
- Usually one to three 18-gauge needle passes are required to obtain an adequate pathology sample.
- Smaller caliber needles (20-gauge core biopsy needles) and larger caliber needles (16-gauge core biopsy needles) may require more needle passes or fewer needle passes, respectively.

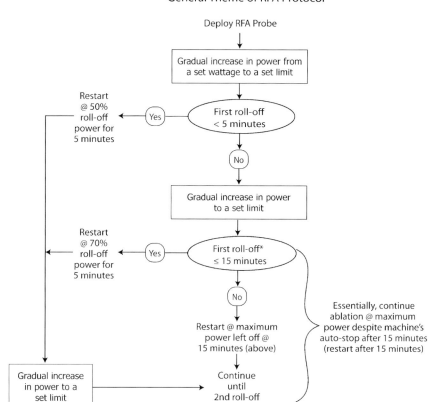

General Theme of RFA Protocol

Fig. 19.5 Flowchart demonstrating the general theme of an impedance-based ablative system; specifically the LeVeen radiofrequency ablation (RFA) probe.

• Grossly evaluating the core sample with the naked eye of the operator. The operator's judgment is used to determine when to stop making core biopsy needle passes (after the first, second, or third needle pass). This assertion is anecdotal and is not based on evidence-based research.

Endpoint of Ablation

• Adequate positioning of the probe during the procedure is key. Immediate endpoints that are image-based are difficult to make by ultrasound (shadow artifact precluding visualization) (**Figs. 19.1 and 19.2**).
• Immediate CT imaging would demonstrate
  ○ A low attenuation area over the lesion with possible air bubbles in the parenchyma secondary to cavitation (**Fig. 19.3**)
  ○ Air in the adjacent biliary segments (**Fig. 19.3**)
  ○ Possibly are in adjacent vessels such as portal vein branches
• Subcapsular hematomas can be seen. Treat the patient for pain and provide hemodynamic stability.
• The true endpoint is on delayed imaging.
  ○ A 24- to 48-hour CT scan would show complete coagulative necrosis of the lesion and a safety margin (**Fig. 19.3**).

  ○ A 24- to 48-hour CT is performed to evaluate technical success and look for complications.
  ○ The procedure is considered a success if there is a lack of enhancement consistent with no recurrence/residual tumor (see below).
• Follow-up
  ○ A 24- to 48-hour CT scan would show complete coagulative necrosis of the lesion and a safety margin (**Fig. 19.3**).
  ○ Follow-up cross-sectional imaging looking for a lack of enhancement consistent with no recurrence/residual tumor is required to consider the procedure a success (**Fig. 19.1**).
  ○ Cross-sectional imaging every 3–4 months includes
    • Conventional
      ○ Contrast-enhanced CT
      ○ Contrast-enhanced magnetic resonance imaging (MRI)
    • Unconventional
      ○ Positron emission tomography (PET) CT
      ○ Diffusion weighted imaging (DWI)
      ○ Ultrasound contrast (Europe)
      ○ Ultrasound elastography (experimental)
  ○ Serum carcinoembryonic antigen (CEA) follow-up in cases of ablation of hepatic colorectal metastases

General Theme of RFA Protocol

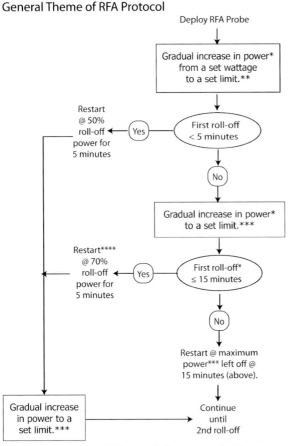

Table 2

RFA Probe Size	* Rate of gradual incremental increase in power at any level	** Initial start power to initial set limit at 5 minutes	*** Maximum power at or above 15 minutes prior to or after first roll-off
2.0 cm	10 Watts / 60 seconds	30 to 60 Watts	60 Watts
3.0 cm	10 Watts / 30 seconds	40 to 80 Watts	150 Watts
3.5 cm	10 Watts / 30 seconds	50 to 90 Watts	180 Watts
4.0 cm	10 Watts / 30 seconds	80 to 130 Watts	190 Watts
5.0 cm	10 Watts / 30 seconds	100 to 150 Watts	200 Watts

*, **, and *** asterisks refer to certain locations on the radiofrequency ablation flow chart.

Table 3

**** Power at which roll-off was achieved	70% of Power to restart RFA
50 w	35 w
60 w	42 w
70 w	49 w
80 w	56 w
90 w	63 w
100 w	70 w
110 w	77 w
120 w	84 w
130 w	91 w
140 w	98 w
150 w	105 w
160 w	112 w
170 w	119 w
180 w	126 w
190 w	133 w
200 w	140 w

**** Asterisks refer to certain locations on the radiofrequency ablation flow chart.

*Gradual increase in power 10 Watts/min. for 2 cm probe and 10 Watts/30 secs for probes > 3 cm (see Table 2).
** See Table 2.
*** See Table 2.
**** See Table 3.

Fig. 19.6 Flowchart demonstrating the ablation protocol of the LeVeen radiofrequency ablation probe.

Postprocedural Evaluation and Management

Initial Postprocedural Observation Period and Admission

- Postprocedural stay varies from one practice to another.
- Postliver RFA patients are kept under closer observation for 3–4 hours after the ablative procedure.
- Almost all practices admit the patient for at least 24 hours/overnight stay.

Intravenous Fluid and Diet

- IV access should be kept until just prior to discharge.
- Institutions that practice moderate sedation start with a clear liquid diet and advance it as tolerated. This helps to offset patients' nausea and vomiting.

- Other institutions/operators commence a clear liquid diet after a period of abstinence of oral intake. This period could be one hour, for example.
- Give IV fluid until oral intake is adequate.

Activity

- Bed rest for the period for which the patient is being observed closely (1–4 hours postablation)
- Activity is then as tolerated by patient.

Pain Management

- The patient may have mild to moderate pain for 2–5 days postprocedure.
- Narcotics are usually not required during the postablation stay of the patient prior to discharge. Occasionally, some patients require oral narcotic analgesics such as

acetaminophen and hydrocodone combination medication. Rarely does a patient require IV narcotics such as fentanyl.

- Pain radiating to the left shoulder would further support chemical/irritant peritonitis. However, if coupled with shortness of breath and desaturation (not splinting), one should suspect a significant pneumothorax; a chest x-ray is warranted.
- On discharge, patients usually tolerate the procedure well and do not require analgesics more potent than over-the-counter medications.

Medications

- Medication for pain management is described above.
- Anti-emetics are given if patients are symptomatic and can be expected to be given for 24 hours.
- Antibiotics (Flagyl [metronidazole]; Pfizer Pharmaceuticals, New York, NY) are given by some institutions for 5–7 days.

Monitoring Vital Signs

- Vital sign monitoring includes blood pressure and heart rate. Occasionally, oxygen saturation monitoring is required in cases of shortness of breath and/or chest pain.
- Institutions/operators that practice conscious sedation may record a softer blood pressure than a patient's baseline blood pressure after the hepatic ablation. This is most likely due to sedation with or without dehydration. The patient usually responds in time with hydration, particularly as the sedatives wear off.
- Continued hypotension and more importantly a rise in heart rate are of concern for hypovolemia (bleeding). If signs of hypovolemia occur, an IV volume bolus is given and a noncontrast CT exam is performed to confirm the clinical suspicion of bleeding.

Laboratory Evaluation

- Most institutions routinely perform a set of laboratory evaluations within 24 hours (just prior to discharge).
- These include
  - Liver function tests (LFTs)
  - Complete blood count (CBC)
  - Coagulopathy tests (prothrombin time, INR)

Complications and Their Management

Please see **Table 19.1** for a list of types of complications and their incidence following liver ablation. It should be noted that most complications, particularly life-threatening

complications, are clinically unmasked within 3 hours for the liver biopsy.

Management of Pain and Pain-Related Morbidity

- Patients may have mild to moderate pain for 2–5 days postprocedure.
- Narcotics are usually not required during the posthepatic ablation stay of the patient prior to discharge. Occasionally, some patients require oral narcotic analgesics such as acetaminophen and hydrocodone combination medication. Rarely does a patient require IV narcotics such as fentanyl.
- Continued pain requires further clinical and possibly imaging evaluation. Signs of peritonitis may denote chemical peritonitis from intraperitoneal bleeding or bile leak. The degree of pain does not correlate with the degree of bleeding. However, changes in vital signs do signify a significant bleed.
- Occasionally, operators respond to continued pain by performing a diagnostic imaging exam.
  - A limited ultrasound examination at the site to evaluate for a capsular hematoma
  - A more global exam such as a noncontrast abdominal CT exam. Remember, ultimately the decisive factor for determining significant bleeding is the patient's stability (vital signs) and not what you see on the images.

Management of Bleeding Complications

- IV access should be kept until just after discharge in case fluid resuscitation is required.
- Bleeding can take several forms and have different sources.
  - Skin bleeding (external)
  - Intercostal bleeding (hemothorax, external skin bleeding, or hemoperitoneum)
  - Hepatic parenchyma/capsule (hemoperitoneum if not contained, capsular hematoma if contained).
  - Hemobilia (gastrointestinal bleeding)
- Significant bleeding affecting vital signs and patient stability should be managed by
  - Fluid resuscitation starting with crystalloid fluid bolus
  - Type and cross
  - Repeat hematocrit to compare with baseline
  - Blood transfusion to maintain hematocrit at or above 30%
    - 75% of major bleeding requires a blood transfusion only
    - 25% of major bleeding requires additional surgery or hepatic artery embolization
  - Surgical/interventional radiology consult

- Interventional radiology offers
  - Hepatic arteriography with super-selective arterial embolization if bleeding or a pseudoaneurysm is seen.
  - Hepatic arteriography with global arterial Gelfoam embolization to reduce arterial perfusion in the liver if bleeding or a pseudoaneurysm is not seen. One should be cautious about globally embolizing the hepatic artery in a patient who has had a liver ablation. There is a good chance that the patient may be cirrhotic. Patients with cirrhosis may have a higher incidence of hepatic infarction after global arterial embolization.
- In cases of severe uncontrolled bleeding, a surgical consultation may offer open surgery, exploration, and local hemostasis of surface bleeding.

Management of Pleural/Thoracic Complications

- One must be able to differentiate clinically:
  - Referred shoulder pain from irritant peritonitis versus pleurisy from a hemo- and/or pneumothorax
  - Reduced oxygen saturation from poor inspiratory effort secondary to pain-related respiratory splinting versus reduced oxygenation due to hemo- and/or pneumothorax
- If chest pain with or without reduced oxygen saturation is encountered, a chest x-ray should be obtained to rule out pneumothorax or hemothorax. This is particularly true of liver ablations using an intercostals-approach.
- Right-sided pleural effusion can occur in up to 1.4–2.0% of cases. If it is not symptomatic, there is no need for further treatment.
- Clinically significant hemo- and/or pneumothorax require chest tube placement, increased nasal cannula oxygenation, and fluid resuscitation/bleeding management in the case of the former (see above section, Management of Bleeding Complications).

Management of Puncture of Adjacent Organs

- With image guidance, this is a rare complication.
- Even when transgression of adjacent organs occurs, the result is clinically inconsequential. The problem is incidental and does not rise to the level of a minor clinical complication, let alone a major complication.
- Bile leak from inadvertent puncture of the gallbladder (rare) would require percutaneous drainage of the resultant biloma and perhaps cholecystectomy.

Bowel Perforation

- Occurs in 0.3–0.5% of cases
- It is more of a delayed perforation from thermal injury rather than a direct mechanical puncture (needle transgression).
- The colon is more susceptible to thermal injury than the small bowel or stomach.

- A surgical consult should be sought
  - If the abdomen is "nonsurgical"
    - Supportive therapy
    - Antibiotics (against enterococci and anaerobes)
    - Repeat imaging (CT), diagnostic colonoscopy to assess injury
  - If abdomen is "surgical" (peritoneal signs)
    - Hemicolectomy

Abscess Formation

- Occurs in 0.3–2.0% of cases
- Must differentiate tumor necrosis from a true abscess
  - Abscess is larger than the original tumor.
  - Abscess is associated with persistent high-grade fever.
- Antibiotics (against enterococci and anaerobes) should be given and then according to culture and sensitivity
- Two-thirds (67%) of abscesses require surgical evacuation or percutaneous drainage. Percutaneous drainage is the first-line therapy.
- The hepatic/perihepatic abscess can be from
  - Tumor necrosis with super-added infection
  - Bile leak, biloma formation (may require additional biliary drainage: endoscopic retrograde cholangiopancreatogram [ERCP], percutaneous transhepatic cholangiography [PTC], and percutaneous biliary drain)
  - Bowel infarction with delayed bowel leak (may require hemicolectomy)
  - Most common in patients following
    - Biliary duct manipulations such as
      - ERCP with stent placement
      - Biliary drainage
    - Whipple procedure
    - Sphincterotomy

Liver Failure/Hepatic Decompensation

- Occurs in 0.04–0.3% of cases
- Can be transient and does well with supportive therapy
- 0.04% of cases can develop into fulminant hepatic failure and death.
- Obtain hepatology and liver transplant consult
- Supportive therapy is provided and hospital stay continued.
- Contemplate liver transplantation if the patient is a candidate (Mayo End-Stage Liver Disease [MELD] score)

Needle Tract Tumor Seeding

- Occurs in 0.3–0.5% of hepatic ablative cases
- Can be managed
  - Tract ablation
  - Surgical resection
  - Palliative therapy if there are distant metastases
- Report to liver transplant service – the patient may no longer be a transplant candidate

Cholecystitis

- Occurs in 0.04% of hepatic ablative cases
- Usually transient, treated with antibiotics

- Can be managed
  - Antibiotics ± cholecystostomy
  - Cholecystectomy

Further Reading

Bruix J, Sherman M; Practice Guidelines Committee, American Association for the Study of Liver Diseases. Management of hepatocellular carcinoma. Hepatology 2005;42(5):1208–1236

Cheung L, Livraghi T, Solbiati L, et al. Complications of tumor ablation. In: van Sonnenberg E, McMullen W, Solbiati L, eds. Tumor Ablation: Principles and Practice. New York: Springer; 2005:440–458

Crum CD, van Sonnenberg E, Silverman SG, Morrison PR, Tuncali K. Cryotherapy of liver tumors. In: Mauro M, Murphy K, Thomson K, Venbrux A, Zollikofer C, eds. Image Guided Interventions. Philadelphia: Saunders; 2008:1516–1522

de Baère T, Risse O, Kuoch V, et al. Adverse events during radiofrequency treatment of 582 hepatic tumors. AJR Am J Roentgenol 2003;181(3):695–700

Fahy BN, Jarnagin WR. Evolving techniques in the treatment of liver colorectal metastases: role of laparoscopy, radiofrequency ablation, microwave coagulation, hepatic arterial chemotherapy, indications and contraindications for resection, role of transplantation, and timing of chemotherapy. Surg Clin North Am 2006; 86(4):1005–1022

Lencioni R, Crocetti L, Bozzi E, Bartolozzi C. Thermal (heat) ablation of hepatocellular cancer. In: Mauro M, Murphy K, Thomson K, Venbrux A, Zollikofer C, eds. Image Guided Interventions. Philadelphia: Saunders; 2008:1491–1504

Lencioni R, Della Pina C, Bartolozzi C. Percutaneous image-guided radiofrequency ablation in the therapeutic management of hepatocellular carcinoma. Abdom Imaging 2005;30(4):401–408

Livraghi T, Solbiati L, Meloni MF, Gazelle GS, Halpern EF, Goldberg SN. Treatment of focal liver tumors with percutaneous radio-frequency ablation: complications encountered in a multicenter study. Radiology 2003;226(2):441–451

Solbiati L, Lerace T, Cova L, Zaid S. Thermal (heat) ablation of other liver lesions. In: Mauro M, Murphy K, Thomson K, Venbrux A, Zollikofer C, eds. Image Guided Interventions. Philadelphia: Saunders; 2008:1505–1515

Solbiati L, Lerace T, Tonolini M, Cova L. Ablation of liver metastasis. In: van Sonnenberg E, McMullen W, Solbiati L, eds. Tumor Ablation: Principles and Practice. New York, Springer; 2005: 311–321

20 Thermal Ablation of Renal Lesion

Wael E. A. Saad and Daniel B. Brown

Classification and Indications

This book deals with ultrasound-guided procedures. The majority of institutions/operators utilize computed tomography (CT-) guidance, not ultrasound guidance, for renal ablation. This is for several reasons.

- Although ultrasound guidance provides real-time imaging and can be helpful during needle placement, its advantage is lost once radiofrequency ablation (RFA)/cryoablation begins due to the increased echogenicity/visualization of the lead edge of the ice-ball during cryoablation.
- Not all lesions can be visualized easily with ultrasound to the extent that an operator may not be comfortable that he or she is in a good position for a complete ablation. This is particularly true in patients with large body habitus. Almost all masses can be seen, assessed, and treated with CT guidance. For the sake of streamlining the process and not tailoring guidance requirements to each lesion/patient, many institutions adopt "get-them-all" guidance.
- CT provides a global image of the surrounding structures ("a lay of the land") and accurately assesses distances between the probe and adjacent structures, particularly the colon. It is easier to assess colon distance (with reproducibility) by CT particularly for lesions that are at a higher risk for being closer to the colon – lower pole and posterior lesions.
- For the reason noted above, CT rather than with ultrasound is more accurate (with reproducibility) in assessing bowel displacement techniques because it helps the operator to maintain a safe distance between bowel and the ablative probe before and after displacement.

The increasing use of cross-sectional imaging over the past two decades has led to the discovery of more incidental early-stage renal tumors. In addition, the trend for managing early stage – less than 3-to 4-cm diameter – renal masses has been away from nephrectomy and toward nephron-sparing surgeries. Percutaneous thermal ablation of renal tumors with its reduced morbidity is a further step in the progression of this trend.

The rising "incidence," or rather, discovery of renal masses and the minimally invasive treatment trend drive percutaneous ablation of renal tumors. However, the lack of randomized control trials and/or long-term follow-up data (especially when we are dealing with renal cell carcinoma [RCC] with tumor size <3–4 cm, which usually has a long-term survival rate without patient treatment) make it difficult to clearly define indications for image-guided renal mass ablation. Therefore, this chapter will discuss patient candidates/lesion selection rather than indications. Patient selection should be multidisciplinary.

Indications Based on Pathology

- Small (<3–4 cm) solid renal cell mass confined to the kidney
- Renal arteriovenous malformation (AVM) with gross hematuria that is inaccessible by endoluminal means

Indications Based on Pathology for Ablative Modality

A lot of device selection is going to come down to operator preference.
- Radiofrequency ablation
  - Small solid lesions
  - Exophytic lesions
- Cryoablation (heat-sump problems for RFA)
  - Central lesions closer to collecting system (pelvicalyceal system)
  - Cystic lesions
  - Solid lesions adjacent to cysts
  - Cryoablation is less painful and may be more appropriate for patients undergoing ablation under sedation only (no general anesthesia).

Image-Guidance Ablation Candidates

- Patients with high medical comorbidities (nonsurgical candidates)
- Very elderly patients with small (<3 cm) RCC (life expectancy)
- Patients who refuse surgery
- Patients requiring the highest nephron-sparing procedure available
  - Multifocal RCC whether
    - Metachronous lesions: Recurrent multifocal RCC after an initial nephrectomy/partial nephrectomy

- Synchronous: Multiple lesions at the same time making surgery not feasible or requiring multiple surgeries where the surgical morbidities rise higher than their norm (risk versus benefit: percutaneous ablation has less morbidity)
  - Von Hippel-Lindau disease patients (metachronous and synchronous lesions and other comorbidities)
  - RCC in solitary native kidneys
  - RCC in transplanted kidney
  - Borderline poor renal function (on the brink of dialysis)

Ultrasound-Guidance Ablation Candidates

- See the introduction to this chapter
- Lesions seen by ultrasound – especially lesions that are intraparenchymal and are appreciated by ultrasound (differentiated from surrounding normal parenchyma) and not by unenhanced CT
- Lesions found by preprocedural cross-sectional imaging that are clearly at a distance (>2 cm) from the colon

Contraindications

Absolute Contraindications

- Uncorrected coagulopathy
- Suggested coagulation parameters
  - International normalized ratio (INR): ≤1.4
  - Platelets (PLT): ≥50,000
  - Activated partial thromboplastin time (aPTT): ≤65 seconds

Relative Contraindications

- Renal ablation should be performed electively unless hematuria is the cause of instability or is adding to the instability, which is not common).
- Sepsis (can be treated first, unless you are dealing with gross hematuria requiring a blood transfusion)
- Patient instability (can stabilize first, unless you are dealing with gross hematuria requiring a blood transfusion)

Noncandidates

- Lesions that are anterior on the kidney that require access percutaneously via normal kidney (transrenal approach) are probably better candidates for laparoscopic ablation and not image-guided percutaneous ablation.
- Lesions that are anteromedial and adjacent to the ureteropelvic junction (UPJ) or proximal ureter (particularly in the lower pole) have a higher risk of causing UPJ/ureteric injury such as
  - Ureteric obstruction/stenosis
  - Urine leaks
- Disease not confined to kidney (extrarenal dissemination)
  - Distant metastasis (unless you are treating hematuria)
  - Large lesion extending to surrounding structures outside Gerota's fascia
- Vascular invasion (renal venous tumor thrombus)
- Location related: Lesions that are close to adjacent structures especially bowel in cases where bowel displacement techniques have failed

Preprocedural Evaluation

Evaluate Prior Cross-Sectional Imaging

- Characterize the lesion
  - Make sure that this is a legitimate lesion. Fat inside the lesion may indicate that it is an angiomyolipoma and not a malignant lesion that needs to be ablated.
  - Cystic lesions may rupture, and thus change shape, characteristics, and size on deploying the ablative probe. Be prepared for that; think of using cryotherapy.
  - Some institutions/operators tailor the ablative modality depending on lesion characteristics (alternate cryoablation and radiofrequency).
    - Cystic and/or central lesions get cryoablation.
    - Exophytic and/or solid lesions get cryoablation.
  - Lesion size: Ideal lesion size is <3 cm. The smaller the better, if you can see it.
  - Lesions that are anterior on the kidney that require access percutaneously via normal kidney (transrenal approach) are probably better candidates for laparoscopic cryotherapy and not image-guided percutaneous ablation.
  - Small central and intraparenchymal lesions may not be appreciated by noncontrast CT.
    - See if you can identify and access the lesion by ultrasound
    - Carefully examine intrarenal landmarks that do not rely on intravenous (IV) contrast to attempt to identify its location to ablate the region of the lesion ("vicinity ablation")
- Look for adjacent organs that can be inadvertently traversed or are close enough that they can be thermally injured
  - This helps plan the needle trajectory (ablative approach).
  - This can help reduce transgression of adjacent organs with subsequent potential major complications.

- Particular organs that may be traversed include colon, spleen, lung (pleura), stomach, and less likely small bowel.
  - Small bowel is more likely an issue in transplanted kidneys or anterior lesions.
  - Transhepatic ablation is not necessarily a problem (intentional or inadvertent).
- Thermal ablation injury concerns and avoidance planning
  - The colon is the organ causing the most concern.
    - The colon is more vulnerable than other segments of the gastrointestinal tract (stomach and small bowel).
    - Injuring the edge of solid organs, such as liver or spleen, is not a great concern.
  - Lesions that are anteromedial and adjacent to the UPJ or proximal ureter have a higher risk of causing UPJ/ureteric injury (urine obstruction/leak).
  - The thermal safety margin is ~10–20 mm.
  - When planning bowel displacement, convert the procedure/plan for the procedure to be CT guided.
  - Need to identify patient positioning for both the ablation probe and the saline displacement probe
  - Need to plan needle trajectory for hydrodisplacement (saline injection) between the colon and the lesion
  - Remember that the relative position of the colon and other nontarget structures in relation to the renal mass may change when the patient is prone for the ablation in comparison with the typical supine position used for working-up tumors
- Size and identify the shape of the lesion for probe sizing
  - Ablation should involve the lesion in its entirety with a 5- to 10-mm normal parenchymal margin.
  - Longitudinal/egg-shaped lesions should be treated with the intent of ablating at multiple overlapping stations with a probe access along the longitudinal axis of the lesion.

Evaluate Preablative Laboratory Values

- Laboratory value evaluation to rule out coagulopathy. Suggested coagulopathy thresholds are
  - INR: <1.4
  - PLT: ≥70,000
  - aPTT: ≤65 seconds
- Obtain a baseline serum creatinine value especially in nephron-sparing situations

Obtain Informed Consent

- Indications
  - Local control of malignant renal disease

- Local control of malignant liver disease can be with the intention of
  - Cure
  - Temporizing and local control
  - Palliation (hematuria)
- Result summary for percutaneous thermal ablation of RCC
  - Local tumor control (technical success): 80–100% (usually >90%)
  - Technical success/local control depend on tumor location/morphology: Lesions that are more amenable to ablation are those that are exophytic – even if they are large (up to 5 cm), they can be treated successfully.
  - Technical success/local control also depend on tumor size.
    - <3 cm tumor: 100% success rate
    - 3–5 cm tumor: 92% success rate
    - <4 cm tumor
      - 92% first session
      - 100% by the second session
    - >5 cm tumor: 25%
  - Recurrence rate for RFA is 1.3–5.3% (up to 3% in partial nephrectomy).
  - Recurrence rate for cryotherapy is not as clear and is probably the same. A quoted recurrence rate is 3.6%.
- Alternatives
  - There is no firm evidence to establish the optimal first-line treatment of early-stage RCC because of the lack of randomized controlled trials.
  - The lack of randomized control trials and/or long-term follow-up data (especially because we are dealing with RCC with a tumor size of <3–4 cm, which has a long-term survival rate without treatment) make it difficult to clearly define indications for image-guided renal mass ablation.
  - To refuse the percutaneous ablation or any other therapy
  - Surgery nephrectomy, partial nephrectomy
    - Traditional treatment of choice
  - Laparoscopic-guided thermal ablation
    - Applicable to anterior lesions that can be identified and are accessible laparoscopically
    - Ability to displace/remove bowel away from the target lesion
- Advantages of percutaneous thermal ablation
  - Can be performed on nonsurgical candidates
  - Can be performed on postoperative patients
  - Is nephron-sparing
  - Repeatability of treatment if initial treatments are incomplete
  - Can be used with regional and systemic chemotherapy
  - Minimally invasive
    - Limited complications
    - Usually preserves renal function
    - Limited hospital stay/outpatient

- Limited procedural cost
- Can be performed on nonsurgical candidates or postoperative cases
- Procedural risks
  - Mortality is rare.
  - Major complications occur in 0–8.3% of cases and include
    - Bleeding
      - Most common complication
      - More common with central lesion
      - Can present with
        - Renal capsular hematomas
          - Minor ones can be seen in up to 43% of cases.
          - Larger ones can be seen in 1.9–12.5% of cases.
          - Subcapsular hematomas and/or extrarenal retroperitoneal hematomas (bellow) requiring blood transfusion occur in 0.8–4.2% of cases.
        - Extrarenal retroperitoneal bleeding (drop in hematocrit)
        - Gross hematuria
    - Infection
      - Wound infection (more common)
      - Retroperitoneal abscess (not common)
      - It is more common with cryoablation and is reported in 1.0–4.3% of cryoablation cases.
    - Pneumothorax, hemothorax requiring chest tube
      - Not common
      - More common with upper pole lesion
      - More common with intercostal approach
    - Grounding pad burns (second- or third-degree burns)
    - Pelvicalyceal/ureteric injury
      - Leaks
      - Strictures
      - Obstruction
    - Early: Clotted gross hematuria (1.9%)
    - Late: Ureteric stricture (0.0–8.3%)
    - Focal hydrocalyx (0.0–2.5%)
- Minor complications
  - Occur in 2.5–12.5% of cases
  - Usually include
    - Postablative syndrome (fever) seen in up to 70% of patients
    - Flank pain seen in up to 10% of patients 24 hours from the procedure
    - Transient hematuria not requiring a blood transfusion
    - Incidental perirenal hematuria
    - Paresthesia (transient)
    - Minor wound infection
- Tumor seeding
  - Can occur in up to 1.7–2.6% of cases

Equipment

Ultrasound Guidance

- Ultrasound machine with Doppler capability
- Multiarray 4–5 MHz ultrasound transducer
- Transducer guide bracket
- Sterile transducer cover

Standard Surgical Preparation and Draping

- Chlorhexidine skin preparation/cleansing fluid
- Fenestrated drape

Local Infiltrative Analgesia Administration

- 21-gauge infiltration needle
- 10–20 mL 1% lidocaine syringe

Sharp Access

- 11-blade incision scalpel
- Coaxial access needle
  - Some thermal probes are introduced through coaxial needles.
  - Coaxial needles allow coaxial biopsy needle placement followed by ablative probe placement without losing access.
  - A coaxial needle may reduce the risk of tract seeding (anecdotal).
- Thermal ablative probes

Thermal Ablation Probes

The probes currently in use are summarized below.
- RFA systems
  - The radiofrequency generator and the patient are the main components of an electric circuit.
  - The generator is the source of the alternating current and the patient's body is the resistor.
  - The resistance in the tissue (*impedance*) to the radiofrequency current is what generates heat and creates a thermal ablation effect.
  - The thermal ablative (radiofrequency) electrode enters the body and an alternating electric current passes directly into the body. However, a return connection to the generator is required. This return is established by grounding pads usually placed on the patient's thighs.
  - RFA systems include
    - Radionics RFA Probe (Cool-Tip Radionics, Burlington, MA)
      - This is a monopolar RFA electrode needle.
      - Single 17-gauge needle

- ○ Cluster design of three 17-gauge needles
- ○ Cooled by continued flow of cold water that is not deposited in the body
- LeVeen Needle Electrode (Boston Scientific Corp., Natick, MA) (**Fig. 20.1**)
  - ○ This is an array monopolar RFA electrode.
  - ○ It is a single needle with 10 tines that splay radially and arch back in a "palm tree" appearance (**Fig. 20.1**).

- ○ The array diameters (2.0, 3.0, 3.5, 4.0, and 5.0 cm) can be selected to match the tumor size.
- ○ The unique feature of this system is its impedance feedback mechanism. No measure of temperature is made by this device.
- RITA StarBurst RFA Probe (RITA Medical, Mountain View, CA)
  - ○ This is an array monopolar RFA electrode.

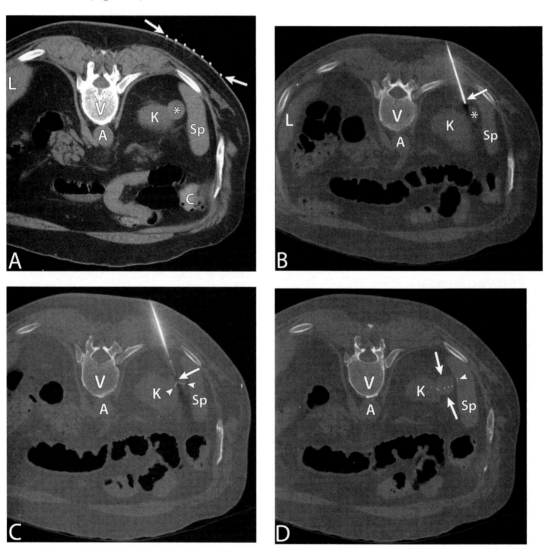

Fig. 20.1 Computed tomography (CT-) guided radiofrequency ablation (RFA) of an exophytic left renal mass. **(A)** Noncontrast axial CT image of the abdomen while the patient is prone. Seven markers have been placed over the patient's left flank (*between arrows*). A spherical exophytic mass (* *in center*) is seen between the upper pole of the left kidney (K) and the spleen (Sp) (V, vertebra; A, aorta; L, liver; C, colon). **(B)** Noncontrast axial CT image of the abdomen while the patient is prone. The operator has passed a diamond-tip coaxial needle (*arrow*) toward the exophytic renal mass (* *in center*). At this moment in the procedure, the operator takes the inner stylet of the needle and obtains an 18-gauge biopsy from the periphery of the mass K, upper pole of left kidney (Sp, spleen; V, vertebra; A, aorta; L, liver). **(C)** Noncontrast axial CT image of the abdomen while the patient is prone. The operator has obtained the biopsy and has now deployed the tines of the LeVeen probe (*arrowheads*) through the coaxial needle. Note, the tip of the coaxial needle is in the center of the exophytic renal mass (*arrow*) (K, upper pole of left kidney; Sp, spleen; V, vertebra; A, aorta). **(D)** Noncontrast axial CT image of the abdomen while the patient is prone. Again, noted are the tines of the LeVeen probe, which have been deployed through the coaxial needle and into the renal mass (*between arrows*). Note that at least one of the tines (*arrowhead*) is through the splenic capsule: this is usually not a problem (same goes for liver) (K, upper pole of left kidney; Sp, spleen; V, vertebra; A, aorta).

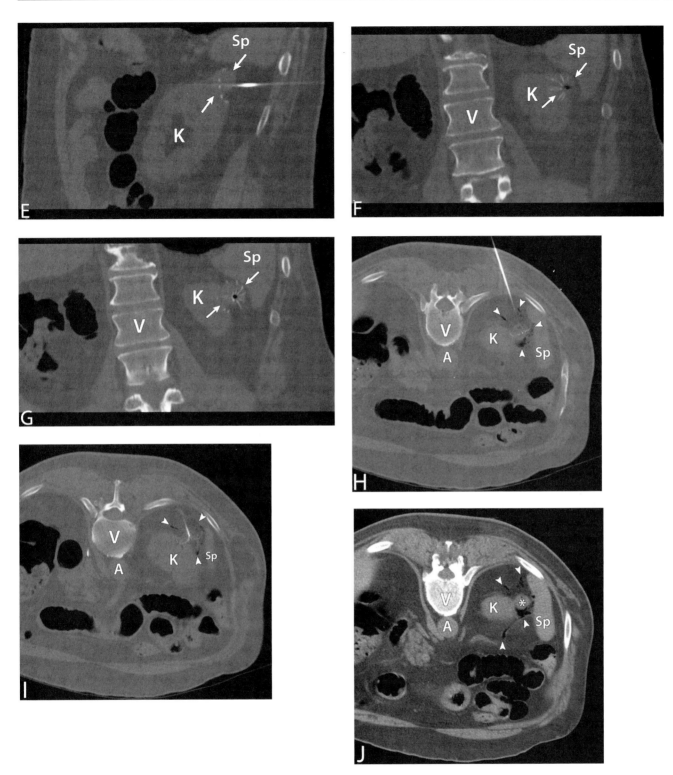

Fig. 20.1 *(Continued)* **(E)** Noncontrast sagittal CT reconstruction of the abdomen of the same patient. In one image the location and deployment of the probe and its tines, respectively, are seen. The tines are well deployed in the upper pole exophytic mass (*between arrows*) (K, left kidney; Sp, spleen). **(F,G)** Noncontrast coronal CT reconstruction images of the abdomen of the same patient. Again seen are tines that are well deployed in the upper pole exophytic mass (*between arrows*) (K, left kidney; Sp, spleen; V, vertebral column). **(H,I)** Noncontrast axial CT images of the abdomen of the same patient after undergoing RFA. The probe is still is place. Air pockets as a result of the RFA are seen (*arrowheads*) (K, left kidney; Sp, spleen; V, vertebral column; A, aorta). **(J)** Noncontrast axial CT image of the abdomen of the same patient after undergoing RFA. The probe has been removed. Air pockets as a result of the RFA are seen in the perinephric fat (*arrowheads*) (K, left kidney; Sp, spleen; V, vertebral column; A, aorta).

- It is a single needle with 7– 9 tines, which splay forward and radially in a "starburst" appearance.
- The array diameters (2–5 cm) can be selected to match the tumor size (7-tine array for diameters 2–3 cm and 9-tine array for 3–5 cm).
- The unique features of this system are its ability to measure temperature and then infuse saline through select elements of the array.
- The StarBurst array probe is composed of a 14-gauge trocar.
- Other radiofrequency ablation systems include
  - Celon ProSurge applicators (Celon AG Medical Instruments, Berlin, Germany)
  - Berchtold HiTT electrode (Berchtold, GmbH, Tuttlingen, Germany)
- Cryoablation systems include
  - Galil-CryoHit ablation system (Galil Medical, Westbury, NY)
    - Gas-based probe that uses argon and helium
    - Up to seven probes can be used at once
    - Temperatures include a freeze temperature of –180°C and a thaw temperature of +35°C.
    - A "stick mode" temperature is usually set at –20°C. This provides a limited freeze to the probe, so that the probe adheres (anchors) to the immediate tissue and prevents migration of the probe while other probes are placed.
    - The operator has to add a separate thermistor needle to get real-time temperature measurements during ablation.
    - Cryoablation treatments are composed of a timed freeze (usually 15 minutes) with a thaw, with or without an additional freeze.
  - CRYOcare System (Endocare, Inc., Irvine, CA)
    - Gas-based probe that uses argon and helium
    - Up to eight probes can be used at once
    - Temperatures include variable freeze temperature ranging from –130 to –150°C and a thaw temperature of +40°C.
    - A "stick mode" temperature is usually set at –10°C. This provides a limited freeze to the probe, so that the probe adheres (anchors) to the immediate tissue and prevents migration of the probe while other probes are placed.
    - Cryoablation treatments are composed of a timed freeze with a thaw, with or without additional freeze.

Technique

Intravenous Access

- Required for moderate sedation administration or for administration of muscle relaxants and general anesthesia

- Moderate sedation versus general anesthesia is operator/institution dependent.
- When tailoring general anesthesia versus moderate sedation
  - General anesthesia may be more commonly used in patients who
    - Are uncooperative, nervous
    - Have large lesions (longer procedure)
  - Moderate sedation may be more commonly used in patients who
    - Have small (<2 cm) lesions
    - Are at risk of increased comorbidity – high risk for general anesthesia
- IV access is required in case of any complication (including pain-related complications), or if the need arises to administer sedation.

Standard Surgical Preparation and Draping

- Skin preparation/cleansing in the region that was chosen as an ultrasound imaging portal and a needle access needle portal
- Place a fenestrated drape at the chosen and prepared skin region

Local Infiltrative Analgesia Administration

- Utilizing a 21-gauge (by at least a 3.7-cm-long) infiltration needle, 1% lidocaine infiltration is performed.

Sharp Access

- An incision is made utilizing an 11-blade scalpel usually by a 3-mm-depth stab of the 11-blade.
- A coaxial access needle can be passed under real-time ultrasound guidance/CT-guidance.
- The coaxial access needle
  - Allows biopsy acquisition/sampling, followed by ablation without reaccessing (**Fig. 20.1B**)
  - May reduce tumor seeding of the tract
  - Embolization of the tract in patients with coagulopathy

Pathology Sample Acquisition (Preablation Biopsy)

- An automated spring-loaded core biopsy needle is passed to the end of a coaxial needle and "fired" (automatically deployed) and withdrawn.
- Usually one to two core (18-gauge) biopsy needle passes/deployments are made.

Thermal Ablation

- The thermal ablation probe is connected to its thermal generator (see the above subsection *Thermal Ablation Probes* under Equipment).

- The thermal ablation probe is advanced under real-time ultrasound. The probe's positioning depends on
  - The type of probe
    - A cryo-probe requires its probe tip to be placed past the center of the target lesion (on the deep-end of the lesion) because the ice-ball forms at the tip and is usually longitudinal along the axis/shaft of the probe (**Fig. 20.2**).
    - A RFA LeVeen probe requires its probe tip to be placed at, or just short-of, the center of the target lesion because the secondary probes (tines) open at the level of the probe tip or slightly forward (**Figs. 20.1 and 20.3**).

- A RFA Rita probe requires its probe tip to be placed at the superficial aspect of the target lesion because the secondary probes (tines) open forward (deeper to the probe/needle tip).
  - The number of probes (if manufactured in clusters)
  - The size of the ablation area
  - The shape of ablation area
  - The shape and size of the lesion and how to tailor the size and shape of the proposed ablation area of the probe
- As an example, details of the RFA system that utilizes the LeVeen needle electrode are given in the section below.
- The RFA LeVeen probe is advanced into the target lesion. The probe placement is

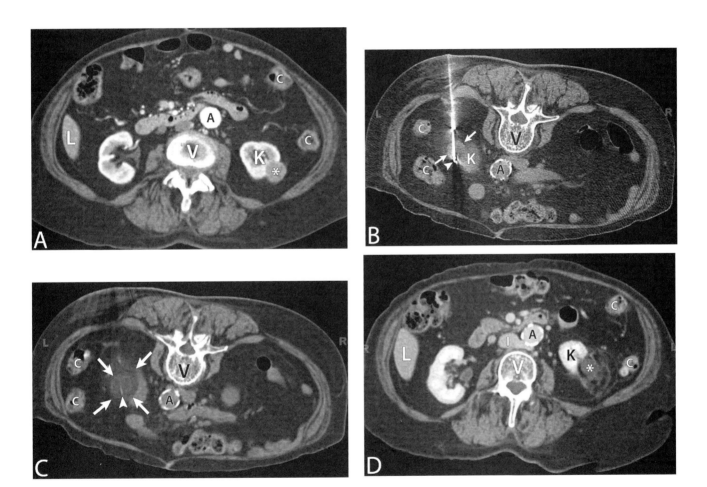

Fig. 20.2 Computed tomography (CT-) guided cryoablation of a left renal mass. **(A)** Contrast-enhanced axial CT image of the abdomen while the patient is supine. A spherical exophytic mass (* *in center*) is seen in the upper pole of the left kidney (K). The colon (C) is more than 2 cm from the mass edge (V, vertebra; A, aorta; L, liver). **(B)** Noncontrast axial CT image of the abdomen while the patient is prone. The operator has passed the cryo-probe needle (*arrowhead at tip*). Notice, that the needle tip (*arrowhead*) is on the deep end of the lesion (*between arrows*). Cryo-probes, unlike radiofrequency ablation (RFA) probes, need to have their tips on the deep end of the lesion and not in the center of the lesion (compare with **Fig. 20.1**). At this moment in the proce- dure the operator will start ablating the mass (K, upper pole of left kidney; C, colon; V, vertebra; A, aorta). **(C)** Noncontrast axial CT image of the abdomen while the patient is prone. The operator has cryoablated the lesion (*arrowhead at probe tip*). Notice the low attenuation ice-ball (*arrows*) (K, upper pole of left kidney; C, colon; V, vertebra; A, aorta). **(D)** Contrast-enhanced axial CT image of the abdomen while the patient is supine. This is an 8-month follow-up exam demonstrating no enhancement of the ablated lesion (*) at the upper pole of the left kidney (K, upper pole of left kidney; L, liver; V, vertebra; A, aorta; I, inferior vena cava [IVC]; C, colon).

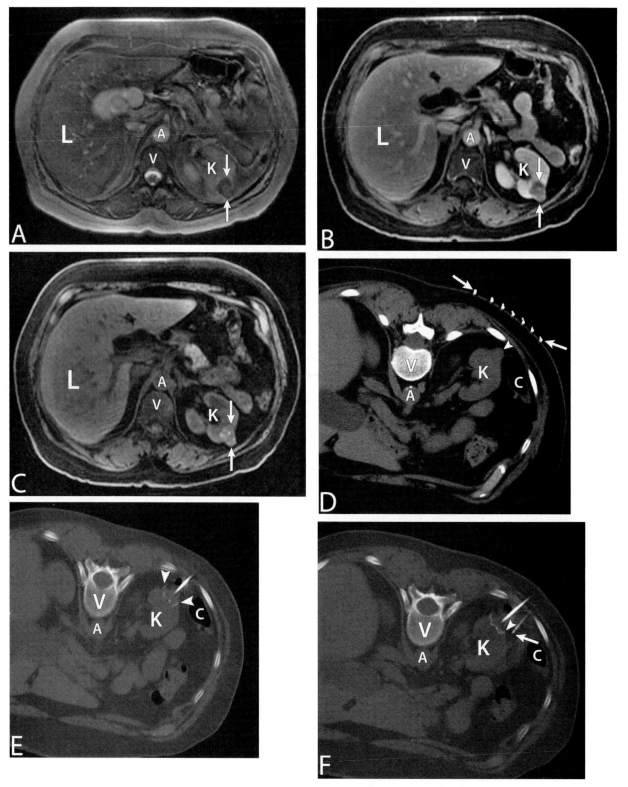

Fig. 20.3 Computed tomography (CT-) guided radiofrequency ablation (RFA) of a left renal mass with tract seeding. **(A,B,C)** Magnetic resonance images (MRIs) demonstrating a solid renal mass (*between arrows*) in the midportion of the left kidney (K). (V, vertebra; A, aorta; L, liver). **(D)** Noncontrast axial CT image of the abdomen while the patient is prone. Seven markers have been placed over the patients left flank (between arrows). A partly exophytic mass (*arrowhead*) is again seen in midportion of the left kidney (K) (V, vertebra; A, aorta; L, liver; C, colon). **(E)** Noncontrast axial CT image of the abdomen while the patient is prone. The operator has passed and deployed a RFA-probe into the left renal mass (*arrowheads pointing to outer tines*). The most lateral tines are within a centimeter of the left hemicolon (C) (K, Upper pole of left kidney; V, vertebra; A, aorta). **(F)** Noncontrast axial CT image of the abdomen while the patient is prone. The operator has now passed a 19-gauge needle between the RFA-probe tines and the left hemicolon (C) (*arrow points to 19-gauge needle*). The distance between the left hemicolon (C) and the nearest tine (*arrowhead*) is not greater than 2 cm. It is now safer for the operator to start ablating (K, left kidney; V, vertebra; A, aorta).

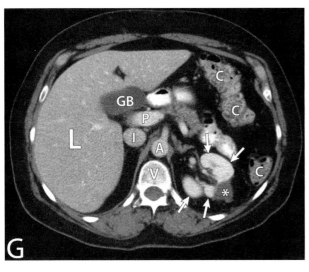

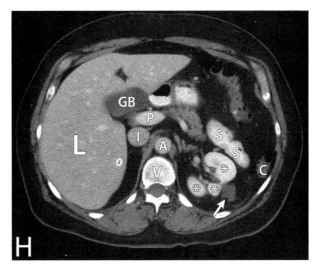

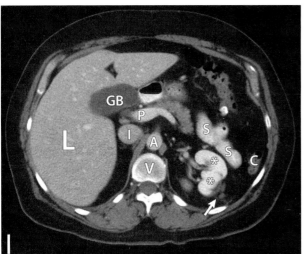

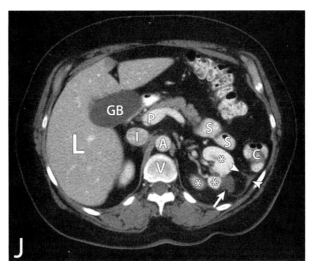

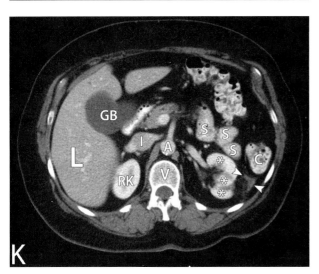

Fig. 20.3 *(Continued)* **(G)** Postablation 3-month contrast-enhanced axial CT image of the abdomen while the patient is supine. Contrast is enhancing the normal parenchyma of the left kidney (*arrows*). The lesion is not enhancing (*). The perinephric fat between the lesion and the left hemicolon (C) is clear ("clean"); compare with **Figs. 20.3J and 20.3K** (V, vertebra; A, aorta; I, inferior vena cava [IVC]; L, liver; GB, gallbladder; P, portal vein). **(H,I)** Two postablation 9-month contrast-enhanced axial CT images of the abdomen while the patient is supine. Contrast is enhancing the normal parenchyma of the left kidney (*). The lesion is not enhancing (*arrow*). The perinephric fat between the lesion and the left hemicolon (C) is clear ("clean"); compare with **Figs. 20.3J and 20.3K** (S, small bowel; V, vertebra; A, aorta; I, inferior vena cava [IVC], L, liver; GB, gallbladder; P, portal vein). **(J,K)** Two postablation 15-month contrast-enhanced axial CT images of the abdomen while the patient is supine. Contrast is enhancing the normal parenchyma of the left kidney (*) and the right kidney (RK). The perinephric fat between the lesion and the left hemicolon (C) is now occupied by a triangular-shaped enhancing soft tissue mass (*between arrowheads*); compare with **Figs. 20.3H and 20.3I**. This perinephric soft tissue enhances by ~35–45 Hounsfield units (HU) (S, small bowel; V, vertebra; A, aorta; I, inferior vena cava [IVC]; L, liver; GB, gallbladder; P, portal vein).

- At the center of small lesions using smaller probes (≤3 cm)
- Just short of the center of the target lesion/probe size (>3 cm)
- If the lesion is egg-shaped and the operator is passing the RFA probe along the long axis of a lesion (diameter of ablation more than short axis diameter of lesion, but less than the long access of the lesion):
  - A multiple station ablation is required.
  - The probe is deployed on the deep-end of the lesion and is then pulled back with a lesion overlap.
  - Pulling back the probe requires a retraction of the tines, withdrawal of the probe with a lesion overlap, and redeployment of the tines.
  - Using CT from the beginning of the procedure precludes a change in modality later.
- RFA protocol utilizing the LeVeen probe is summarized in **Figs. 20.4 and 20.5**.

Immediate Postablation Ultrasound Imaging

- Immediate postablation ultrasound imaging is usually nondiagnostic as far as the lesion is concerned due to shadowing artifact (unless the lesion was missed).
- However, it can be used for documentation and obtaining a baseline image of a capsular or subcapsular hematoma.

- Visualizing a renal capsular hematoma does not alter postprocedural care or management.

Endpoints

Endpoint of Target Renal Biopsy

- Usually one to two 18-gauge needle passes are required to obtain an adequate pathology sample.
- Smaller caliber needles (20-gauge core biopsy needles) and larger caliber needles (16-gauge core biopsy needles) may require more needle passes or fewer needle passes, respectively.

Endpoint of Ablation

- Adequate positioning of the probe during the procedure is key. Immediate endpoints that are image-based are difficult to make by ultrasound (shadow artifact precluding visualization). Immediate CT imaging would demonstrate
  - A low attenuation area over the lesion with possible air bubbles in the parenchyma secondary to cavitation (**Figs. 20.1H, 20.1I, 20.1J**)
  - Air in the adjacent perirenal fat (**Figs. 20.1H, 20.1I, 20.1J**)

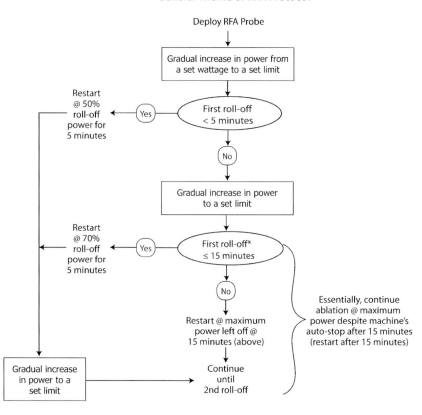

General Theme of RFA Protocol

Fig. 20.4 Flowchart demonstrating the general theme of an impedance-based ablative system, specifically the LeVeen radiofrequency ablation probe.

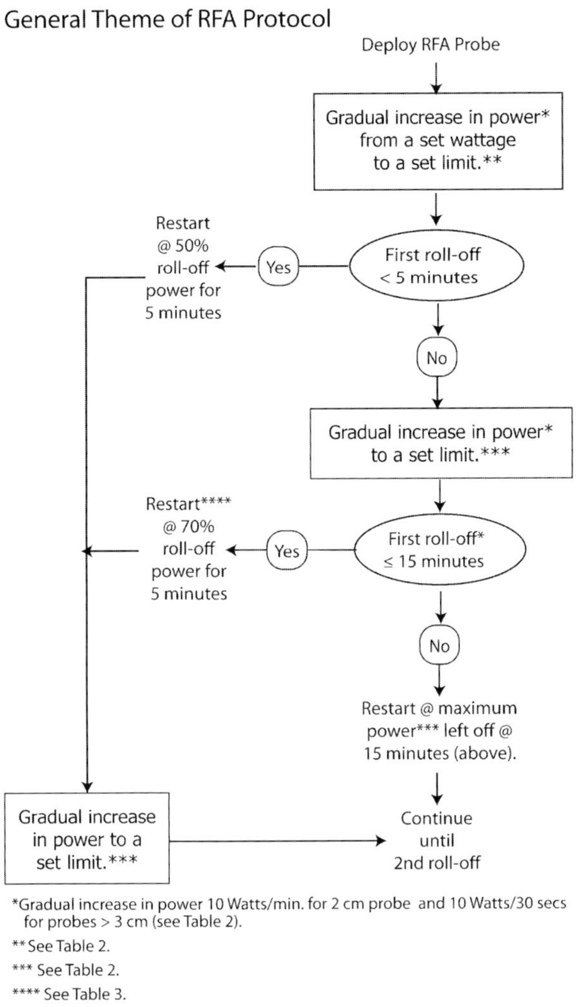

General Theme of RFA Protocol

Fig. 20.5 Flowchart demonstrating the ablation protocol of the LeVeen radiofrequency ablation probe.

Table 2

RFA Probe Size	* Rate of gradual incremental increase in power at any level	** Initial start power to initial set limit at 5 minutes	*** Maximum power at or above 15 minutes prior to or after first roll-off
2.0 cm	10 Watts / 60 seconds	30 to 60 Watts	60 Watts
3.0 cm	10 Watts / 30 seconds	40 to 80 Watts	150 Watts
3.5 cm	10 Watts / 30 seconds	50 to 90 Watts	180 Watts
4.0 cm	10 Watts / 30 seconds	80 to 130 Watts	190 Watts
5.0 cm	10 Watts / 30 seconds	100 to 150 Watts	200 Watts

*, **, and *** asterisks refer to certain locations on the radiofrequency ablation flow chart.

Table 3

**** Power at which roll-off was achieved	70% of Power to restart RFA
50 w	35 w
60 w	42 w
70 w	49 w
80 w	56 w
90 w	63 w
100 w	70 w
110 w	77 w
120 w	84 w
130 w	91 w
140 w	98 w
150 w	105 w
160 w	112 w
170 w	119 w
180 w	126 w
190 w	133 w
200 w	140 w

**** Asterisks refer to certain locations on the radiofrequency ablation flow chart.

*Gradual increase in power 10 Watts/min. for 2 cm probe and 10 Watts/30 secs for probes > 3 cm (see Table 2).

** See Table 2.

*** See Table 2.

**** See Table 3.

- ○ In cases of cryoablation, a low attenuation ice-ball is seen over the ablated mass at the end of the probe (**Fig. 20.2C**).
- Subcapsular hematomas can be seen. Treat the patient for pain and provide hemodynamic stability.
- The true endpoint is on delayed imaging.
  - ○ A postprocedure 24- to 48-hour CT scan would show complete coagulative necrosis of the lesion and a safety margin.
  - ○ A postprocedure 24- to 48-hour CT scan should be done to evaluate technical success and look for complications.
  - ○ The procedure is considered a success if there is a lack of enhancement consistent with no recurrence/residual tumor (see below).
- Follow-up
  - ○ A postprocedure 24- to 48-hour CT scan would show complete coagulative necrosis of the lesion and a safety margin.

- ○ Follow-up cross-sectional imaging looking for lack of enhancement consistent with no recurrence/residual tumor is required to consider complete success.
- ○ Cross-sectional imaging at 1, 3, 6, and 12 months and annually thereafter includes
  - Contrast-enhanced CT (**Figs. 20.6, 20.7, 20.8**)
  - Contrast-enhanced magnetic resonance imaging (MRI)
  - Ultrasound contrast (Europe/experimental)
- ○ A minimal zone of contrast enhancement (enhancing rim) with an enhancement of <20 Hounsfield units (HU) can be seen.
  - This can be normal post-RFA.
  - May represent vascular/capillary leakage

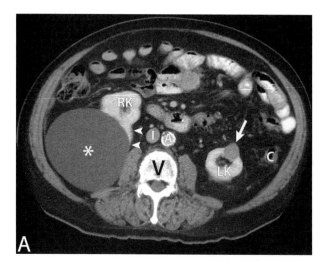

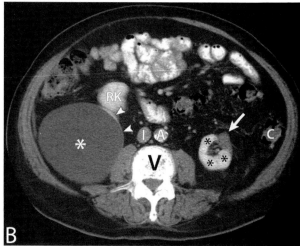

Fig. 20.6 (A) Contrast-enhanced axial computed tomography (CT) image of the abdomen while the patient is supine. A partly exophytic mass (*arrow*) is seen in the anterior left kidney (LK). Incidentally, a large cyst is seen coming off the right kidney (RK). Notice the "claw sign" of the right kidney (*arrowheads*) (V, vertebra; A, aorta; I, inferior vena cava [IVC]; C, left hemicolon). **(B)** Postablation 9-month contrast-enhanced axial CT image of the abdomen while the patient is supine. Contrast is enhancing the normal parenchyma of the left kidney (*). The lesion is not enhancing (*arrow*). Incidentally, a large cyst is seen coming off the right kidney (RK). Notice the "claw sign" of the right kidney (*arrowheads*) (V, vertebra; A, aorta I, inferior vena cava (IVC); C, left hemicolon; RK, right kidney).

Postprocedural Evaluation and Management

Initial Postprocedural Observation Period and Admission

- The postprocedural stay varies from one practice to the other. Patients should be observed closely during the anesthesia recovery period.

- Almost all practices admit the patient for at least 24 hours/overnight stay.

Intravenous Fluid and Diet

- Institutions that practice moderate sedation start with a clear liquid diet and advance it as tolerated. This helps to offset patients' nausea and vomiting.

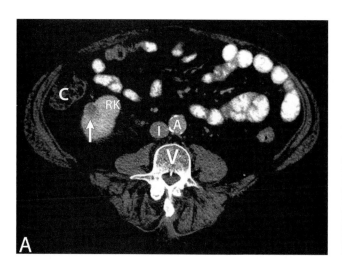

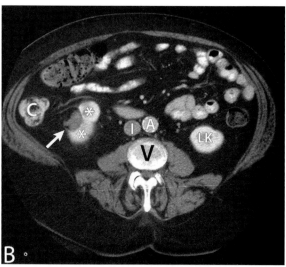

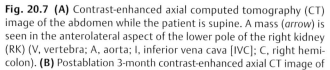

Fig. 20.7 (A) Contrast-enhanced axial computed tomography (CT) image of the abdomen while the patient is supine. A mass (*arrow*) is seen in the anterolateral aspect of the lower pole of the right kidney (RK) (V, vertebra; A, aorta; I, inferior vena cava [IVC]; C, right hemicolon). **(B)** Postablation 3-month contrast-enhanced axial CT image of the abdomen while the patient is supine. Contrast is enhancing the normal parenchyma of the right kidney (*). The lesion is not enhancing (*arrow*) (V, vertebra; A, aorta; I, Inferior vena cava (IVC); C, left hemicolon; LK, lower pole of left kidney).

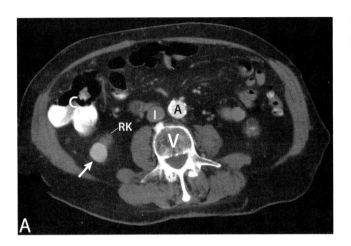 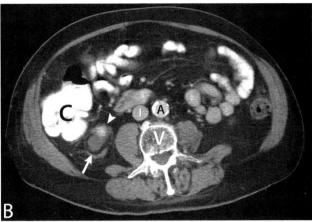

Fig. 20.8 **(A)** Contrast-enhanced axial computed tomography (CT-) image of the abdomen while the patient is supine. An exophytic mass (*arrow*) off the lowermost aspect of the lower pole of the right kidney (RK) is seen enhancing even more so than the lower pole of the right kidney (V, vertebra; A, aorta; I, inferior vena cava [IVC]; C, right hemicolon). **(B)** Postablation 3-month contrast-enhanced axial CT image of the abdomen while the patient is supine. Contrast is enhancing the normal parenchyma of the right kidney (*arrowhead*). The lesion is not enhancing (*arrow*) (V, vertebra; A, aorta; I, inferior vena cava [IVC]; C, right hemicolon).

- Other institutions/operators commence a clear liquid diet after a period of abstinence of oral intake. This period could be one hour, for example.
- Give IV fluid until oral intake is adequate.
- Make sure the patient voids urine and that it is clear (no gross hematuria).

Activity

- Bed rest for the period for which the patient is being observed closely (1–4 hours postablation)
- Activity is then as tolerated by the patient.

Pain Management

- Mild to moderate pain is not uncommon for the first 2 days postprocedure.
- Narcotics are usually not required during the postablation stay of the patient prior to discharge. Occasionally, some patients require oral narcotic analgesics such as acetaminophen and hydrocodone combination medication. Rarely does a patient require IV narcotics such as morphine or fentanyl.
- Continued back pain may prompt a retroperitoneal CT scan (noncontrast) to rule out retroperitoneal bleeding.
- On discharge, patients usually tolerate the procedure well and do not require analgesics more potent than over-the-counter medications.

Monitoring Vital Signs

- Vital sign monitoring includes blood pressure and heart rate. Occasionally, oxygen saturation monitoring

is required in cases of shortness of breath and/or chest pain.

- Institutions/operators that practice conscious sedation may record a softer blood pressure than a patient's baseline blood pressure after the hepatic ablation. This is most likely due to sedation with or without dehydration. The patient usually responds in time with hydration, particularly as the sedatives wear off.
- Continued hypotension and, more importantly, a rise in heart rate are concerning for hypovolemia (bleeding). If signs of hypovolemia occur, an IV volume bolus is given and a noncontrast CT exam is performed to confirm the clinical suspicion of bleeding.
- Make sure the patient voids urine and that it is clear (no gross hematuria).

Complications and Their Management

Please see **Table 20.1** for a list of complications and their incidence following renal ablation.

Management of Pain and Pain-Related Morbidity

- Mild to moderate pain is not uncommon for 48 hours postprocedure.
- Narcotics are usually not required during the posthepatic ablation stay of the patient prior to discharge. Occasionally, some patients require oral narcotic analgesics such as acetaminophen and hydrocodone combination medication. Rarely does a patient require IV narcotics such as fentanyl.
- Continued pain requires further clinical and possibly imaging evaluation.

Table 20.1   Complications of Renal Radiofrequency Ablation (RFA)

Complication	Incidence
Fever (post-RFA syndrome)	Up to 70%
Flank pain >24 hours,with no retroperitoneal bleeding	Up to 10%
Pericapsular hematoma	1.9–12.5%
Retroperitoneal bleeding including hematoma requiring blood transfusion	0.8–4.2%
Hematuria	0.0–3.7%*
Wound infection/abscess formation	0.0–3.7%†
Hemo- and/or pneumothorax	0.0–4.1%†
Grounding pad burns	0.0–1.7%†
Tumor seeding of RFA needle tract	up to 1.7–2.6%†
Paresthesia	2.0–3.3%†
Ureteric injury/stricture	0.0–8.3%†
Focal polar hydrocalyx	0.0–2.5%
Bowel perforation	Rare
Mortality	Rare

Source: Data from Aron M, Gill IS. Renal tumor ablation. Curr Opin Urol 2005;15(5):298–305; Breen DJ, Rutherford EE, Stedman B, et al. Management of renal tumors by image-guided radiofrequency ablation: experience in 105 tumors. Cardiovasc Intervent Radiol 2007;30(5):936–942; Gervais DA, Arellano RS, McGovern FJ, McDougal WS, Mueller PR. Radiofrequency ablation of renal cell carcinoma: part 2, Lessons learned with ablation of 100 tumors. AJR Am J Roentgenol 2005;185(1):72–80; Gervais DA, Arellano RS, Mueller P. Percutaneous ablation of kidney tumors in nonsurgical candidates. Oncology (Williston Park) 2005; 19(11, Suppl 4):6–11; Gervais DA, McGovern FJ, Arellano RS, McDougal WS, Mueller PR. Renal cell carcinoma: clinical experience and technical success with radio-frequency ablation of 42 tumors. Radiology 2003;226(2):417–424; Goldberg SN, Grassi CJ, Cardella JF, et al; Society of Interventional Radiology Technology Assessment Committee. Image-guided tumor ablation: standardization of terminology and reporting criteria. J Vasc Interv Radiol 2005;16(6):765–778; Mayo-Smith WW, Dupuy DE, Parikh PM, et al. Imaging-guided percutaneous radiofrequency ablation of solid renal masses: Techniques and outcomes of 38 treatments in 32 consecutive patients. AJR Am J Roentgenol 2003;180:1503–1508; Wallace MJ, Ahrar K. Thermal ablation of the kidney. In: Mauro M, Murphy K, Thomson K, Venbrux A, Zollikofer C, eds. Image Guided Interventions. Philadelphia: Saunders; 2008:1597–1605; Zagoria RJ, Traver MA, Werle DM, Perini M, Hayasaka S, Clark PE. Oncologic efficacy of CT-guided percutaneous radiofrequency ablation of renal cell carcinomas. AJR Am J Roentgenol 2007;189(2):429–436; Zagoria RJ. Percutaneous image-guided radiofrequency ablation of renal malignancies. Radiol Clin North Am 2003;41(5):1067–1075.

*Hematuria causing urinary obstruction found in up to 1.9% of cases.

†From authors' institutions' unpublished data.

○ Continued back pain may represent the symptoms of an expanding retroperitoneal hematoma.
○ Back pain can also represent thermal injury to the paraspinal or psoas muscles, especially if there is associated neuropathy.
○ However, changes in vital signs do signify a significant bleed.
○ Remember, ultimately the decisive factor for determining if there is significant bleeding is the patient's stability (vitals) – not what you see on the images.

Management of Bleeding Complications

- IV access should be kept until just before discharge in case fluid resuscitation is required.

- Bleeding can take two forms (internal, intraperitoneal or extraperitoneal, external, access site or hematuria) and has different sources:
  ○ Skin bleeding (external)
  ○ Retroperitoneal bleeding (renal source, posterior abdominal wall, paravertebral muscles)
  ○ Subcapsular hematoma with Paige kidney
  ○ Intercostal bleeding, which is rare (hemothorax, external skin bleeding, or hemoperitoneum)
  ○ Gross hematuria with or without urinary obstruction
- Significant bleeding affecting vital signs and patient stability should be managed by
  ○ Fluid resuscitation starting with crystalloid fluid bolus
  ○ Type and cross
  ○ Repeat hematocrit to compare with baseline
  ○ Blood transfusion to maintain hematocrit at or above 30%
  ○ Surgical consult/interventional radiology consult

- Interventional radiology offers
  - Renal and/or retroperitoneal (including lumbar) arteriography with super-selective arterial embolization if bleeding or a pseudoaneurysm is seen
- In cases of severe uncontrolled bleeding, a surgical consultation may offer open surgery, exploration, and local hemostasis of surface bleeding.

Management of Pleural/Thoracic Complications

- If chest pain with or without reduced oxygen saturation is encountered, a chest x-ray should be obtained to rule out pneumothorax or hemothorax. This is particularly true of an intercostals-approach renal ablation.
- Clinically significant hemo- and/or pneumothorax require chest tube placement, increased nasal cannula oxygenation, and fluid resuscitation/bleeding management in case of the former (see above).

Management of Puncture of Adjacent Organs

- With image guidance, this is a rare complication.
- Even when transgression of adjacent organs occurs, the result is clinically inconsequential. The problem is incidental and does not really rise to the level of a minor clinical complication, let alone a major complication.

Bowel Perforation

- It is more of a delayed perforation from thermal injury rather than a direct mechanical puncture (needle transgression).
- The colon is more susceptible to thermal injury than the small bowel or stomach.
- Surgical consult should be sought.
  - If the abdomen is "nonsurgical"
    - Supportive therapy
    - Antibiotics (against enterococci and anaerobes)
    - Repeat imaging (CT), diagnostic colonoscopy to assess injury
  - If abdomen is "surgical" (peritoneal signs)
    - Hemicolectomy

Wound Infection or Abscess Formation

- Must differentiate tumor necrosis from a true abscess
  - The abscess is larger than the original tumor.
  - The abscess is associated with persistent high-grade fever.
- Antibiotics (against anaerobes) should be given imperially, then according to the culture and sensitivity of organisms cultured from the blood, if any.

Needle Tract Tumor Seeding

- Can occur in up to 1.7–2.6% of renal ablative cases (**Fig. 20.3**)
- Can be managed
  - Tract ablation
  - Surgical resection
  - Report to liver transplant/heart transplant service. The patient may no longer be a transplant candidate.

Paresthesia

- Can occur in up to 3.4% of cases
- Usually transient
  - Reassurance
  - Supportive therapy

Gross Hematuria

- Can develop into urinary obstruction
- If severe
  - Can cause drop in hematocrit requiring a blood transfusion
  - Can cause patient instability requiring a blood transfusion and intervention (surgery or embolization)

Further Reading

Aron M, Gill IS. Renal tumor ablation. Curr Opin Urol 2005;15(5):298–305

Breen DJ, Rutherford EE, Stedman B, et al. Management of renal tumors by image-guided radiofrequency ablation: experience in 105 tumors. Cardiovasc Intervent Radiol 2007;30(5):936–942

Fotiadis NI, Sabharwal T, Morales JP, Hodgson DJ, O'Brien TS, Adam A. Combined percutaneous radiofrequency ablation and ethanol injection of renal tumours: midterm results. Eur Urol 2007;52(3):777–784

Gervais DA, Arellano RS, McGovern FJ, McDougal WS, Mueller PR. Radiofrequency ablation of renal cell carcinoma: part 2, lessons learned with ablation of 100 tumors. AJR Am J Roentgenol 2005;185(1):72–80

Gervais DA, Arellano RS, Mueller P. Percutaneous ablation of kidney tumors in nonsurgical candidates. Oncology (Williston Park) 2005;19(11, Suppl 4): 6–11

Gervais DA, McGovern FJ, Arellano RS, McDougal WS, Mueller PR. Renal cell carcinoma: clinical experience and technical success with radio-frequency ablation of 42 tumors. Radiology 2003; 226(2):417–424

Goldberg SN, Grassi CJ, Cardella JF, et al; Society of Interventional Radiology Technology Assessment Committee. Image-guided tumor ablation: standardization of terminology and reporting criteria. J Vasc Interv Radiol 2005;16(6):765–778

Mayo-Smith WW, Dupuy DE, Parikh PM, et al. Imaging-guided percutaneous radiofrequency ablation of solid renal masses: techniques and outcomes of 38 treatments in 32 consecutive patients. AJR Am J Roentgenol 2003;180:1503–1508

Mouraviev V, Joniau S, Van Poppel H, Polascik TJ. Current status of minimally invasive ablative techniques in the treatment of small renal tumors. Eur Urol 2007;51:328–336

Memarsadeghi M, Schmook T, Remzi M, et al. Percutaneous radiofrequency ablation of renal tumors: midterm results in 16 patients. Eur J Radiol 2006;59(2):183–189

Wah TM, Arellano RS, Gervais DA, et al. Image-guided percutaneous radiofrequency ablation and incidence of post-radiofrequency ablation syndrome: prospective survey. Radiology 2005;237(3): 1097–1102

Wallace MJ, Ahrar K. Thermal ablation of the kidney. In: Mauro M, Murphy K, Thomson K, Venbrux A, Zollikofer C, eds. Image Guided Interventions. Philadelphia: Saunders; 2008: 1597–1605

Zagoria RJ, Traver MA, Werle DM, Perini M, Hayasaka S, Clark PE. Oncologic efficacy of CT-guided percutaneous radiofrequency ablation of renal cell carcinomas. AJR Am J Roentgenol 2007;189(2):429–436

Zagoria RJ. Percutaneous image-guided radiofrequency ablation of renal malignancies. Radiol Clin North Am 2003;41(5):1067–1075

21 Direct Percutaneous Sclerosis of Vascular Malformation

Wael E.A. Saad

Classification and Indication

Vascular malformations are classified into hemangiomas and vascular malformations proper. With respect to ultrasound-guided procedures, vascular malformations are classified here into high-flow and low-flow vascular malformations.

Numerous methods, with technical variants within each method, for the management of vascular malformations have been described. However, the focus of this chapter is ultrasound-guided direct percutaneous sclerosis of vascular malformations. Transcatheter/endoluminal techniques in managing vascular malformations are not addressed in this chapter.

Here the indications for treating arteriovenous malformation (AVM) in general are provided, as well as guidelines for the use of direct percutaneous sclerosis techniques over transcatheter/endoluminal techniques. The ideal features of particular AVMs more amenable to direct percutaneous ultrasound-guided needle access and sclerotherapy are described.

Indications for Treating Vascular Malformations

- Cardiovascular symptoms
  - A drop in heart rate is caused by a complete or partial interruption of the blood flow in a vascular malformation (for subclinical high-flow AVMs).
  - Tachycardia and hyperdynamic circulation excluding other causes of hyperdynamic circulation
    - Hyperthyroidism and endocrine conditions that exhibit hyperthyroidism
    - Pregnancy
    - Arteriovenous fistulas
    - Other AVMs
  - Congestive right-sided heart failure
- Loss of function/disability
  - Mass effect on extremities
  - Arterial steel phenomenon
- Pain
  - Minimum: Annoying pain not responding to over-the-counter pain medication
  - Maximum: Debilitating pain

- Deformity
  - Minimum: Simple aesthetic purposes
  - Maximum: Help control and/or curb significant disfigurement

Indications for Ultrasound-Guided Direct Percutaneous Vascular Malformation Sclerosis

My preference is to treat vascular malformations via an endoluminal approach when possible rather than a direct percutaneous approach. The ultrasound-guided direct percutaneous approach is reserved for vascular malformations that are poorly accessible by endoluminal means.

- Slow-flow vascular malformations
  - Numerous vascular malformations are slow-flow vascular malformations that are commonly not accessible or have limited access by endoluminal means.
  - The slow-flow vascular malformations include
    - Venous malformations
    - Lymphatic malformations (lymphangiomas, cystic hygromas)
    - Lymphovenous mixed vascular malformations
- High-flow vascular malformations
  - The majority of high-flow vascular malformations are more commonly accessible by endoluminal means.
  - Ultrasound-guided direct percutaneous approach is reserved for high-flow vascular malformations that are poorly accessible by endoluminal means.
    - Tortuous native arterial blood supply making the nidus of the vascular malformation inaccessible
    - Prior endoluminal or surgical interventions that have partly occluded arterial endoluminal access to the nidus of the high-flow vascular malformation

Contraindications
Relative Contraindication

- Uncorrected coagulopathy. Relative versus absolute contraindication depends on the degree of coagulopathy. Remember that rarely is there urgency to perform a vascular malformation sclerosis.

- Diffuse involvement of a closed space such as muscle compartment (concerns for compartment syndrome)

Absolute Contraindication

- Infected overlying soft tissue or overlying skin erosion/breakdown
- Ulcerated overlying skin
- Associated arteriovenous fistulous component that cannot be occluded with concerns for venous embolizations
  - Especially in the setting of patent foramen ovale (PFO)
  - Emissary veins leading to cavernous sinus in head and face vascular malformations

Preprocedural Evaluation

Evaluate Prior Cross-Sectional Imaging

- Look for radiographic findings to support the diagnosis of vascular malformation
  - Contrast-enhanced magnetic resonance imaging (MRI) and magnetic resonance angiography (MRA)
    - These are the primary diagnostic modalities in most institutions.
    - Contrast-filled tuft of abnormal vessels and/or flow voids in high-flow vascular malformations – small soft tissue mass relative to the overall mass effect created by vascular malformations (see findings below under Contrast-enhanced computed tomography [CT] and computed tomography angiography [CTA])

- Lymphangiomas (**Fig. 21.1A**)
  - May have varying MRI signals on T1- and T2-weighted images depending on the degree of proteinaceous fluid within the cysts and presence/age of hemorrhage within the cystic components of the lymphangiomas
  - Remember, that soft tissue components may evolve into complex lymphangiomas.
  - One can categorize, based on MRI, whether lymphangiomas are microcytic, macrocytic, or mixed. This helps with the prognosis of determining response to percutaneous therapy (microcytic are most refractory to percutaneous therapy)
- If a large soft tissue and/or fat component is seen, the lesion may not be a true vascular malformation, but a soft tissue tumor with a vascular component.
- MRI and MRA provide reproducible examinations that can be used as a baseline comparative exam after treatment.
  - Contrast-enhanced computed tomography (CT) and computed tomography angiography (CTA)
    - These are not the primary diagnostic modalities, but they are used as baseline studies. This is because CT/CTA is the most reproducible and most available cross-sectional study (more reproducible

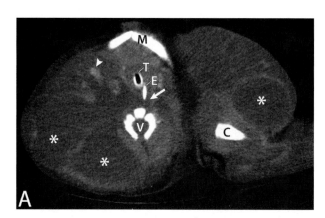
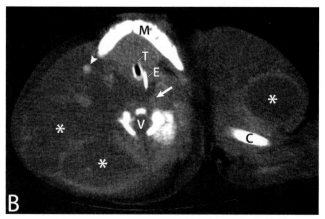

Fig. 21.1 Lymphangioma (cystic hygroma): imaging and therapy. **(A)** Axial computed tomography (CT) image of the upper neck at the level of the mentum (M, mentum/mandible) of a neonate with Klippel-Trenaunay syndrome exhibiting multiple neck, axillary, and chest lymphangiomas. The low-density areas are the cystic lymphangiomas. Asterisks mark some of the clearly defined cysts. The lymphangiomas are seen dissecting deep around the carotid artery (*arrowhead*), which seems suspended in the lymphangioma. In this image, the lymphangioma is seen dissecting deep and crossing the midline (from right to left) posterior to the trachea (T) with an endotracheal tube in it and the esophagus (E) with an nasogastric tube in it and anterior to the vertebral (V) column. The left clavicular (C) head is incidentally seen in this axial

image. **(B)** Axial CT image of the upper neck at a higher (more cephalad) level than in **Fig. 21.1A** (despite this, the clavicle, C, is seen in its shaft because the left shoulder girdle is raised due to left axillary lymphangiomas which are not seen in this image). Again, seen in the low-density areas are the cystic lymphangiomas. Asterisks mark the continuum of the clearly defined cysts marked in **Fig. 21.1A**. The lymphangiomas are seen dissecting deep around the carotid artery (*arrowhead*), which seems suspended in the lymphangioma. In this image, the lymphangioma is seen dissecting deep and crossing the midline (*from right to left*) posterior to the trachea (T) with an endotracheal tube in it and the esophagus (E) with an nasogastric tube in it and anterior to the vertebral (V) column.

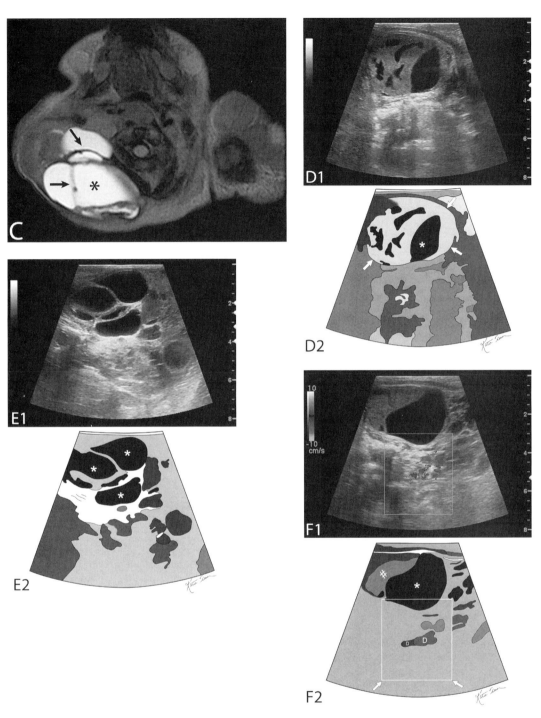

Fig. 21.1 *(Continued)* **(C)** Axial T2-weighted magnetic resonance (MR) image of the neck of the same neonate with Klippel-Trenaunay syndrome. Again seen are the cystic components of the lymphangiomas with their high T2-weighted signal intensity. Low signal intensity septa are seen (*arrows*) traversing the macrocytic part of the lymphangioma. An asterisk marks one of the larger simple cystic components of the lymphangioma. **(D)** Gray-scale ultrasound image (*top*) and schematic sketch (*bottom*) of the lymphangiomas of the right neck of the same neonate as in **Figs 21.1A–21.1C**. The complexity of the lymphangiomas (*between arrows*) now is more apparent that what was conveyed in the axial CT and MR images. An asterisk marks one of the larger cystic components of the lymphangioma. Around it is the sponge-like appearance of the soft tissue component of the malformation (*arrows pointing to lymphangioma*). **(E)** Gray-scale ultrasound image (*top*) and schematic sketch (*bottom*) of the same lymphangioma of the right neck as in **Fig. 21.1D**. More cystic compartments (*) with traversing septa are seen in this part of the lymphangioma. **(F)** Doppler image (*top*) (*arrow pointing to Doppler box*) and schematic sketch (*bottom*) of the same lymphangioma as in **Figs. 21.1A–21.1E**. The carotid vessels (D, Doppler) are seen deep to this particular cystic component of the lymphangioma. The asterisk and the # sign mark the cystic and soft tissue aspects of the visualized lymphangioma component, respectively.   *(Continued on page 284)*

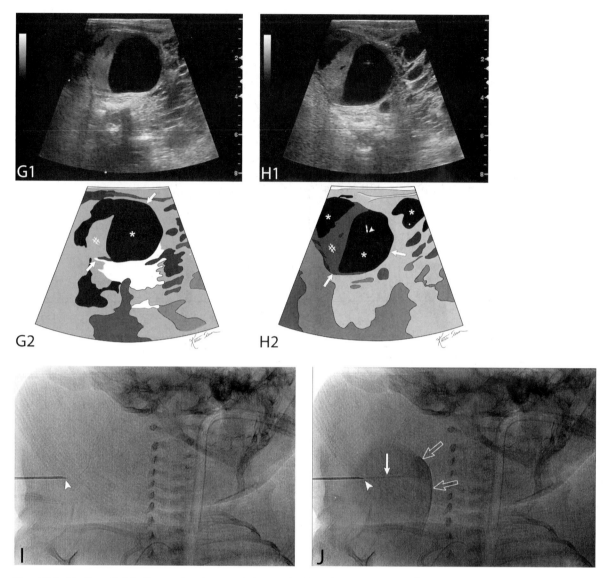

Fig. 21.1 *(Continued)* **(G)** Gray-scale ultrasound image *(top)* and schematic sketch *(bottom)* of the lymphangiomas of the right neck of the same neonate just prior to accessing the cyst for direct percutaneous sclerotherapy. The asterisk and the # sign mark the cystic and soft tissue aspects of the visualized lymphangioma *(between arrows)* component, respectively. **(H)** Gray-scale ultrasound image *(top)* and schematic sketch *(bottom)* of the lymphangiomas of the right neck after accessing a cystic locule with a 21-gauge needle *(arrowhead)*. The asterisks and the # sign mark the cystic and soft tissue aspects of the visualized lymphangioma *(between arrows)* component, respectively. At this time, the procedure is converted from real-time ultrasound guidance to real-time fluoroscopic guidance. **(I)** Fluoroscopic spot image with the 21-gauge needle in the cystic component of the lymphangioma *(arrowhead at needle tip)*. **(J)** Fluoroscopic spot image during contrast injection through the 21-gauge needle in the cystic component of the lymphangioma *(arrowhead at needle tip)*. Notice the jet of contrast *(solid arrow)* as it traverses the cyst and hits the back wall *(hollow arrows)* of the cystic locule.**(K)** Fluoroscopic spot image after contrast injection through the 21-gauge needle in the cystic component (*) of the lymphangioma *(arrowhead at needle tip)*. There is no communication with vital cavities or draining veins. It is safe to inject the sclerosant. The operators prefer to use a catheter or sheath and not a needle especially as a sclerosant such as doxycycline is used, which requires a long sclerosant dwell time 30–60 minutes prior to aspiration. **(L)** Fluoroscopic spot image with the 21-gauge needle in the cystic component of the lymphangioma *(arrowhead at needle tip)*. A 0.018-inch wire has been passed through the needle and is coiling in the cystic locule *(arrows)*. **(M)** Fluoroscopic spot image with a 5-French short micropuncture sheath in the collection *(arrows)*. The contrast in the cyst has been partly aspirated prior to the doxycycline concoction administration. **(N)** Fluoroscopic spot image as the 5-French short micropuncture sheath in the collection is being pulled back *(arrows)*. The operator is aspirating the contrast as the sheath is being pulled back, but not completely out *(arrowheads)*. Blunt (sheath) access is to be maintained to administer the doxycycline mixture (300 mg of doxycycline powder reconstituted by 15 cc of normal saline and 5 cc of 1% lidocaine). **(O)** Gray-scale ultrasound image *(top)* and schematic sketch *(bottom)* of the lymphangiomas of the right neck after the doxycycline mixture (300 mg of doxycycline powder reconstituted by 15 cc of normal saline and 5 cc of 1% lidocaine) has been administered through the 5-French sheath *(arrowhead at tip of 5-French sheath)* into the target locule *(arrows)*. Notice the isoechoic fluid mixture, which is more echogenic due to small bubbles suspended within the doxycycline. Superficial to the target locule is an untreated (not accessed) adjacent cyst (*). **(P)** Fluoroscopic spot image with the 5-French short micropuncture sheath in the collection *(arrows)*. The doxycycline mixture (300 mg of doxycycline powder reconstituted by 15 cc of normal saline and 5 cc of 1% lidocaine) has been dwelling in the cyst *(arrowheads)* for 30–40 minutes.

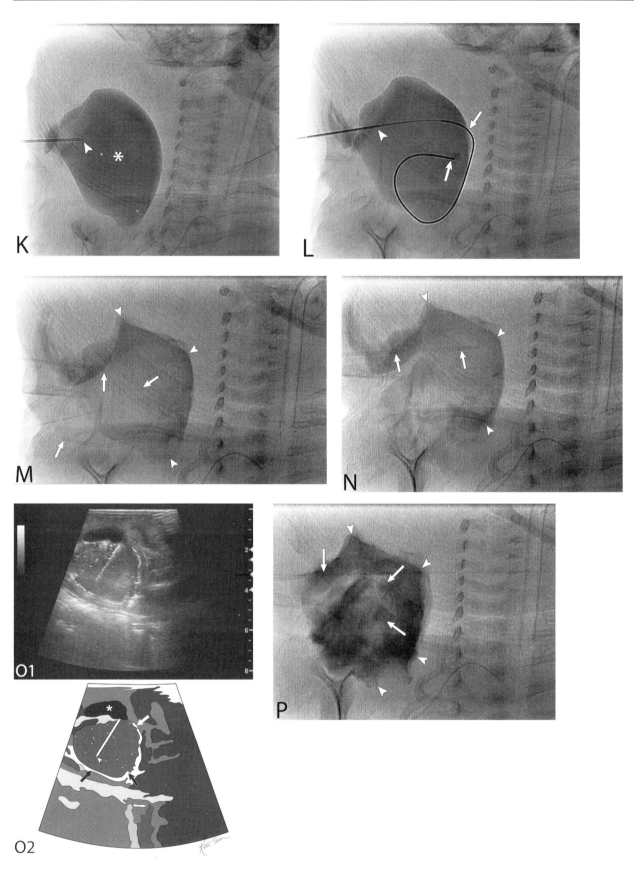

Fig. 21.1 *(Continued)*

and more available than MRI/MRA especially when repeated in between treatment sessions).

- This is particularly true after treatments commence because hemorrhage and postsclerosis inflammation may confuse the diagnosis or mask the positive response to treatment when evaluating posttherapy vascular malformations with MRI/MRA (an anecdote).
- Findings
  - Contrast-filled tuft of abnormal vessels
  - Delayed images may be required in slower flowing vascular malformations
  - Feeding vessel(s) if any/if seen
    - Should be seen in high-flow vascular malformations
    - Can be single (simple vascular malformation) or multiple (complex vascular malformation)
  - Draining vessel(s) if any/if seen
    - Should be seen in high-flow vascular malformations
    - Can be large caliber and meandering especially in high-flow vascular malformations

  - Small soft tissue mass relative to the overall mass effect created by vascular malformations
- CT is a reliable modality to get the "lay of the land." It can identify underlying and overlying structures. CT/CTA will clarify the orientation of the vascular malformation relative to surrounding/associated structures and organs (**Figs. 21.1B and 21.1C**).
  - Underlying structures can be potentially injured.
  - Overlying structures can be inadvertently transgressed (injured), intentionally transgressed, or avoided if possible.
- Doppler ultrasound
  - This is not the primary diagnostic modality, but it is valuable particularly when contemplating a direct percutaneous approach.
  - Low-flow vascular malformations may not be detected (may not "light-up") by Doppler ultrasound. The flow may be so slow it is undetectable even by power Doppler, which is sensitive in detecting vascular flow (**Fig. 21.2**).

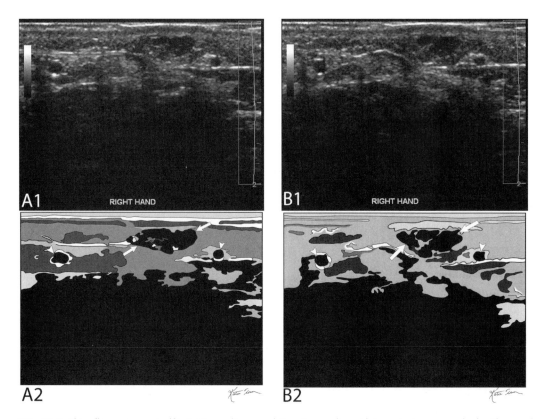

Fig. 21.2 Slow-flow venous malformation: ultrasound imaging and therapy. **(A)** Gray-scale ultrasound image of a superficial and small slow-flow venous malformation in the palm (hypothenar eminence) of a young woman's hand (*top*) and schematic sketch of it (*bottom*). The *arrows* point to the localized hypoechoic tuft of vessels. Adjacent palmar arteries are marked with *arrowheads*. **(B)** Gray-scale ultrasound image of the same superficial slow-flow venous malformation in the palm (*top*) at an adjacent site and schematic sketch of it (*bottom*). The *arrows* point to the localized hypoechoic tuft of vessels. Adjacent palmar arteries are marked with *arrowheads*.

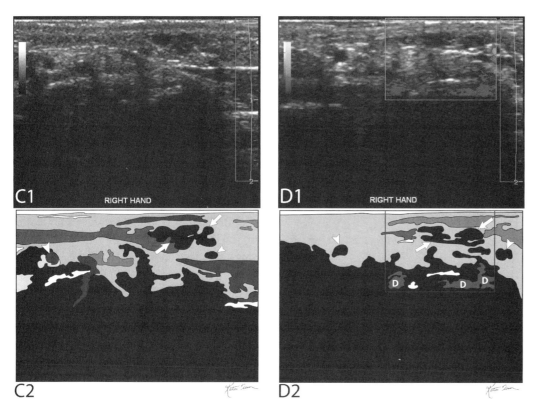

Fig. 21.2 *(Continued)* **(C)** Gray-scale ultrasound image of the same superficial slow-flow venous malformation in the palm (*top*) at an adjacent site and schematic sketch of it (*bottom*). The *arrows* point to the localized hypoechoic tuft of vessels. Adjacent palmar arteries are marked with *arrowheads*. **(D)** Doppler image (*top*) and schematic sketch of it (*bottom*) of the same venous malformation (*arrows*) as in **Figs. 21.2A–21.2C**. Power Doppler ultrasound coloring (D) deep to the venous malformation is seen. However, power Doppler is not able to detect flow within the venous malformation. This is typical of slow-flow venous and lymphangiovenous malformation where blood flow is so slow that it is not picked up by color Doppler or even the more sensitive power Doppler. Adjacent palmar arteries are marked with *arrowheads*. *(Continued on page 287)*

- Aliasing can be seen in very high-flow components of the vascular malformation or with high-flow arteriovenous shunting.
- Complex high-flow vascular malformations can be confusing by Doppler with numerous feeders, tortuosity, and numerous draining veins.
- Doppler ultrasound is valuable in diagnosing and determining the rate of flow of the vascular malformation (high-flow, slow-venous flow, undetectable flow, etc.).
○ Conventional angiography
  - This is the traditional gold standard imaging diagnosis of vascular malformations especially high-flow vascular malformations. MRI/MRA has become the gold standard for low-flow vascular malformations.
  - Contrast is seen filling tortuous vessels with draining veins (**Figs. 21.3, 21.4, 21.5**). A central tuft of abnormal vessels is probably the nidus or vessels around the nidus.
  - Venous slow-flow malformations may not be evident on digital subtraction angiography due to

very slow flow (**Fig. 21.4**). They maybe detected by delayed fluoroscopic spot images.
- Look for and study overlying organs and/or structures.
  ○ Plan to avoid overlying structures
  ○ Plan to transgress overlying structures/organs intentionally
  ○ Identify overlying vessels and adjacent vessels to avoid traversing them or misidentifying them by Doppler ultrasound as being part of the vascular malformation (avoid nontarget embolization/sclerosis)

Evaluate Pretreatment Laboratory Values

- Laboratory value evaluation mostly revolves around ruling out coagulopathy.
- Acceptable coagulopathy parameters are not set.
  ○ Suggested coagulopathy thresholds for superficial vascular malformations are
    - International normalized ratio (INR): ≤1.7–1.8
    - Platelets (PLT): ≥40,000
    - Activated partial thromboplastin time (aPTT): ≤65 seconds

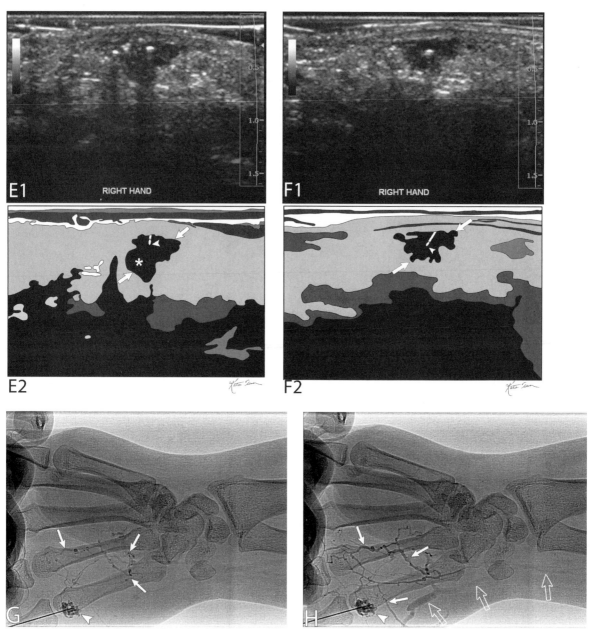

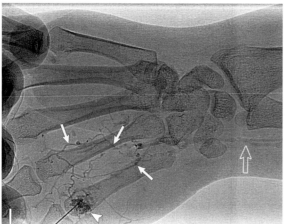

Fig. 21.2 *(Continued)* **(E)** Gray-scale ultrasound image of the same superficial slow-flow venous malformation in the palm *(top)* at an adjacent site and schematic sketch of it *(bottom)*. The venous malformation (* = *tuft of abnormal veins*) has been accessed using a 23-gauge butterfly needle *(arrowhead at needle tip)*. The *arrows* point to the outer confines of the tuft of abnormal venous vessels. **(F)** Gray-scale ultrasound image of the same superficial slow-flow venous malformation in the palm *(top)* at an adjacent site and schematic sketch of it *(bottom)*. The venous malformation has been accessed using a 23-gauge butterfly needle *(arrowhead at needle tip)*. The *arrows* point to the outer confines of the tuft of abnormal venous vessels. At this time, the procedure is converted from real-time ultrasound guidance to real-time fluoroscopic guidance. **(G,H,I)** Fluoroscopic spot images in series with the 23-gauge butterfly needle in the tuft of abnormal vessels *(arrowhead)*. A tangle of abnormal draining veins *(solid arrows)* is seen leading to normal draining ulnar veins *(hollow arrows)*. This is followed by 98–99% absolute alcohol injection through the 23-gauge needle under real-time fluoroscopy as the operator sees the contrast being displaced with alcohol and washed away in the draining veins.

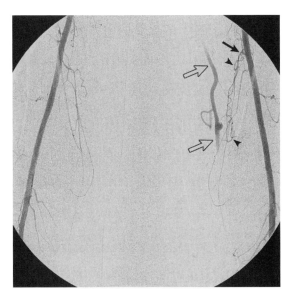

Fig. 21.3 Lower extremity angiogram demonstrating a left midthigh arteriovenous malformation (AVM) (*arrowheads*). The AVM is supplied by branches (*solid arrow*) from left superficial femoral artery (SFA) and is being drained by an early draining vein (*hollow arrows*).

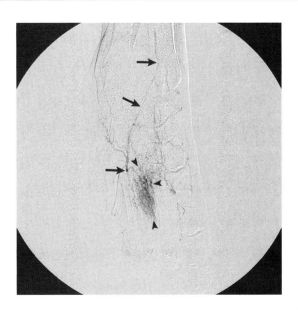

Fig. 21.4 Lower extremity angiogram demonstrating a right foot arteriovenous malformation (AVM) (*arrowheads*). The AVM is supplied by arterial branches (*solid arrows*) from dorsalis pedis artery. No draining vein is seen.

○ Suggested coagulopathy thresholds for deep vascular malformations and/or possible transgression of viscera are
  • INR: ≤1.4
  • PLT: ≥50,000
  • aPTT: ≤65 seconds

• Thrombocytopenia may be a feature of large vascular malformations that may break up platelets and reduce their count (consumption coagulopathy: Kasselbach-Merritt syndrome). In this situation, it is best to transfuse platelets during the procedure. Transfusing platelets before the procedure may not raise the

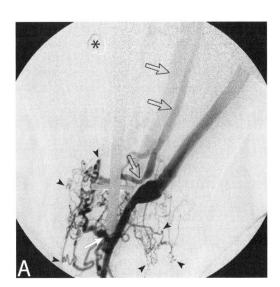

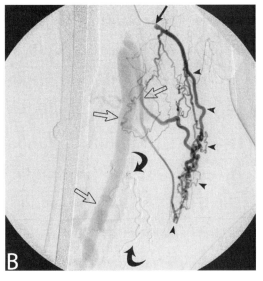

Fig. 21.5 (A) Lower extremity angiogram demonstrating a right midthigh high-throughput arteriovenous malformation (AVM) (*arrowheads*) in a man status postgunshot wound in his distant past (** over subtracted bullet fragment*). The AVM is supplied by branches (*solid arrow*) from the right superficial femoral artery (SFA) and is being drained by an early draining vein (*hollow arrows*). **(B)** Lower extremity angiogram demonstrating another component of the right midthigh high-throughput arteriovenous malformation (AVM) (*arrowheads*). This AVM component is more selectively catheterized by a 5-French vertebral catheter (*solid arrow*). Again, noted is an early draining vein (*hollow arrows*). The operator is in position to inject n-butyl-2-cyanoacrylate (glue). Notice the subtracted glue in an adjacent AVM component (*curved arrows*). (Continued on page 290)

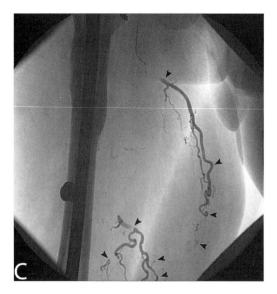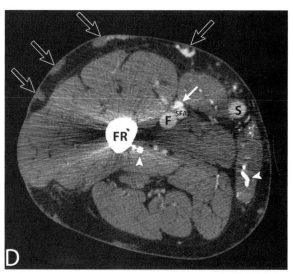

Fig. 21.5 *(Continued)* **(C)** Fluoroscopic spot image of the right thigh after two *n*-butyl-2-cyanoacrylate (glue) injections in two different AVM arborized components (*arrowheads*). The 5-French catheter is still in position for a posttreatment angiogram. The glue that is "casting" the upper AVM component was injected through a microcatheter, which was placed coaxially through the 5-French catheter and "yanked" quickly at the end of the glue injection. **(D)** Axial contrast-enhanced computed tomography (CT) image of the right thigh of the patient in **Figs. 21.5A–21.5C** after glue therapy of some components of this complex high-flow AVM. High-density glue cast in deep and superficial AVM vessels is seen (*arrowheads*). Dilated early enhancing greater saphenous vein (S) and femoral vein (F) are seen reflecting the high-throughput fistulous aspect of the AVM. A hypertrophied branch off the right superficial femoral artery (SFA) is seen (*solid arrow*), which feeds the more superficial AVM (*hollow arrows*). Notice the varying enhancement levels of the superficial AVM components (*hollow arrows*), which reflect varying throughputs (flow velocities) and represent different distances from the feeding arteries (more enhancing may be closer to the feeding artery, more on the arterial side, whereas less enhancing may be further for the feeding artery and more on the venous side). The beam hardening artifact is from the intramedullary metal rod in the femoral shaft (FR).

platelet count above its required threshold (40–50,000 platelets/mm³).

Obtain Informed Consent

The most important part of the procedure in managing vascular malformations is counseling patients and their families. The patient should have realistic expectations and should understand the risks versus the benefit of these procedures. A "cure" is usually not achieved. Treating vascular malformations is a balance between achieving therapeutic response and avoiding complications (collateral damage). Learn from your complications. When repeating treatment sessions, reduce the extent of "aggression" that was used on the prior session, which led to the complication.

- Indications
  - Be conservative in your consent
    - Be cautiously optimistic
    - You will not cure or completely resolve the problem.
    - You are attempting to reduce or relieve the symptoms.
    - If symptoms resolve after the procedure, they may recur in the long-term.
    - To help reduce the pain, deformity, and mass effect
    - Improvement in symptoms is difficult to gauge objectively; however, a common percentage of improvement that is quoted is 70–75%.
- Alternatives
  - To refuse the procedure (observation). Not unreasonable for asymptomatic vascular malformations
  - Surgical
    - Reasonable when the entire involved region is removed and the vascular malformation within it is removed completely
    - Partial surgical removal will cause recurrences and may preclude, if not make more difficult, endoluminal therapy.
    - Surgery may be enlisted for the rapid debulking of lesions.
  - Intralesional laser photocoagulation
    - Applied through catheters or large cannulas
    - More applicable to longitudinally oriented malformations
    - Less swelling and inflammation postprocedure and faster recovery when compared with direct percutaneous sclerosis
    - Best results obtained when combined with direct percutaneous sclerosis

- Procedural risks
  - Overall, 12% of procedures will have complications (range: 10–30%).
  - As repeated therapies are more likely required, the cumulative risk to the individual patient increases (up to 30% of patients may eventually sustain at least one complication).
- Major complications are
  - Cardiovascular collapse (more in children)
  - Pulmonary emboli
  - Morbid swelling
    - Compartment syndrome (denervation and ischemia)
    - Compression of airway if in neck (more in children)
    - Problems with swallowing (more in neck lesions in children)
- Minor complications are
  - Swelling without space-occupying secondary complications (common)
  - Skin blistering (common)
  - Nonhealing ulceration (considered major if in head and neck)
  - Nerve injury
    - 1% of procedures and 10% of patients
    - Usually minor or self-limiting

Equipment

Ultrasound Guidance and Compression

- Ultrasound machine with Doppler capability
- Linear 7–9 MHz ultrasound transducer
- Some operators use high-frequency transducers (7.5–12 MHz)
- A guidance bracket (needle guide) is usually not necessary for superficial vascular malformations. In fact, needle access, once placed, can be tenuous and disengaging the needle from the guide may result in the needle falling out of the vascular malformation.
- Sterile transducer cover

Standard Surgical Preparation and Draping

- Chlorhexidine skin preparation/cleansing fluid
- Fenestrated drape

Local Infiltrative Analgesia Administration

- 21-gauge infiltration needle
- 5–10 mL 1% lidocaine syringe for a deep vascular malformation
- If superficial anesthesia and general anesthesia are used, lidocaine may not necessarily be employed.

Sharp Access

- 20- to 25-gauge needle
- 21- to 25-gauge butterfly needles for superficial vascular malformations are preferred.
- For lymphangiomatous malformations (lymphangiomas, cystic hygromas) with large volumes of cystic fluid to be aspirated, larger bore needles are used (20- to 21-gauge needles).

Sclerosant Administration Reservoir

- 1 to 10 mL syringe depending on the sclerosant used
  - Alcohol usually requires 1–3 mL fortified syringe.
  - Doxycycline for larger macrocytic lymphangiomas requires larger syringes (not necessarily fortified syringes).
- Connector tube to connect between the needle and the syringe. This allows flexibility and nimble manipulating of the needle while being ready to respond by injecting thrombin.

Sclerosants Used

Various sclerosants have been used to treat vascular malformations.
- 95–98% Alcohol (ETOH)
  - The more traditional sclerosant
  - Used for endoluminal and direct percutaneous techniques
  - Used for all types of vascular malformations
  - Edema and inflammation more common with alcohol
  - Requires general anesthesia
    - For intraprocedural exquisite pain management
    - Cardiopulmonary support especially in
      - Children
      - Poor cardiopulmonary reserve patients
      - Pulmonary hypertension (considered a contraindication by some)
      - High doses of alcohol will be used.
  - Maximum alcohol dose
    - 0.5– 1.0 mL/kilogram body weight (kg BW) with a ceiling of 40 mL total per session
    - >0.5 mL/kg BW has a risk of cardiopulmonary collapse. Consider maximum dose of 0.5 mL/kg BW for high-risk cardiopulmonary collapse patients
      - Children
      - Poor cardiopulmonary reserve patients
      - Pulmonary hypertension (considered a contraindication by some)
- Sodium tetradecyl sulfate (STS; detergent)
  - Used for slow-flow vascular malformation
  - Usually not used for lymphangiomatous malformations
  - Maximum dose for STS: 0.5 mL/kg BW with a ceiling of 20 mL total per session

- Doxycycline
  - Used primarily for slow-flow vascular malformation
  - Usually used for lymphangiomatous malformations
  - Can be mixed with water-soluble contrast for fluoroscopic visualization

Technique

Intravenous Access

- The necessity for moderate sedation or general anesthesia (administered intravenously)
- Intravenous access is required for cardiopulmonary support.

Pretreatment Clinical Exam

- Evaluate the overlying skin for necrosis and/or infection
- If possible, may want to avoid the most superficial aspect of the vascular malformation (may reduce local ulcerations at the access site)
- Determine the baseline distal arterial status (pulses, ankle-brachial indices [ABIs])

Pretreatment Ultrasound Exam

- Determine the overall size of the vascular malformation, its dimensions, and its hemodynamics
- Determine the relation of the vascular malformation with adjacent normal-appearing vessels
- Evaluate for arteriovenous shunting; try to keep needle access away from shunting sites
- If possible, may want to avoid the most superficial aspect of the vascular malformation (may reduce local ulcerations at the access site)
- Make sure there are no vessels or structures between the skin and the vascular malformation. These vessels should be avoided.
  - They may be injured in the process by the access needle.
  - They may be thrombosed/sclerosed or their distal aspects embolized by inadvertent sclerosant injection.
- Based on the ultrasound exam findings and the status of the overlying skin findings, depth of lesion, adjacent vessels and/or structures, the decision to proceed with the treatment and the ideal needle access site and approach are determined.

Standard Surgical Preparation and Draping

- Skin preparation/cleansing in the region that was chosen as an ultrasound imaging portal and a needle access needle portal

- Place a fenestrated drape at the chosen and prepared skin region

Local Infiltrative Analgesia Administration

- Utilizing a 21-gauge infiltration needle, 1% lidocaine infiltration is performed.
- Do not enter the vascular malformation. A superficial wheal is enough.
- Some operators do not use lidocaine infiltration (no local anesthetic), especially if the lesion is very superficial and the patient is heavily sedated or under general anesthesia.

Sharp Access

- The Doppler ultrasound is switched to gray-scale ultrasound mode for real-time guidance.
- Real-time gray-scale ultrasound is used to image the needle tip.
- Needle ranges: 21- to 25-gauge
- Use free-hand ultrasound guidance of the needle (**Figs. 21.1, 21.2, and 21.6**)
- Once the needle tip is in an adequate position in the vascular malformation, the procedure is converted to fluoroscopic guidance (**Figs. 21.1, 21.2, 21.6, and 21.7**).

Sclerosant Administration

- Alcohol sclerosant
  - Technical variant 1
    - Contrast can be injected through the butterfly needle to evaluate for
      - Adequate placement of the needle into the vascular malformation
      - Volume required to fill vascular malformation
      - Rate of injection (flow) required to gently fill the vascular malformation
      - Rule out high-flow shunting to see if it is safe for sclerosis (high-flow shunting may be embolized with coils to slow them down to increase "dwell time" of the alcohol)
      - Identify the draining vein(s) and test if you can occlude them by compressing them. If so, rehearse it.
    - Alcohol is then injected at the same volume and rate as the prior contrast injection. The contrast is observed as it washes out (displaced) by the alcohol. If possible, compress the draining vein to shut or minimize the outflow and maximize the dwell time of the alcohol in the vascular malformation.

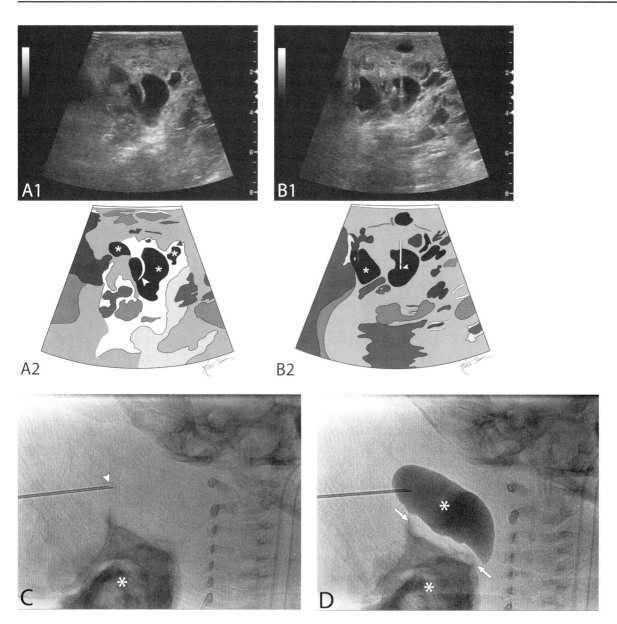

Fig. 21.6 Lymphangioma (cystic hygroma) ultrasound-guided direct percutaneous therapy with doxycycline. **(A)** Gray-scale ultrasound image (*top*) and schematic sketch (*bottom*) of the lymphangiomas of the right neck of the same neonate as in **Fig. 21.1**. The complexity of the lymphangiomas is noted where multiple cystic components are identified (*) interrupted by soft tissue and septa (*arrowhead*). The operator obtained this image just prior to accessing the cyst for direct percutaneous sclerotherapy. **(B)** Gray-scale ultrasound image (*top*) and schematic sketch (*bottom*) of the lymphangiomas of the right neck after accessing a cystic locule with a 21-gauge needle (*arrowhead*). The asterisk marks an adjacent cystic locule that was not accessed. At this time, the procedure is converted from real-time ultrasound guidance to real-time fluoroscopic guidance. **(C)** Fluoroscopic spot image with the

21-gauge needle in the cystic component of the lymphangioma (*arrowhead at needle tip*). The asterisk is in an adjacent cystic cavity that was treated with doxycycline in **Fig. 21.1**. **(D)** Fluoroscopic spot image after contrast injection through the 21-gauge needle in the cystic component (*upper asterisk*) of the lymphangioma. Notice the wide irregular soft tissue septum that stands between the accessed cyst (*upper asterisk*) and the prior treated cyst (*lower asterisk*). There is no communication with vital cavities or draining veins. It is safe to inject the sclerosant. The operators prefer to use a catheter or sheath and not a needle especially if a sclerosant such as doxycycline is used, which requires a long sclerosant dwell time (30–60 minutes) prior to aspiration. *(Continued on page 294)*

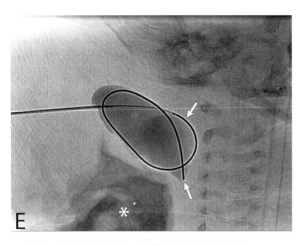

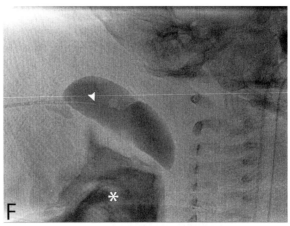

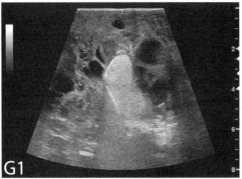

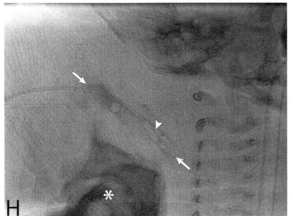

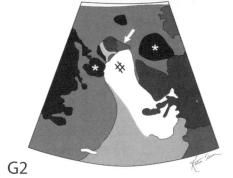

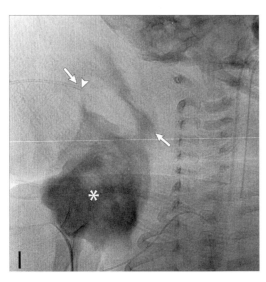

Fig. 21.6 *(Continued)* **(E)** Fluoroscopic spot image with the 21-gauge needle in the cystic component of the lymphangioma. A 0.018-inch wire has been passed through the needle and is coiling in the cystic locule (*arrows*). The asterisk marks the adjacent, treated cyst that has residual contrast and doxycycline that have not been completely aspirated from the prior treatment. **(F)** Fluoroscopic spot image with a 5-French short micropuncture sheath in the collection (*arrowhead*). The contrast in the cyst is about to be aspirated prior to the doxycycline mixture administration. The asterisk is in an adjacent cystic cavity, which was treated with doxycycline in **Fig. 21.1**. **(G)** Gray-scale ultrasound image (*top*) and schematic sketch (*bottom*) of the lymphangiomas of the right neck after the doxycycline mixture (300 mg of doxycycline powder reconstituted by 15 cc of normal saline and 5 cc of 1% lidocaine) has been administered through the 5-French sheath into the target locule. Notice the hyperechoic fluid concoction with shadowing (#). This hyperechogenicity is due to numerous microbubbles in the doxycycline emulsion (just like ultrasound contrast microbubbles). Superficial to the target locule is a partly untreated adjacent cyst (*arrow*). Adjacent cysts that are not accessed are marked with asterisks. **(H)** Fluoroscopic spot image with the 5-French short micropuncture sheath in the collection (*arrowhead at sheath tip*). The doxycycline mixture (300 mg of doxycycline powder reconstituted by 15 cc of normal saline and 5 cc of 1% lidocaine) has been aspirated almost completely after it had dwelled in the cyst for 40 minutes. The cyst has almost completely collapsed (*between arrows*) and has air bubbles within it. The asterisk marks the adjacent, treated cyst that has residual contrast and doxycycline that have not been completely aspirated from the prior treatment (**Fig. 21.1**). Not all cysts can be aspirated completely of the sclerosant, especially irregular complex cysts with irregular mural soft tissue components. **(I)** Fluoroscopic spot image, which is an overview of **Fig. 21.6H**, with the 5-French short micropuncture sheath in the collection (*arrowhead at sheath tip*). The doxycycline mixture (300 mg of doxycycline powder reconstituted by 15 cc of normal saline and 5 cc of 1% lidocaine) has been aspirated almost completely after it had dwelled in the cyst for 40 minutes. The cyst has almost completely collapsed (*between arrows*).

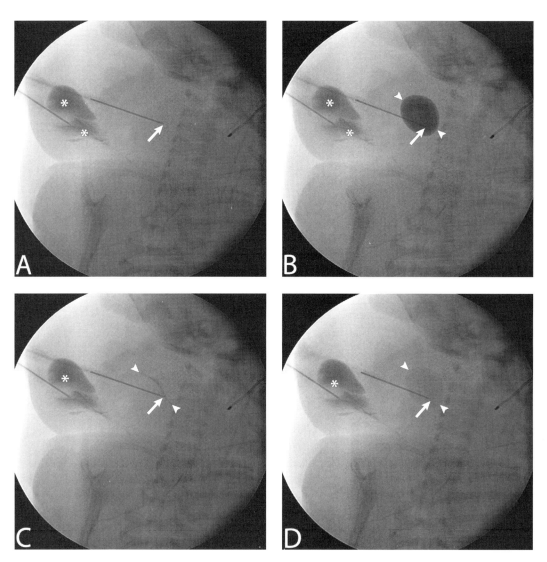

Fig. 21.7 Lymphangioma (cystic hygroma) ultrasound-guided direct percutaneous therapy with absolute alcohol. **(A)** Fluoroscopic spot image with the 21-gauge needle in a cystic component of the lymphangioma (*arrow at needle tip*). The asterisks are in an adjacent cystic cavity, which was treated with absolute (98–99%) alcohol. The 21-gauge needle was placed in this smaller simple cystic component via real-time ultrasound guidance. **(B)** Fluoroscopic spot image with the 21-gauge needle in a cystic component of the lymphangioma (*arrow at needle tip*). Contrast has been injected to fill the cyst (*between arrowheads*). There are no communications with adjacent vital cavities or vessels. The asterisks are in an adjacent cystic cavity, which was treated with absolute (98–99%) alcohol. The 21-gauge needle was placed in this smaller simple cystic component via real-time ultrasound guidance. **(C)** Fluoroscopic spot image with the 21-gauge needle in a cystic component of the lymphangioma (*arrow at needle tip*). Contrast that had been injected to fill the cyst depicted in **Fig. 21.7B** has been aspirated (*between arrowheads*). Only a wisp of contrast is seen in the collapsed cavity (*between arrowheads*). At this time, the operator is ready to refill the cavity/cyst by replacing the contrast volume aspirated with the same volume of absolute alcohol. The asterisks are in an adjacent cystic cavity, which was treated with absolute (98–99%) alcohol. **(D)** Fluoroscopic spot image with the 21-gauge needle in a cystic component of the lymphangioma (*arrow at needle tip*). The operator has refilled the cavity/cyst by replacing the contrast volume aspirated with the same volume of absolute alcohol. The asterisks are in an adjacent cystic cavity, which was treated with absolute (98–99%) alcohol. The absolute alcohol is allowed to dwell for 10–15 minutes, then it is aspirated out as much as possible.

- This can be repeated.
- Be cautious that the patient must be in deep general anesthesia. If not in deep anesthesia, the patient may retract the extremity as a flexor reflex response to pain and you may lose needle access.

  ○ Technical variant 2
  - The alcohol can be admixed with lipid-based contrast (lipiodol, ethiodol) to visualize the alcohol as it is administered.
  - Water-soluble contrast cannot be used because it precipitates with the alcohol.

- STS
  - Administered in similar techniques to alcohol (see above)
  - STS has a foam consistency.
  - If admixed with contrast, it can be admixed (unlike alcohol) with either water or fat-soluble contrast agents.
  - When admixed with contrast, it is in a ratio of 1:10 to 3:10 (contrast to sclerosant).
  - STS is injected gently as to occupy the entire vascular malformation.
  - STS injection can be repeated after 5 minutes.
  - Operator stops injection when
    - The lesion is firm to palpation.
    - No additional blood returns when aspirating from the access needle.
    - Ultrasonography demonstrates adequate filling of the entire visualized lesion.
    - The lesion blanches or becomes pale.
- *n*-butyl-2-cyanoacrylate (NBCA; glue)
  - For direct percutaneous treatment of vascular malformations – rarely used
  - More likely used in endoluminal techniques
  - Some operators will not use it by any means (endoluminal nor direct percutaneous) because they believe that it recannulates and does not truly sclerose the abnormal endothelium of the vascular malformation.
  - Not used by me for the direct percutaneous treatment of vascular malformations, but I do use it for endoluminal therapy of vascular malformations (**Fig. 21.5**)

Immediate Posttreatment Ultrasound Imaging

- Ultrasound is not very effective in evaluating the following points especially if it is a very slow-flow vascular malformation.
- Helps determine endpoint (success), which is the filling of the vascular malformation with sclerosant
- Evaluate for residual flow by Doppler ultrasound, especially residual pockets of flow in the vascular malformation

Endpoints

Therapeutic Response

- Technical endpoints
  - Firmness of the lesion and swelling. This is a good sign that a therapeutic clinical response will ensue barring a complication.
  - Blanching of the lesion
- Clinical endpoints of success in the long-term
  - Occur in 70–75% of cases
  - Difficult to gauge because they are subjective and usually require patient questionnaires

- They include
  - Improved limb function
  - Reduced pain
  - Reduced deformity or disfigurement

No Immediate Complications

- Skin blistering to skin sloughing to chronic ulceration
  - Blanching or dusky color of overlying skin is not uncommon. Ulceration may not develop.
  - Placing cold compresses may reduce the risk of ulceration.
  - More likely to occur with alcohol
- Swelling is not uncommon.
  - Sign of good therapeutic response
  - Swelling is more common with alcohol.
  - Swelling may case compartment syndrome (see below).
- Pulmonary emboli
  - May occur when tourniquets are removed or the patient ambulates
- See below for detailed management of complications.

Postprocedural Evaluation and Management

Most institutions perform direct percutaneous treatment of vascular malformations on adults on an outpatient basis. Infants and small children are usually admitted. Discharge is based upon sedation/anesthesia protocol usually.

Postprocedural Observation Period

- Postprocedural stay varies from one practice to the other.
- If patients are to stay briefly before discharge, they should stay for ~2 hours after treatment.
- During this period
  - The lesion is inspected for early signs of acute skin injury.
  - Cold compresses can be applied if significant discoloration is evident.
  - In cases of high-flow vascular malformations (arterial involvement), repeat distal arterial evaluation is made and compared with the baseline arterial evaluation.
- The first dose of steroids should have been given during the procedure. If not, give it during this period.

Intravenous Fluid and Diet

- Intravenous (IV) access should be kept until just prior discharge or after adequate oral intake for inpatients.
- Start clear liquid diet immediately and advance it as tolerated.

Activity

- Bed rest usually
- The region of the vascular malformation should be grossly immobilized.

Pain Management

- Narcotics are usually not required during the postbiopsy stay of the patient prior to discharge. Occasionally, some patients require oral narcotic analgesics such as acetaminophen and hydrocodone combination medication.
- On discharge, patients usually tolerate the procedure well and do not require analgesics more potent than over-the-counter medications.

Monitoring Vital Signs

- Vital sign monitoring includes blood pressure and heart rate.
- Due to conscious sedation/general anesthesia, a softer blood pressure than a patient's baseline blood pressure may be encountered after the vascular malformation treatment. This is the most likely due to sedation with or without dehydration. Patients usually respond with time by hydration and particularly as the sedatives wear off.

Complications and Their Management

The overall complication rate per procedure is 10–12%. The complication rate for the patient with multiple treatment sessions involved (cumulative risk of complications) is 28–30%. Treating vascular malformations is a balance between achieving therapeutic response and avoiding complications (collateral damage). Learn from your complications. When repeating treatment sessions, reduce the extent of "aggression" that led to the complication.

Management of Nerve Injury

- Incidence
  - Occurs after 1% of procedures
  - Occurs in 10% of patients (cumulatively with multiple sessions)
- More common with alcohol ablation
- Must rule out that is due to direct injury and not a sign of compartment syndrome
- Usually self-limiting and requires reassurance
- Usually requires supportive therapy

Management of Run-Away Swelling and Inflammatory Pain

- Common, especially if alcohol was used
- Sign of good therapeutic response

- Swelling may cause compartment syndrome (see below).
- If in the neck, swelling may affect breathing and swallowing.
- Management
  - Steroids (Solu-Medrol; Pfizer Pharmaceuticals, New York, NY)
    - Should be given prophylactically
    - First steroid dose should be given intraprocedurally
    - Continuation of the Solu-Medrol pack should be given as indicated by the manufacturer.
  - Cold compresses can be given.
  - Rule out compartment syndrome (see below)
  - If there is swelling in the neck and breathing difficulty, intubation may be required.

Management of Compartment Syndrome

- Not common, especially if operators are weary to avoid extensive treatment of vascular malformations in closed spaces (closed compartments) such as the orbit or muscle groups
- Usually due to significant inflammation and swelling – more common with alcohol
- Management
  - Early realization of the symptoms of the complication (early diagnosis)
    - Edema
    - Cold extremities
    - Compromised distal pulses
    - Numbness and tingling
  - Compartment pressures confirm the diagnosis
  - Surgical consult to confirm diagnosis and to perform fasciotomy is usually required.

Management of Overlying Skin Breakdown

- Skin breakdown is a collective description of various skin conditions including
  - Skin blistering
  - Skin necrosis and sloughing
  - Chronic ulceration with bleeding
- Skin blistering is not uncommon and usually heals uneventfully. It may be prevented with cold compresses at a stage when the overlying skin becomes extremely dusky or pale (blanched).
- Necrosis and sloughing and with chronicity, ulceration
  - Can occur in up to 10–15% of patients
  - Request a plastic surgery consult
  - Be patient and council the patient for a long healing process with scarring (may take months)
  - If a large area is involved, skin grafting may be required (plastic surgery consult).
  - Do not repeat treatment sessions during the healing process

○ Treating vascular malformations is a balance between achieving therapeutic response and avoiding complications (collateral damage). Learn from your complications. When repeating treatment sessions, reduce the extent of "aggression" that led to the complication.

Management of Distal Embolization

- If distal embolization is subclinical and only encountered by reduction in ABI
  ○ The patient should receive anticoagulation therapy.
  ○ Surgical consult
  ○ Serial ABI, pulse checks
  ○ If the situation becomes clinically evident, surgery is required.
- If an embolic event is clinically evident, an angiogram is performed with or without thrombolysis. Surgical thrombectomy is an alternative with or without a prior failed transcatheter thrombolysis.

- If tissue loss and necrosis occur, a plastic surgery consult may be required.

Management of Pulmonary Embolization

- Pulmonary embolization occurs
  ○ Immediately intraprocedurally
  ○ On removal of tourniquets
  ○ On patient ambulation
  ○ After discharge to home
- Symptoms depend on the severity of the pulmonary emboli (embolic burden) and the underlying cardiopulmonary reserve.
- Symptoms include
  ○ Asymptomatic
  ○ Stitching pleuritic pain
  ○ Shortness of breath
  ○ Cardiopulmonary collapse with or without myocardial infarction

Further Reading

Burrows PE, Alomari A. Management of low-flow vascular malformations. In: Mauro M, Murphy K, Thomson K, Venbrux A, Zollikofer C, eds. Image Guided Interventions. Philadelphia: Saunders; 2008:573–584

Burrows PE, Mason KP. Percutaneous treatment of low flow vascular malformations. J Vasc Interv Radiol 2004;15(5):431–445

Rosen RJ, Blei F. Interventional management of hemangiomas, arterio-venous fistulas and vascular malformations. In: Mauro M,

Murphy K, Thomson K, Venbrux A, Zollikofer C, eds. Image Guided Interventions. Philadelphia: Saunders; 2008:585–604

Yakes WF, Haas DK, Parker SH, et al. Symptomatic vascular malformations: ethanol embolotherapy. Radiology 1989;170(3 Pt 2):1059–1066

Yakes WF, Rossi P, Odink H. How I do it. Arteriovenous malformation management. Cardiovasc Intervent Radiol 1996;19(2):65–71

22 Management of Postcatheterization Pseudoaneurysm

Wael E.A. Saad and Christine O. Menias

Classification

Arterial pseudoaneurysms are the most common complication (61%) of femoral artery catheterization and are associated with increased morbidity. The overall incidence of postcatheterization pseudoaneurysms ranges from 0.11 to 1.52%. The incidence of access of pseudoaneurysms increases with transcatheter therapeutic interventions (3.5–5.5%) compared with studies confined to diagnostic arterial catheterizations (0.1–1.1%). Due to the ongoing paradigm shift in transcatheter endoluminal interventions as opposed to traditional open surgical interventions, the incidence of postcatheterization pseudoaneurysms is on the rise with ~15,000 femoral pseudoaneurysms diagnosed in the United States annually as of the year 2000.

Numerous methods, with variants within each method, for the management of postcatheterization pseudoaneurysms have been described. For the purposes of this chapter, the two most commonly described approaches (pseudoaneurysm compression and direct percutaneous thrombin injection) and their variant techniques will be discussed.

Indications

Due to the high success rate and low complication rate (see below) with the risk–benefit ratio largely in favor of treatment, the indication for treatment of postcatheterization access pseudoaneurysms is broad and involves almost all patients. However, it is particularly indicated if the postcatheterization access pseudoaneurysms are

- Painful
- Affecting ambulation
- Growing
- Larger than 1.8–2.0 cm in diameter (>6 cm in volume)

The following are lists that describe the ideal features that make each patient/pseudoaneurysm ideal for either ultrasound-guided compression therapy or direct ultrasound-guided percutaneous thrombin injection.

Pseudoaneurysm Compression

- Small pseudoaneurysms
- Long accessible necks (superficial)
- Intact overlying skin
- Patients not on anticoagulants

Direct Percutaneous Thrombin Injection

- Almost all patients with the exception of uncommon contraindications (see below)

Contraindications

Pseudoaneurysm Compression

Poor candidates for compression represent ~10% of all patients and 50% of intent-to-treat technical failures.

- Pain intolerance/painful pseudoaneurysms (25–34% of failures)
- Morbid obesity (13% of failures)
- Large pseudoaneurysms obliterating adjacent vascular structures (19% of failures)
- Associated arteriovenous fistulous (AVF) component (1–2% of pseudoaneurysms)
- Super-added infection or overlying skin breakdown
- Unstable patients (2% of failures)

Direct Percutaneous Thrombin Injection

The contraindications to direct percutaneous thrombin injection therapy include
- Infected pseudoaneurysms or overlying skin erosion/breakdown
- Ruptured pseudoaneurysms
- Associated AVF component
- Associated ipsilateral deep venous thrombosis (DVT)
- Previous treatment/exposure to bovine thrombin due to concerns for allergic reactions (relative contraindication)
- Documented allergic reaction to bovine thrombin

Preprocedural Evaluation

Evaluate Prior Cross-Sectional Imaging

- Look for radiographic findings to support the diagnosis of postcatheterization access pseudoaneurysm
  - ○ Real-time gray-scale ultrasound
    - Hypoechoic lesion/mass in the groin (**Figs. 22.1 and 22.2**)
    - Pulsatile hypoechoic mass especially when gentle pressure is applied by the transducer
    - A hypoechoic (vessel-like) neck communicating between the donor (mother) artery and the pseudoaneurysm (**Fig. 22.2A**)
    - Concentric layers of hematoma can be seen around the pseudoaneurysm (**Fig. 22.3**).
  - ○ Doppler ultrasound
    - This is the primary diagnostic modality.
    - A to-and-fro-flow (red and blue color) on Doppler is seen within the pseudoaneurysm (yin–yang sign) (**Figs. 22.1B, 22.1C, 22.2B, and 22.4**).
    - Aliasing can be seen at the neck of the pseudoaneurysm (**Fig. 22.2B**) or varying colors (red and blue without aliasing) (**Figs. 22.1C and 22.4B**).

- Doppler tracing wave form over the pseudoaneurysm neck typically shows high velocity bidirectional flow (**Figs. 22.2C and 22.3A**).
- Complex pseudoaneurysms may have multiple lobulations or components to them.
- Evaluate if there is an AVF component to the pseudoaneurysm (arterialization of the femoral vein, aliasing at the AVF site)
- The donor or mother artery can be
  - ○ Common femoral artery
  - ○ Superficial femoral artery (most common)
  - ○ Profunda femoris artery
  - ○ Branches from the above branches such as circumflex iliac branches or circumflex femoral branches
  - ○ Contrast-enhanced computed tomography (CT)
    - This is not the primary diagnostic modality.
    - Contrast-filled out-pouching from the donor artery is seen. Concentric hematoma around the out-pouching (pseudoaneurysm) with stranding (ecchymosis) can be seen in the groin.
    - Contrast-enhanced CT (with or without maximized intensity projections [MIPS]) is a good

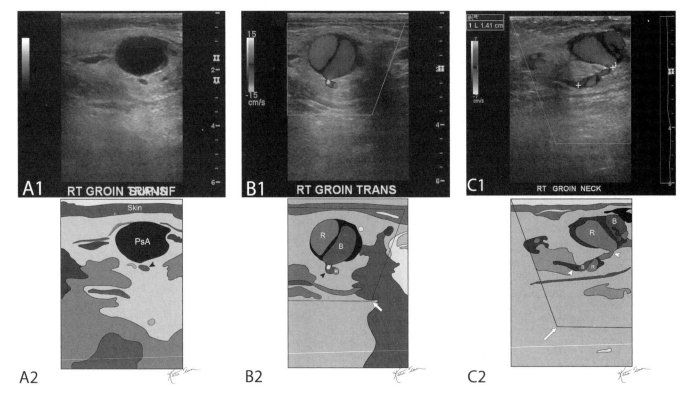

Fig. 22.1 (A) Doppler ultrasound evaluation of a femoral pseudoaneurysm gray-scale ultrasound image (*top*) and schematic sketch (*bottom*) of a femoral pseudoaneurysm (PsA) demonstrating a hypoechoic spherical structure, which pulsates in real-time. The pseudoaneurysm (PsA) is superficial (under 1 cm from the overlying skin). **(B)** Doppler image (*top*) and schematic sketch (*bottom*; *arrow pointing to Doppler box*) of the same pseudoaneurysm as in **Fig. 22.1A**, showing the typical yin–yang appearance with half of the pseudoaneurysm coloring in red (R), and the other half in blue (B). **(C)** Doppler image (*top*) and schematic sketch (*bottom*; *arrow pointing to Doppler box*) of the same pseudoaneurysm as in **Figs. 22.1A and 22.1B**. The image is along the longitudinal axis of the pseudoaneurysm neck (*between arrowheads*). Again, the typical yin–yang appearance with half of the pseudoaneurysm coloring in red (R), and the other half in blue (B). Coloring of the pseudoaneurysm neck is also in red and blue (R and B, respectively). The pseudoaneurysm neck measures at least 1.4 cm in length.

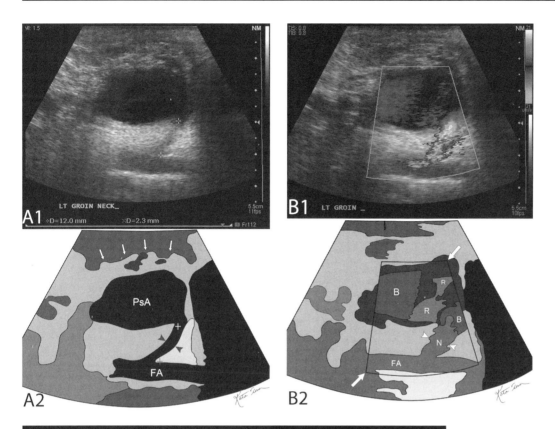

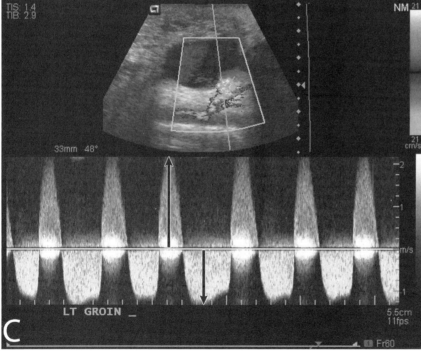

Fig. 22.2 (A) Gray-scale ultrasound image of a femoral pseudoaneurysm (PsA) (*top*) and schematic sketch (*bottom*) demonstrating a hypoechoic spherical structure, which pulsates in real-time. The image is along the longitudinal axis of the pseudoaneurysm neck (*between arrowheads, and cursor crosses/calipers*) and the femoral artery (FA). The pseudoaneurysm neck is also hypoechoic like the femoral artery and the pseudoaneurysm and measures 1.2 cm in length. **(B)** Doppler image (*top*) and schematic sketch (*bottom; arrow pointing to Doppler box*) of the same pseudoaneurysm as in **Fig. 22.2A**, showing the yin–yang appearance with half of the pseudoaneurysm coloring in red (R), and the other half would be colored blue (B). The image is along the longitudinal axis of the neck (*N: in between arrowheads*), which exhibits aliasing. Also note the injured femoral artery. **(C)** Doppler spectral waveform analysis sampling at the neck demonstrating bidirectional high velocity flow. In one direction (*above the line*), flow is in excess of 220 cm/second and in the other direction (*below the line*) flow is in excess of 120 cm/second.

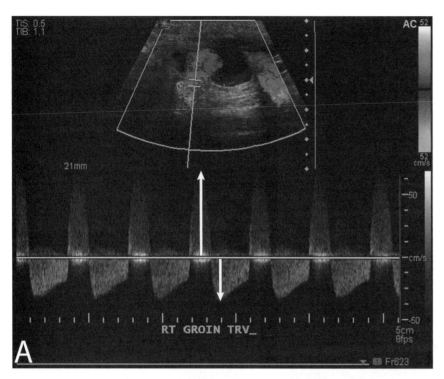

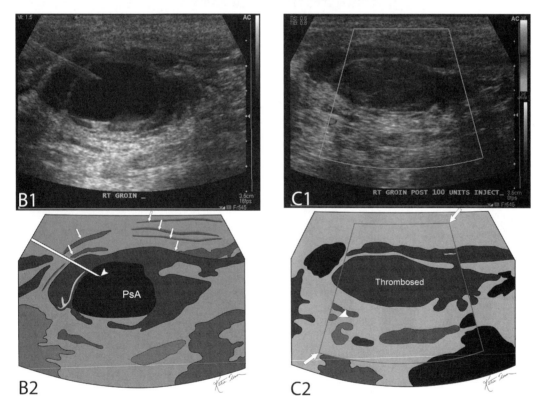

Fig. 22.3 **(A)** Direct percutaneous thrombin injection of a femoral pseudoaneurysm. Doppler spectral waveform analysis sampling at the neck of a pseudoaneurysm demonstrating bidirectional high-velocity flow. In one direction (*above the line*), flow is in excess of 60 cm/second and in the other direction (*below the line*) flow is in excess of 30 cm/ second. **(B)** Gray-scale ultrasound image (*top*) and schematic sketch (*bottom*) during needle placement into the pseudoaneurysm (PsA). The needle tip is seen in the hypoechoic pseudoaneurysm (PsA). *Arrows* point to the different layers of the pseudoaneurysm and the compression of surrounding tissue plains. **(C)** Doppler image (*top*) and schematic sketch (*bottom*; *arrows pointing to Doppler box*) of the same pseudoaneurysm as in **Figs. 22.3A and 22.3B**, demonstrating no color/flow in the pseudoaneurysm. This indicates successful treatment of the pseudoaneurysm. The *arrowhead* points to an adjacent vessel with color/flow within it.

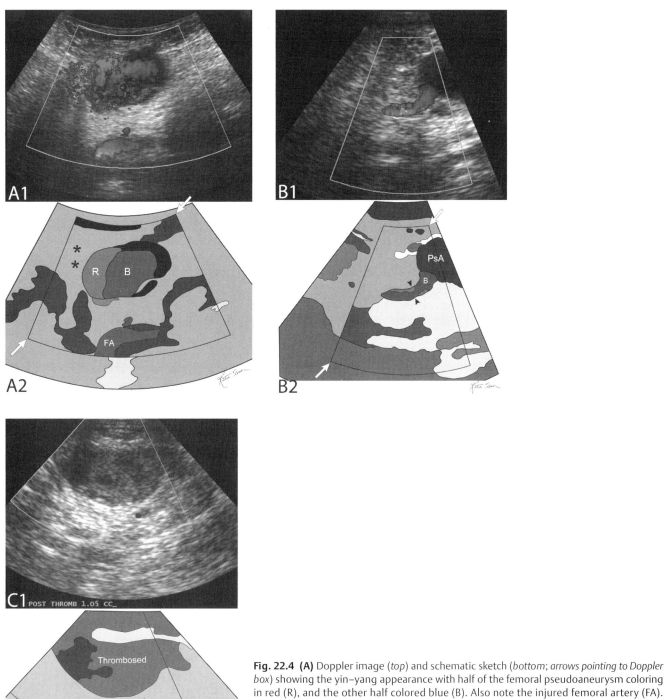

Fig. 22.4 **(A)** Doppler image (*top*) and schematic sketch (*bottom*; *arrows pointing to Doppler box*) showing the yin–yang appearance with half of the femoral pseudoaneurysm coloring in red (R), and the other half colored blue (B). Also note the injured femoral artery (FA). The area of mottled coloring (*labeled as* *) is due to motion from the pulsation and thrill/vibration of the adjacent pseudoaneurysm. **(B)** Doppler image (*top*) and schematic sketch (*bottom*; *arrows pointing to Doppler box*) of the same pseudoaneurysm (PsA) as in **Fig. 22.4A**. The image is along the longitudinal axis of the neck (*between arrowheads*), which exhibits blue coloring (B). **(C)** Doppler image (*top*) and schematic sketch (*bottom*; *arrows pointing to Doppler box*) of the same pseudoaneurysm as in **Figs. 22.4A and 22.4B**, demonstrating no color/flow in the pseudoaneurysm. This indicates successful treatment of the pseudoaneurysm. The *arrowhead* points to an adjacent vessel with color/flow within it.

modality to evaluate the orientation of the pseudoaneurysm relative to the surrounding arteries.
  ○ Is the pseudoaneurysm deep to or superficial to the donor arteries?
  ○ Are there vessels superficial to the pseudoaneurysm that may hinder percutaneous needle access or compression?
○ Contrast-enhanced magnetic resonance imaging (MRI)
  • This is not the primary diagnostic modality.
  • Contrast-filled out-pouching from the donor artery is seen. Concentric hematoma around the out-pouching (pseudoaneurysm) with varying degrees of signal intensity depending on the age of the hematoma (usually acute and subacute phase)
  • Similar advantages to contrast-enhanced CT (see above)
○ Conventional angiography
  • This is the traditional gold standard imaging diagnosis of pseudoaneurysms. Doppler ultrasound has become the primary imaging modality for the evaluation of postcatheterization access pseudoaneurysms.
  • Contrast is seen filling an irregular or globular out-pouching from the donor artery. A wash-out (slower than the wash-in) of contrast is seen lagging behind the donor artery segmental angiogram.
  • Fistulous communication with adjacent veins is more evident than any other modality including Doppler ultrasound (this is true especially if the arteriovenous component of the pseudoaneurysm is small).

Evaluate Pretreatment Laboratory Values

• Laboratory value evaluation mostly revolves around ruling out coagulopathy.
  ○ Suggested coagulopathy thresholds are not set. There are no real coagulopathy-related contraindications.
  ○ Coagulopathy, however, is a predictor of success especially for compression therapy. Coagulopathic patients are less likely to respond to compression therapy than they are to respond to direct percutaneous thrombin injection.

Obtain Informed Consent

• Indications
  ○ To resolve/treat the arterial injury
  ○ To help ambulation
  ○ To reduce the risk of rupture and bleeding
  ○ The expected success rate for compression is 73% for the first attempt with an ultimate success (>1 attempt) of 80% (**Table 22.1**).

Table 22.1 Percentage of Candidacy and Success for Ultrasound-Guided Compression versus Ultrasound-Guided Direct Percutaneous Thrombin Injection

Results and Candidacy		Compression (%)	Thrombin Injection (%)
Rate of noncandidates		10	<2
Success rate	Ultimate success*	80	97
	First attempt success	73	89
	% of ultimate successes requiring >1 session	13	8

*Irrespective of the number of attempts.

○ The expected success rate for direct percutaneous thrombin injection is 89% for the first attempt with an ultimate success (>1 attempt) of 97% (**Table 22.1**).
• Alternatives
  ○ To refuse the procedure (observation). Not unreasonable for
    • Asymptomatic pseudoaneurysms
    • Under 1.8–2.0 cm and not growing
    • No anticoagulation therapy
  ○ Endoluminal coiling
    • Usually applied to branch vessels (profunda femoris branches or circumflex branches) and not the larger vessels
    • Causes a hard lump that does not resolve (more of a problem with thin patients)
  ○ Temporary endoluminal neck occlusion using a balloon placed across the neck
    • Not commonly performed
    • Used in wide and short neck pseudoaneurysms
  ○ Surgical
    • Historic standard management (no longer the treatment of choice)
    • Currently required when
      ○ Minimally invasive methods (see above) fail.
      ○ There is associated infection and/or overlying skin breakdown.
      ○ The injury is complex with an AVF component.
• Procedural risks
  ○ Overall, <1.5% of cases whether compression or thrombin injection
  ○ Major and minor complications occur in <0.5% and <1.0% of cases, respectively, whether compression therapy or thrombin injection.
  ○ See **Tables 22.2 and 22.3** for details of complications of both ultrasound-guided compression therapy and ultrasound-guided direct percutaneous thrombin injection

Table 22.2 Complications Encountered with Ultrasound-Guided Compression Management of Postcatheterization Pseudoaneurysms

Complications		Range Incidence of Complications (%)	Average Incidence of Complications (%)
All complications	Overall	0.0–5.5	1.3
	Major		0.5
	Minor		0.8
Pain-associated complications	Overall	0.0–4.1	0.7
	Major (angina/atrial fibrillation)		0.2
	Minor (vasovagal/hypertension)		0.5
Pseudoaneurysm rupture		0.0–0.9	0.2
Distal arterial embolization		0.0–0.8	0.1
Deep venous thrombosis		0.0–0.3	0.1
Pulmonary embolism		Rare	0.0

Equipment

For Ultrasound Guidance and Compression

- Ultrasound machine with Doppler capability
- Multiarray 7–9 MHz ultrasound transducer
- If compression is by the ultrasound transducer itself or by manual digital compression, then the above is all that is needed.
- If the ultrasound transducer is for guidance and not compression, a compression device (vice-like mechanical compression) is sometimes used. Such a device is the FemoStop device (Femoral Compression System, RADI Medical Systems AB, Uppsala, Sweden, distributed by Radi Medical Systems, Inc., Reading, MA).

For Ultrasound Guidance and Direct Percutaneous Thrombin Injection

- Ultrasound machine with Doppler capability
- Multiarray 5–7.5 MHz linear array ultrasound transducer
- Some operators use high-frequency transducers (7.5–12 MHz)
- Transducer guide bracket (not necessary, can be performed free-hand)
- Sterile transducer cover

Standard Surgical Preparation and Draping

- Chlorhexidine skin preparation/cleansing fluid
- Fenestrated drape

Table 22.3 Complications Encountered with Ultrasound-Guided Direct Percutaneous Thrombin Injection Management of Postcatheterization Pseudoaneurysms

Complications		Range Incidence of Complications (%)	Average Incidence of Complications (%)
All complications	Overall	0.0–3.5	1.4
	Major		0.4
	Minor		1.0
Distal arterial embolization	Overall	0.0–2.6	1.0
	Major (requiring intervention)	0.0–1.5	0.3
	Minor (transient / self limiting)	0.0–2.6	0.7
Allergic reaction		0.0–0.4	0.1
Infection		0.0–0.9	0.1
Pseudoaneurysm rupture		0.0–0.8	0.1
Pain ± vasovagal reaction		0.0–0.4	0.1
Hypotension and bradycardia		Rare	0.0
Deep venous thrombosis		Rare	0.0

Local Infiltrative Analgesia Administration

- 21-gauge infiltration needle
- 10–20 mL 1% lidocaine syringe

Sharp Access

- 20- to 22-gauge needle
- Use of 19-gauge and 23- to 25-gauge needle has also been described.
- A 21-gauge needle is our preference.

Thrombin Administration Reservoir

- 3 mL syringe
- Connector tube to connect between the needle and the syringe. This allows flexibility and nimble manipulating of the needle while being ready to respond by injecting thrombin.

Thrombin and Tissue Adhesives Used

Varying mixtures of thrombin, fibrinogen, and fibrin have been used. The following are some of the more commonly used products.

- Lyophilized, sterilized, and virus-inactivated powdered bovine thrombin to be reconstituted by saline (1000 U/mL and can be diluted to 100 U to 500 U/mL)
  - Recothrom (Gentrac Inc., Johnson and Johnson Medical Inc., Middleton, WI)
  - Thrombin-JMI (Jones Medical Industries, St. Louis, MO)
  - D-Stat Flowable Hemostat (Vascular Solutions, Bochum, Germany)
  - Thrombostat (Park-Davis, Scarborough, Ontario, Canada)
- Sterilized and virus-inactivated human thrombin, tissue sealant to be defrosted (500 U/mL)
  - Tissuecol Duo S 500 (Immuno AG, Vienna, Austria)
  - Tisseal (Baxter Health-care Corp., Glendale, CA)
- Autologous centrifuged and suspended human thrombin
- Fibrinogen, aprotinin, thrombin, and Factor XIII composite tissue adhesive (three doses available: 0.5, 1.0, and 3.9 mL)
  - Beriplast P Combiset (Centeon Pharmaceuticals Ltd., Marburg, Germany)

Technique for Ultrasound-Guided Compression Therapy

Intravenous Access

- The necessity of moderate sedation (administered intravenously [IV]) for compression therapy of pseudoaneurysms varies from one institution to another.

- For those institutions that do not routinely sedate patients, 25–34% of their patients eventually require moderate sedation to tolerate the pseudoaneurysm compression.
- If moderate sedation is not routinely administered, IV access is still reasonable as a standby for any complication (including pain-related complications especially vasovagal reaction).

Pretreatment Clinical Exam

- Evaluate the overlying skin for necrosis and/or infection
- Determine the baseline distal arterial
- Ankle-brachial indices (ABIs) may be calculated.

Pretreatment Ultrasound Exam

- Determine the overall size of the pseudoaneurysm as well as pseudoaneurysm neck location, dimensions, and hemodynamics.
- Determine the relation of the pseudoaneurysm with the supplying femoral artery
- Evaluate for associated arterial injuries such as arteriovenous fistulous components
- Assess the direction required to apply pressure to occlude flow into the pseudoaneurysm sac. The ideal trajectory to apply pressure avoids gross compression of the pseudoaneurysm sac itself as well as the adjacent normal vasculature (femoral vein and artery).

Compression Technique

- The ultrasound probe is positioned directly over the pseudoaneurysm neck and downward pressure is applied until flow into the pseudoaneurysm ceases. Place a fenestrated drape at the prepared skin region.
- The ideal degree of pressure is that which abolishes flow into the pseudoaneurysm, and if possible, avoids compression of the adjacent femoral artery.
- In some patients, temporary occlusion of the femoral artery is unavoidable and there are usually no unexpected sequelae.
- The pseudoaneurysm neck compression is applied intermittently for intervals extending between 6 and 20 minutes.
- It is not uncommon during ultrasound-guided compression to lose the ideal position over the pseudoaneurysm neck, which necessitates adjustment in the ultrasound transducer position.
- Between pressure application intervals, the pseudoaneurysm is evaluated for flow by color Doppler ultrasound.

- If the pseudoaneurysm has thrombosed, the procedure is deemed technically successful.
- If there is still residual flow, a repeat compression interval is performed.
- Most operators will not exceed three or four compression intervals. In addition, it is not uncommon for patients not to tolerate repeat compression intervals/sessions.
- The sum of the duration of compression intervals ranges from 5 minutes to 300 minutes. The average time for compression is ~40 minutes.

Immediate Postcompression Ultrasound Imaging

- Determine endpoint (success), which is thrombosis of the pseudoaneurysm
- Evaluate for residual flow by Doppler ultrasound
- Evaluate for residual AVF flow

Technique for Ultrasound-Guided Direct Percutaneous Thrombin Injection

Intravenous Access

- The necessity of moderate sedation (administered intravenously) for ultrasound-guided direct percutaneous thrombin injection of pseudoaneurysms varies for one institution to the other.
- If moderate sedation is not routinely administered, intravenous access is still reasonable as a standby for any complication.

Pretreatment Clinical Exam

- Evaluate the overlying skin for necrosis and/or infection. Avoiding infected skin or skin breakdown by the needle is preferred.
- Determine the baseline distal arterial pulses
- ABIs may be calculated.

Pretreatment Ultrasound Exam

- Determine the overall size of the pseudoaneurysm as well as pseudoaneurysm neck location, dimensions, and hemodynamics
- Determine the relation of the pseudoaneurysm with the supplying femoral artery
- Evaluate for associated arterial injuries such as AVF components
- Assess the simplicity or complexity of the pseudoaneurysm
  - Simple pseudoaneurysms have one saccule (lobe).
  - Complex pseudoaneurysms have more than one saccule (lobe).

- Make sure there are no vessels between the skin and the pseudoaneurysm. These vessels should be avoided.
  - They may be injured in the process by the access needle.
  - They may be thrombosed or their distal aspects embolized by inadvertent thrombin injection.
- Based on the ultrasound exam findings and the status of the overlying skin findings (location of necrosis and/or infection), the decision to proceed with the treatment and the ideal needle access site and approach are decided upon.

Standard Surgical Preparation and Draping

- Skin preparation/cleansing in the region that was chosen as an ultrasound imaging portal and a needle access needle portal
- Place a fenestrated drape at the chosen and prepared skin region

Local Infiltrative Analgesia Administration

- Utilizing a 21-gauge infiltration needle, 1% lidocaine infiltration is performed.
- Do not enter the pseudoaneurysm. A superficial wheal is enough.
- Some operators do not use lidocaine infiltration (no local anesthetic).

Sharp Access

- The Doppler ultrasound is switched to gray-scale ultrasound mode for real-time guidance.
- Real-time gray-scale ultrasound is used to image the needle tip longitudinally along the needle shaft (**Fig. 22.3B**).
- A 21-gauge needle is our preference (in the literature 19- to 25-gauge needles have been used).
- Use free-hand ultrasound guidance of the needle
- Once the needle tip is in adequate position in the pseudoaneurysm sac, ultrasound is switched to color Doppler with a low-pulse repetition frequency (**Figs. 22.3B and 22.3C**).

Thrombin Injection and Imaging during Its Administration

- Slow and steady thrombin injection ensues under real-time color Doppler ultrasound visualization.
- The rate of injection is enough to gradually form an iso- to hyperechoic thrombus that fills the pseudoaneurysm gradually, but fast enough to not allow it to encase the needle tip. A quoted injection rate is 0.1–0.3 mL of thrombin injection per second.

- If the needle tip becomes encased by a thrombus ball/mound, further injection of thrombin into the thrombin ball/mound can be ineffective. To alleviate this, the needle tip can be gently manipulated to rid the thrombus ball within the pseudoaneurysm lobe and free the needle tip to resume thrombin injection.
- Patients (23%) may experience a local heat sensation.
- Complete or near-complete thrombosis of the entire pseudoaneurysm usually is achieved within seconds.
- **Figure 22.3** demonstrates an actual postcatheterization pseudoaneurysm prior to, during, and after thrombin injection.

Immediate Postcompression Ultrasound Imaging

- Determine endpoint (success), which is thrombosis of the pseudoaneurysm (**Fig. 22.3C**)
- Evaluate for residual flow by Doppler ultrasound, especially residual pockets of flow in the pseudoaneurysm
- Residual pockets identified by Doppler ultrasound
  - Low-flow pockets free of thrombus that are not in communication with the pseudoaneurysm neck are left to thrombose spontaneously.
  - If high-flow pockets are found communicating with the pseudoaneurysm neck (uncommon), they may require additional needle punctures with subsequent thrombin injection.
  - Some operators apply gentle pressure to obliterate such pockets.
- Evaluate for residual AVF flow

Endpoints

Therapeutic Response

- Eventually complete thrombosis of the pseudoaneurysm with preservation of flow in the donor artery
- No hematoma growth and eventual maturation, evolution, and resolution of the hematoma
- Ability of the patient to ambulate (if the groin hematoma/pseudoaneurysm was the impediment to ambulation).

No Distal Complications (Distal Embolization)

- This is more of a problem (10-fold risk) with direct thrombin injection rather than ultrasound-guided compression: 1.0% compared with 0.1%, respectively (**Tables 22.2 and 22.3**).
- Only 30% of documented distal embolizations are clinically significant and require intervention (definition of major complication).

- Due to this, it is standard to repeat the distal arterial evaluation and compare it with the baseline arterial vascular evaluation. This applies to both techniques.
- See below for management of complications.

Postprocedural Evaluation and Management

There is no clear consensus for clinical and imaging follow-up intervals for patients who have undergone successful minimally invasive postcatheterization pseudoaneurysm treatment (whether compression or thrombin injection). As a result, there is no set standard for patient care after pseudoaneurysm therapy regarding whether it should be done on an outpatient or inpatient basis. Some institutions perform access pseudoaneurysm therapy of small pseudoaneurysms on an outpatient basis and admit patients who have "larger" pseudoaneurysms, which cause a hindrance on ambulation, have a higher risk of rupturing, and have a greater chance of requiring more than one treatment session.

Postprocedural Observation Period

- Postprocedural stay varies from one practice to the other (see above).
- If patients are to stay briefly before discharge, they should stay for 4–6 hours after treatment under bed rest.
- During this period
  - Mild to moderate pressure dressing is applied.
  - A repeat distal arterial evaluation is made and compared with the baseline arterial evaluation.
- If the patient is to be discharged
  - A clinical and Doppler ultrasound evaluation is made just prior to discharge (6 hours from the procedure) to confirm continued obliteration of the pseudoaneurysm.
  - The patient usually is required to touch base in 24 hours (next day) or even to return the next day for a 24-hour Doppler ultrasound follow-up evaluation.
- Institutions that do not have a 24-hour Doppler ultrasound evaluation have it at a 3- to 10-day postprocedural interval. As noted earlier, there is no clear consensus for the clinical and imaging follow-up intervals for patients who have undergone successful minimally invasive postcatheterization pseudoaneurysm treatment.

Intravenous Fluid and Diet

- IV access should be kept until just prior to discharge or after adequate oral intake for inpatients.
- Some institutions that give moderate sedation start a clear liquid diet immediately and advance it as tolerated.

- If no moderate sedation was given, there should not be any diet restrictions unless other circumstances present themselves.

Activity

- Bed rest for 4–6 hours
- Mild to moderate pressure dressing is applied.
- Upon discharge, patients are instructed to not engage in strenuous activity for 48 hours post-pseudo-aneurysm obliteration procedure.

Pain Management

- Narcotics are usually not required during the post-biopsy stay of the patient prior to discharge. Occasionally, some patients may require oral narcotic analgesics such as acetaminophen and hydrocodone combination medication.
- On discharge, patients usually tolerate the procedure well and do not require analgesics more potent than over-the-counter medications.

Monitoring Vital Signs

- Vital sign monitoring includes blood pressure and heart rate.
- Institutions/operators that practice conscious sedation may record a softer blood pressure than a patient's baseline blood pressure after the biopsy. This is the most likely due to sedation with or without dehydration. They usually respond with time by hydration and particularly as the sedatives wear off.
- A repeat distal arterial evaluation is made and compared with the baseline arterial evaluation.

Complications and Their Management

Tables 22.2 and 22.3 briefly show the various complications and their incidence after postcatheterization access pseudoaneurysm ablation. The overall complication rate is less than 1.5% whether after compression or thrombin injection. The major and minor complication rate is <0.5 and <1.0%, respectively, again whether after compression or thrombin injection. As can be seen in **Tables 22.2 and 22.3**, the main complication related to ultrasound-guided compression therapy is intraprocedural pain. The main complication related to ultrasound-guided direct thrombin injection therapy is distal arterial embolization.

Management of Pain and Pain-Related Morbidity

- One must classify pain-related morbidity into

  - Intraprocedural pain morbidity
  - Postprocedural pain (usually not morbid)
- Intraprocedural pain is a complication that is primarily related to ultrasound-guided compression therapy and not to direct thrombin injection.
  - Intraprocedural pain can result in
    - Vasovagal reaction
    - Simply pain
    - Cardiovascular response to pain
      - Hypertension
      - Atrial fibrillation
      - Chest angina
  - 17% of these pain and pain-related complications (see above) are considered major complications.
  - Most intraprocedural complications can be avoided by giving patients moderate sedation.
- Postprocedural pain can occur after compression or thrombin injection. It is managed routinely.
  - Narcotics are usually not required during the post-biopsy stay of the patient prior to discharge. Occasionally, some patients require oral narcotic analgesics such as acetaminophen and hydrocodone combination medication.
  - On discharge, patients usually tolerate the procedure well and do not require analgesics more potent than over-the-counter medications.

Management of Bleeding Complications

- Bleeding at the site is related to pseudoaneurysm rupture, which occurs in 0.1 to 0.2% of cases (more likely in compression therapy rather than direct percutaneous thrombin injection treatments).
- Bleeding occurs right at the site
  - Externally, or active extravasation (usually)
  - A growing hematoma
  - Acute and rapid expansion of the pseudoaneurysm (impending rupture), which can occur in up to 1% of cases during compression therapy
- Local control of bleeding
  - Compression over the bleeding site
  - Compression over the donor artery proximal to the pseudoaneurysm (proximal control)
  - Open vascular surgical intervention with proximal and distal control of the donor artery
- Significant bleeding affecting vital signs and patient stability should be managed by
  - Fluid resuscitation starting with crystalloid fluid bolus
  - Type and cross
  - Repeat hematocrit to compare with baseline
  - Blood transfusion to maintain hematocrit at or above 30%
  - Surgical consult/interventional radiology consult

- Interventional radiology offers
  - Pelvic/lower extremity arteriography from the contralateral groin if possible
  - Proximal balloon occlusion to control bleeding until the surgical team is mobilized
  - Possibilities of embolizing or stent placement may be entertained (surgery is preferred if local control of bleeding is achieved).
- Surgical consultation may offer, in the cases of severe uncontrolled bleeding, open surgery, exploration, and local hemostasis (proximal and distal control of bleeding) and repair of the injured vessel.
  - Ligation of bleeding minor branches
  - Primary suturing of important femoral artery
  - Patch angioplasty of femoral artery
  - Bypass if segment is significantly injured
  - Extraanatomic (autologous) bypass if signs of infection are encountered

Management of Distal Embolization

- This complication is more common with direct thrombin injection (1.0%) and is less likely with compression therapy (0.1%).
- 30% of embolic events result in major complications that require intervention.
- If distal embolization is subclinical and only encountered by reduction in ABI
  - The patient should receive anticoagulation therapy
  - Surgical consult
  - Serial ABI, pulse checks
  - If situation becomes clinically evident, surgery is required.
- If an embolic event is clinically evident, an angiogram is performed with or without thrombolysis. Surgical thrombectomy is an alternative with or without a prior failed transcatheter thrombolysis.

Further Reading

Kronzon I. Diagnosis and treatment of iatrogenic femoral artery pseudoaneurysm: a review. J Am Soc Echocardiogr 1997;10(3): 236–245

Middleton WD, Dasyam A, Teefey SA. Diagnosis and treatment of iatrogenic femoral artery pseudoaneurysms. Ultrasound Q 2005; 21(1):3–17

Morgan R, Belli A-M. Current treatment methods for postcatheterization pseudoaneurysms. J Vasc Interv Radiol 2003;14(6):697–710

Saad NEA, Saad WEA, Davies MG, Waldman DL, Fultz PJ, Rubens DJ. Pseudoaneurysms and the role of minimally invasive techniques in their management. Radiographics 2005;25(Suppl 1): S173–S189

Saad NEA, Saad WEA, Rubens DJ, Fultz P. Ultrasound diagnosis of arterial injuries and the role of minimal invasive techniques in their management. Ultrasound Clin N Am, Vascular Ultrasound 2006; 1(1):183–200

Saad WEA, Waldman DL. Management of post-catheterization pseudoaneurysms. In: Mauro M, Murphy K, Thomson K, Venbrux A, Zollikofer C, eds. Image Guided Interventions. Philadelphia: Saunders; 2008: 223–251

IV Sonohysterography

23 Sonohysterography
Chiou Li Ong

Indications

- Abnormal uterine bleeding
  - Postmenopausal
  - Premenopausal
- Abnormal endometrial finding on conventional ultrasonography
  - Abnormal thickening
  - In symptomatic postmenopausal women, endometrial thickness exceeding 5 mm (measurement of the two layers of endometrium)
  - Sonohysterography (SHG) can help to triage patients to "blind" dilatation and curettage, or hysteroscopy and biopsy, depending on whether diffuse or focal abnormalities of the endometrium are found.
  - Criteria for abnormal endometrial thickness in premenopausal and asymptomatic postmenopausal women are less clear.
  - Upper limits for asymptomatic postmenopausal women is around 6–8 mm, and should be correlated with hormonal or tamoxifen therapy.
- Poor visualization of the endometrium
  - May be encountered as a result of the axial orientation of the uterus or previous cesarean section
  - SHG may be indicated in symptomatic patients.
- Leiomyomas with distortion of the endometrium
- Diagnostic workup prior to assisted reproductive techniques
- To confirm presence of retained products of conception

Contraindications

Absolute Contraindications

- Acute pelvic inflammatory disease
- Pregnancy

Relative Contraindications

- Hydrosalpinx
- Bleeding
- Patients with dilated fallopian tubes should have their examinations deferred until they have had an adequate course of antibiotics.

- Although bleeding is not a contraindication to the examination, the presence of blood clots and fibrin strands may present problems in interpretation.

Types of Procedures

Gynecological Pelvic Ultrasound

- Pelvic ultrasonography is the primary imaging modality for the assessment of the endometrium.
- Two main approaches to pelvic ultrasonography: transabdominal for panoramic view and transvaginal for greater resolution and greater diagnostic accuracy
- SHG – a useful adjunct and more specific in diagnosing endometrial pathology

Hysterosalpingography

- X-ray technique that involves ionizing radiation and iodinated contrast medium

Hysteroscopy

- More invasive and may be reserved for patients with focal abnormalities that are found on SHG.

Preprocedural Evaluation and Preparation

- A brief gynecological/medical history is taken.
- Patients with abnormal vaginal discharge suggestive of a pelvic infection should have their examination rescheduled until after the infection has been treated.
- Prophylactic antibiotics are recommended in patients with chronic pelvic inflammation or cardiac valvular problems.
- History of allergy to latex, if latex transducer covers or catheters are used
- Use of a checklist is helpful.
- Nonsteroidal antiinflammatory medication may be given prior to the procedure to minimize cramping.

Timing of Procedure

- It should be performed during the early proliferative phase of the menstrual cycle, typically fourth to sixth day, when the endometrium is thinnest and least likely to produce false-positive results.
- Avoid doing the procedure beyond the 10th day of the patient's cycle
- Patients who have irregular menstrual periods, in whom their real menses cannot be determined, may be given a course of progesterone by the gynecologist to induce "medical curettage" prior to the procedure.

Choice of Catheters

- Nonballoon catheters (examples)
  - Infant feeding tubes (5- to 6-French) usually adequate
  - Intrauterine insemination catheter
- Balloon catheters
  - Foley catheter
  - Commercially available hysterosalpingography catheters

- Choice of catheter
  - Balloon catheters provide a seal on the cervical canal and help prevent rapid expulsion of fluid.
  - Study by Dessole and colleagues found no significant difference among six commonly used catheters.

Technique

- Setup
  - A setup of the procedure tray is shown in **Fig. 23.1**.
- Preliminary ultrasound scans
  - Transabdominal ultrasound for general survey of pelvis
  - Transvaginal ultrasound with patient in lithotomy position, empty urinary bladder, and pelvis elevated by a small sponge block or padding, to allow better maneuver of transducer
  - The uterus, ovaries, and adnexa are evaluated. Documentation is made.
  - The transducer is removed and used sheath discarded.

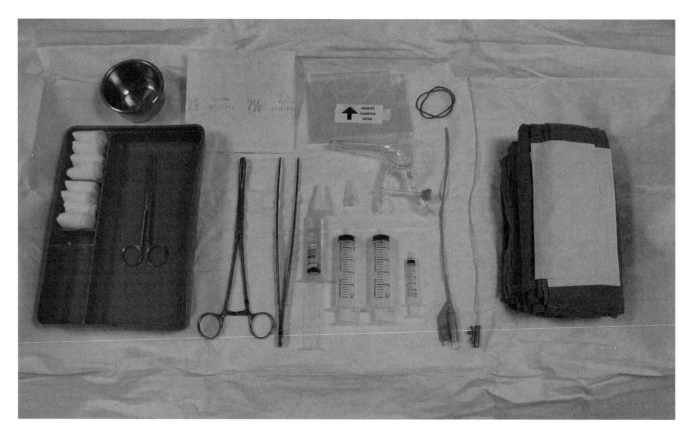

Fig. 23.1 Instruments used for a sonohysterography are shown: plastic tray for cleaning lotions and sponges, ring forceps, long forceps for insertion of catheter, sterile gel, 20-mL syringes, small syringe for balloon catheter, Foley catheter or infant feeding tube, small jar for saline, large-sized gloves for covering transducer, plastic cover for transducer cable.

- Cleansing and draping
  - Cleansing of external genitalia
  - Sterile drapes used to cover patient's legs and thighs
  - Expose vagina, cervix, and external os using sterile vaginal speculum for cleansing
  - Povidone iodine is the most commonly used cleansing lotion, but in cases of patients with an allergy, chlorhexidine and saline may be used depending on institutional practice.
- Insertion of catheter
  - After cleansing, insert saline-filled catheter into the uterine cavity
  - In cases of difficult insertion, a tenaculum may be used, but simple angulation of the cervix by means of the bivalve vaginal speculum can help to facilitate insertion.
  - Use a balloon catheter if a catheter can only reach the level of the cervical canal. In such situations, the catheter should be advanced until the balloon part of the catheter goes past the external os.
  - A recent study comparing intrauterine and intracervical placement of balloon catheters showed that patients experienced less pain when the catheter is placed in the cervical canal.

  - Avoid clamping on the cervix when removing the speculum as this may cause a low-lying catheter to dislodge
  - Remove the speculum after checking that the catheter is firmly in place
- Infusion of saline
  - The vaginal transducer, which has been covered with a sterile sheath (I use a large-sized sterile glove with sterile gel in one of the digits for the transducer, and a long plastic sheath for the cable), is inserted.
  - To avoid obstruction of the field of view, the transducer is placed in front of the catheter if the uterus is anteflexed, and behind it if it is retroflexed (**Fig. 23.2**).
  - With the help of an assistant, saline is injected into the uterine cavity during real-time transvaginal ultrasonography.
  - Avoid overdistension as this could result in cramping
  - An explanation in advance of each step of the procedure to the patient would help to allay her anxiety. (Finer points for improving patient comfort during the procedure may be found in the article by SR Lindheim et al.)

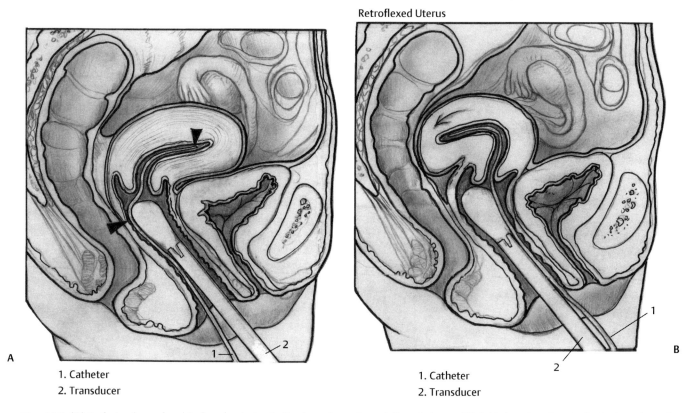

Retroflexed Uterus

A

1. Catheter
2. Transducer

B

1. Catheter
2. Transducer

Fig. 23.2 (A) Catheter (*arrowheads*) placed anterior to the transducer for anteflexed uterus. **(B)** Catheter placed posterior to transducer for retroflexed uterus.

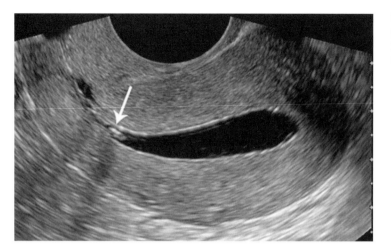

Fig. 23.3 Sagittal ultrasound image of normal-appearing endometrium during early proliferative phase of menstrual cycle in a retroflexed uterus. Catheter tip (*arrow*) is in lower uterine cavity.

- Documentation of imaging
  - Video-recording and snapshots of the endometrial cavity in sagittal and coronal sections
- Normal features and techniques to optimize imaging
  - The whole endometrial cavity must be surveyed.
  - The normal endometrium is smooth and thin in the early proliferative phase of the menstrual cycle (**Fig. 23.3**).
  - The intrauterine catheter may obscure the endometrium (**Fig. 23.4**). The balloon may be deflated to improve visualization.
  - Outline the whole endometrial cavity and cervical canal by continuous infusion while withdrawing the catheter toward the end of study.
  - In cervical catheterization (**Fig. 23.5**), the balloon should be kept distended throughout the study, and deflated only at completion of the examination. Air bubbles may be displaced by turning the patient on her side, or expelled by continued infusion.

- Intravasation of air into the myometrium can result in a pseudolesion that mimics adenomyosis.
- Multiplanar reconstruction of the uterine cavity (**Fig. 23.6**) may be done. This is a useful evaluation for patients with infertility.
- Types of anomalies
  - Endometrial polyps (**Figs. 23.7 and 23.8**)
    - They are the most common anomalies detected on SHG, and often are the anomalies that are missed on conventional ultrasound.
    - The majority are benign, but ~3% may be malignant.
    - Transvaginal ultrasound-guided polypectomy has been described as an extension of SHG.
  - Adhesions
    - May be seen as bridging bands or strands between the walls of the endometrial cavity (**Fig. 23.9**). In severe cases, distension of the endometrial cavity may not be possible.
      - Malignancy

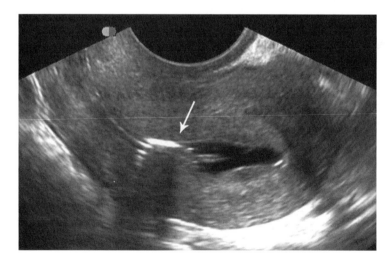

Fig. 23.4 Sagittal ultrasound image showing slightly undulating normal endometrium during the latter part of the proliferative phase. A partially deflated balloon (*arrow*) is obscuring part of the endometrial cavity.

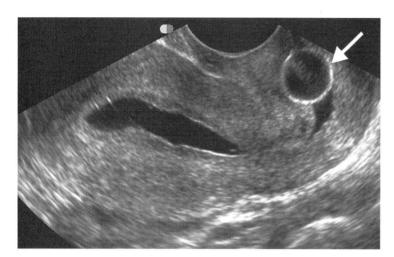

Fig. 23.5 Sagittal sonogram of an anteflexed uterus with balloon catheter (*arrow*) in the cervical canal.

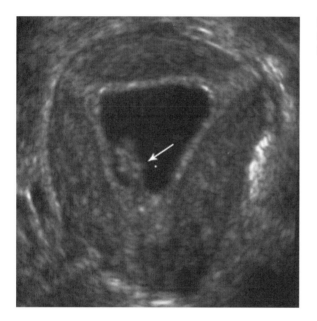

Fig. 23.6 Coronal sonogram of the uterus, using multiplanar reconstruction, showing normal triangular-shaped uterine cavity. Catheter placement shown by *arrow*.

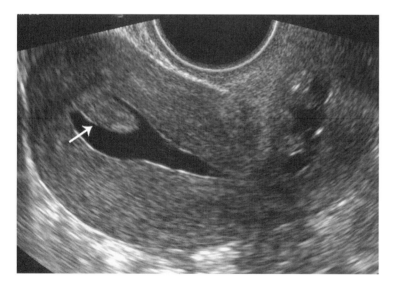

Fig. 23.7 Sagittal sonogram of uterus showing fundal endometrial polyp (*arrow*).

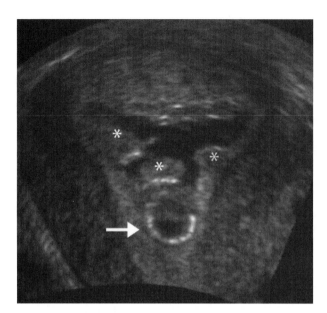

Fig. 23.8 Coronal sonogram of uterus with multiple endometrial polyps (*). Placement of the balloon catheter shown by *arrow*.

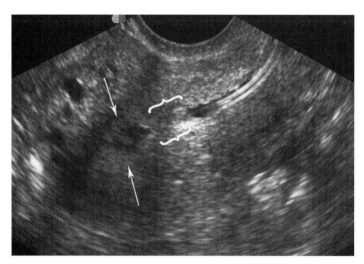

A

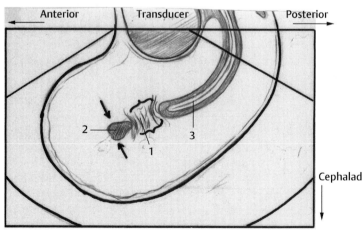

B

1. Length within double brace is the adhesion
2. Black arrow is pointing to small endometrial cavity
3. Tube

Fig. 23.9 (A) Sagittal sonogram of a poorly distended uterine cavity (*long thin arrows*) due to an adhesion/synechia (*double brace*). **(B)** Diagrammatic representation of **Fig. 23.9A**. 1, adhesion/synechia (*double brace*); 2, small distended uterine cavity (*arrows*); 3, catheter.

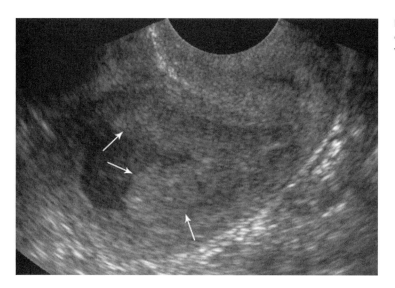

Fig. 23.10 Endometrial carcinoma with irregular thickening of the endometrium (*arrows*). Echogenic endometrial fluid was already present.

- The lesions are usually diffuse and present with uneven thickening of the endometrium (**Fig. 23.10**). Presence of fluid in the endometrial cavity in such cases would preclude the need to perform SHG.
- Poor distensibility of the endometrial cavity may also be a sign of malignancy.
  ○ Submucosal leiomyomas (**Fig. 23.11**)

The ratio of intracavitary to intramural portions of the mass should be assessed as this is helpful in the planning of surgical resection.

Limitations and Complications

- Cervical stenosis
  ○ More common in postmenopausal women

- Not for women unable to undergo transvaginal ultrasonography

Complications

- Low incidence, with infection being the main risk at 1–2%
- Dissemination of malignant cells

A similar situation exists with hysteroscopy and less commonly, hysterosalpingography. At present, there is no evidence to suggest that survival rates would be affected.

SHG is a simple procedure that can help to enhance the diagnostic accuracy of transvaginal ultrasonography. The technique is similar to that of x-ray hysterosalpingography, but the operator needs to be proficient in transvaginal ultrasonography. This can be easily achieved as most pelvic ultrasonography includes transvaginal scanning.

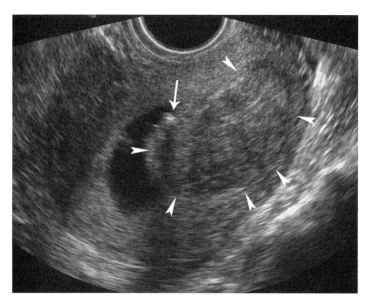

Fig. 23.11 Sagittal sonogram of the uterus showing an intramural leiomyoma (*arrowheads*) with submucosal extension. Catheter placement is indicated by *arrow*.

Further Reading

AIUM practice guideline for the performance of sonohysterography. By the collaborative subcommittees from American Institute of Ultrasound in Medicine (AIUM), American College of Radiology (ACR), and the American College of Obstetricians and Gynecologists (ACOG). Available at http://www.aivm.org. Accessed July 13, 2009

Antunes A Jr, Costa-Paiva L, Arthuso M, Costa JV, Pinto-Neto AM. Endometrial polyps in pre- and postmenopausal women: factors associated with malignancy. Maturitas 2007;57(4):415–421

Ben-Arie A, Goldchmit C, Laviv Y, et al. The malignant potential of endometrial polyps. Eur J Obstet Gynecol Reprod Biol 2004;115(2):206–210

Dessole S, Farina M, Capobianco G, Nadelli GB, Ambrosini G, Meloni GB. Determining the best catheter for sonohysterography. Fertil Steril 2001;76(3):605–609

Devore GR, Schwartz PE, Morris JM. Hysterography: a 5-year follow-up in patients with endometrial carcinoma. Obstet Gynecol 1982;60(3):369–372

Epstein E, Ramirez A, Skoog L, Valentin L. Transvaginal sonography, saline contrast sonohysterography and hysteroscopy for the investigation of women with postmenopausal bleeding and endometrium > 5 mm. Ultrasound Obstet Gynecol 2001;18(2):157–162

Fong K, Kung R, Lytwyn A, et al. Endometrial evaluation with transvaginal US and hysterosonography in asymptomatic postmenopausal women with breast cancer receiving tamoxifen. Radiology 2001;220(3):765–773

Goldberg JM, Falcone T, Attaran M. Sonohysterographic evaluation of uterine abnormalities noted on hysterosalpingography. Hum Reprod 1997;12(10):2151–2153

Goldstein SR. Abnormal uterine bleeding: the role of ultrasound. Radiol Clin North Am 2006;44(6):901–910

Lee C, Ben-Nagi J, Ofili-Yebovi D, Yazbek J, Davies A, Jurkovic D. A new method of transvaginal ultrasound-guided polypectomy: a feasibility study. Ultrasound Obstet Gynecol 2006;27(2):198–201

Lin MC, Gosink BB, Wolf SI, et al. Endometrial thickness after menopause: effect of hormone replacement. Radiology 1991;180(2):427–432

Lindheim SR, Sprague C, Winter TC III. Hysterosalpingography and sonohysterography: lessons in technique. AJR Am J Roentgenol 2006;186(1):24–29

Ors F, Lev-Toaff AS, Bergin D. Echogenic foci mimicking adenomyosis presumably due to air intravasation into the myometrium during sonohysterography. Diagn Interv Radiol 2007;13(1):26–29

Spieldoch RL, Winter TC, Schouweiler C, Ansay S, Evans MD, Lindheim SR. Optimal catheter placement during sonohysterography: a randomized controlled trial comparing cervical to uterine placement. Obstet Gynecol 2008;111(1):15–21

Wolman I, Groutz A, Gordon D, Kuperminc MJ, Lessing JB, Jaffa AJ. Timing of sonohysterography in menstruating women. Gynecol Obstet Invest 1999;48(4):254–258

Index